MEDICINE *for* MOUNTAINEERING

Third Edition

Edited By

JAMES A. WILKERSON, M.D.

Merced Pathology Laboratory
Merced, California

THE MOUNTAINEERS
Seattle, Washington

The Mountaineers: Organized 1906 "...to explore,
study, preserve and enjoy the natural beauty of the
Northwest."

Copyright © 1985 by The Mountaineers
All rights reserved

Published by The Mountaineers
306 Second Avenue West
Seattle, Washington 98117

Published simultaneously in Canada by
Douglas & McIntyre Ltd.
1615 Venables Street, Vancouver, B.C. V5L 2H1

Copyedited by Barbara Chasan

Manufactured in the United States of America

First edition 1967
Second edition 1975
    Second printing March 1978, third printing August
    1979, fourth printing March 1982, fifth printing
    August 1983
Third edition 1985
    First printing April 1985

Library of Congress Cataloging in Publication Data
Main entry under title:

Medicine for mountaineering.

    Includes bibliographies and index.
    1. Mountaineering—Accidents and injuries.
2. Sports medicine. I. Wilkerson, James A., 1934-
[DNLM: 1. Mountaineering. 2. Sports Medicine.
QT 260 M4895]
RC1220.M6M4 1985   617'.1027   85-7180
ISBN 0-89886-086-5

Contributors

C. Kirk Avent, M.D., Professor of Medicine, Infectious Disease Division, The School of Medicine, The University of Alabama in Birmingham, Birmingham, Alabama. (Chapter Twenty-three.)

Earl E. Cammock, M.D., General and Thoracic Surgeon, Mount Vernon, Washington; Clinical Instructor in Surgery, University of Washington School of Medicine, Seattle, Washington. (Chapter Seven.)

Fred T. Darvill, M.D., Internist, Mount Vernon, Washington; Clinical Assistant Professor of Medicine, University of Washington School of Medicine, Seattle, Washington. (Chapter Eighteen.)

Ben Eiseman, M.D. Professor of Surgery, University of Colorado School of Medicine; Chairman, Department of Surgery, Rose Medical Center, Denver, Colorado. (Chapters Ten, Eleven, and Nineteen.)

Charles S. Houston, M.D. Internist and Cardiologist, Burlington, Vermont; Formerly Professor of Medicine, The University of Vermont College of Medicine, Burlington, Vermont. (Chapter Sixteen.)

Herbert N. Hultgren, M.D. Professor of Medicine, Stanford University Medical School; Chief, Cardiology Division, Palo Alto Veterans Administration Medical Center, Palo Alto, California. (Chapters Twelve and Seventeen.)

Thomas O. Nevison, M.D. Anesthesiologist, Denver, Colorado. (Chapter Fourteen.)

Lawrence C. Salvesen, M.D. Psychiatrist, Orono, Maine; Consultant, Eastern Maine Medical Center, Bangor, Maine. (Chapter Four.)

James A. Wilkerson, M.D. Pathologist, Merced, California.

Note: The chapter listings indicate the chapters for which each author was primarily responsible. However, as in the first two editions, the text has been rewritten to provide the uniform approach and consistent style considered desirable for the nonprofessional audience to which this book is directed. The contributors have been most understanding in consenting to such changes in the manuscripts they have submitted.

Table of Contents

Contributors		3
Foreword		7
Preface		9
Acknowledgments		12
Introduction		17

Section One: General Principles

1.	Diagnosis	20
2.	Basic Medical Care and Evacuation	28
3.	Special Problems	40
4.	Psychological Responses to Accidents	60
5.	Preventive Measures	79

Section Two: Traumatic Injuries

6.	Soft Tissue Injuries	94
7.	Fractures and Related Injuries	108
8.	Burns	133
9.	Injuries of the Head and Neck	142
10.	Chest Injuries	154
11.	Abdominal Injuries	164

Section Three: Environmental Injuries

12.	Medical Problems of High Altitude	172
13.	Cold Injuries	199
14.	Heat and Solar Injuries	217
15.	Animal Bites and Stings	230

Section Four: Nontraumatic Diseases

16.	Diseases of the Respiratory System	256
17.	Diseases of the Heart and Blood Vessels	274
18.	Gastrointestinal Diseases	288
19.	Acute Abdominal Pain	314
20.	Genitourinary Disorders	328
21.	Diseases of the Nervous System	341
22.	Disorders of the Eye, Ear, Nose, and Throat	351
23.	Infections	359
24.	Allergies	369

Section Five: Appendixes

A.	Medications	376
B.	Therapeutic Procedures	404
C.	Medical Supplies	418
D.	Legal Considerations	422
E.	Glossary	425
	Index	429

Foreword

Mountaineering: The Freedom of the Hills had been off the press scarcely long enough for copies to traverse the continent to the shores of the Atlantic Ocean when I received a letter from there, commenting on a serious imbalance. The writer, a climber completing his medical education at Johns Hopkins, commented that while the chapters on snowcraft and geology were admirably thorough, the chapter on first aid, though expertly written by climber-physicians, was the barest of elementary outlines. The book told more about the snow under climbers' boots and the rocks in their hands than it did about their bodies.

Given this level of instruction, what could the average wilderness traveler do about pyelonephritis, a pulmonary embolism, a retinal hemorrhage? Could he/she cope with snakebite, a flail chest, a "cafe coronary"? Or for that matter, swollen wisdom tooth, fecal impaction, poison oak?

In the Climbing Course of The Mountaineers, and in a companion course in mountaineering first aid, we went a considerable distance into second aid and urged students to enroll, as well, in a Red Course program. Still, the unspoken rule was: Don't get badly hurt or seriously ill at any distance from civilization unless you have an M.D. in the party. Or, to paraphrase an old Alpine maxim, "When a climber on a weekend trip comes down with the flu or breaks an ankle, he apologizes to his friends. When he gets acute appendicitis three days from the road his friends apologize for him."

Halfway and more through the twentieth century, wilderness mountaineers were recapitulating the frontiering of their nineteenth century ancestors, settlers of lonesome lands where in emergencies they could turn only to themselves and God, and where, ministers and physicians being equally rare visitors, the family library like as not consisted of two volumes — the Bible and the "doctor book."

Our ancestors were better off than we, because they *had* a doctor book. Jim Wilkerson's offer to prepare one was welcomed enthusiastically by those of us who had produced *Freedom of the Hills* yet never in the wildlands been free from submerged anxieties (does that sudden stabbing pain in the abdomen emanate from the appendix? or the salami?), anxieties that erupted as panic when a companion took a hard hit in the head (is it a fracture? a concussion? is blood coming out of the ears? or flowing into them from a cut in the scalp?).

As a non-profit publisher we had no need to consider the potential sales, if any; we expected to sell fewer copies than we gave away to indigent expeditions unable to recruit an M.D. We were content — if on one climb in one mountain range of the world the book ever saved one life it was worth doing. We were certain there would be, over the years, many more than one.

Supposing, though, all the wilderness travelers who ever owned copies were guarded by an incredibly lucky star and never experienced or witnessed mortal peril? Even so the book would be a blessing, for the confidence it gave in copability. To be sure, it could not help a layman remove an inflamed appendix, but it could help him distinguish a dozen feel-alikes from the real thing, and *that* would be a comfort. Those travelers under the incredible star might never turn the pages, yet in all their lucky years would gain peace of mind from having the book in their rucksack.

In the early 1960s we of The Mountaineers book-publishing program took great satisfaction and pride in encouraging Dr. Wilkerson to proceed, and knew the discriminating few would be grateful. What surprised us was that, far from the pages yellowing on the shelves, the book soon was moving out of our warehouse at a rate exceeded only by that of *Freedom* itself. That it has continued to do so and now, after these eighteen years, comes forth in a state-of-the-art third edition shows how wrong publishers can be. Plainly, the merit of the volume has been recognized by the discriminating *many*.

Harvey Manning

Preface

"Anyone who climbs very often for very long must expect sooner or later to be involved in misfortune, if not his own, then someone else's."[1] The outcome of such misfortune often depends on the medical care the victims receive. For mountaineering accidents, which usually occur at a considerable distance from a physician or hospital, ordinary first aid may not be adequate for the victims to recover with minimal permanent disability.

Many first aid texts have been written for a general population in urban surroundings and have been intended primarily to prevent aggravation of existing injuries by well meaning but uninformed individuals. The typical approach has been "what to do until the doctor comes." Such instructions are not sufficient for wilderness situations to which the doctor is not coming.

In addition to injuries resulting from falls or similar accidents, members of mountaineering outings must cope with the problems presented by high terrestrial altitudes and extremes of heat and cold. They must avoid the infectious and parasitic disorders that are always a threat due to inadequate sanitation in undeveloped countries. And they must be prepared to deal with a variety of medical problems usually cared for by physicians. Infectious diseases such as hepatitis and poliomyelitis, noninfectious disorders such as thrombophlebitis or strokes, and surgical problems such as appendicitis have all occurred on mountaineering expeditions in recent years.

Medicine for Mountaineering has been compiled by physicians who are also climbers to provide the information needed to prepare for the medical problems that may be encountered in mountaineering and other wilderness activities. It is a handbook of medicine — not first aid. The treatment described for some conditions includes potent medications or difficult procedures. Such remedies are necessary for optimal care for many disorders but could lead to disaster if used incorrectly. Since the appearance of the first edition, however, extensive experience with emergency medical technicians and paramedics, physician assistants, ski patrolmen, and other medical specialists has clearly demonstrated their ability to perform emergency medical procedures correctly and effectively. Climbers have demonstrated their ability to assimilate such material and use it appropriately.

9

To increase its usefulness and reduce the hazard associated with some of the therapeutic programs, this book has been designed to be used as a reference during the treatment of medical disorders. By referring to the text, the exact details of diagnosis and therapy can be ascertained. Memory is not dependable and should not be relied upon when other sources of information are available. The book can slip into a small pack without adding more than a few ounces.

To reduce potential complications from the use of medications, the doses of drugs usually is not given in the text but is provided only in the appendix where the contraindications and side effects have also been listed. By this expedient a warning of the precautions that must be observed whenever a drug is used has been provided without undue repetition in the text. (Most of the medications can only be obtained by prescription from a physician who should make certain the person obtaining the drugs knows their proper use.)

Because no alternate methods for treating some disorders are available, a few procedures have been included that would be impractical or impossible in many mountaineering circumstances. Intravenous fluid therapy is an example. The solutions and equipment for administering intravenous fluids would almost never be carried by a small climbing party. Even a large expedition might have difficulty keeping such materials in locations where they could be obtained quickly. However, intravenous fluids are the only means for keeping alive patients with some disorders, and instructions for their use have been provided. (In recent years large expeditions have left behind a considerable quantity of medical supplies, and on some popular climbing or trekking routes a significant supply of items such as intravenous fluids is now available.)

The third edition of this book has provided an opportunity to update the contents and to include some new material. The entire text has been rewritten. Larry Salvesen, a new contributor, is a psychiatrist with an uncommon store of "common sense," an experienced climber, and a participant in rescue operations in the Maine wilderness. He has presented the normal and abnormal psychological responses to accidents by both victims and their rescuers — significant material that has been infrequently considered.

To the discussion of immunizations has been added emphasis on techniques to avoid the various types of hepatitis. The description of water disinfection has been expanded to include a discussion of the advantages, the disadvantages, and the (minimal) potential risks of the different iodine methods. The section on traumatic injuries has been extensively rewritten with generous help from Ben Eiseman, but the nonhospital care for such problems has changed little in recent years.

In contrast, much new information about high altitude disorders has been unearthed in the last decade and is included in Herb Hultgren's discussion of these problems. The treatment of cold injuries has been made more understandable by arbitrarily dividing hypothermia into mild and severe forms (with the assistance of Cameron Bangs). Two types of heat stroke, the relatively recently recognized form resulting from vigorous exercise in a hot environment in which heat can not be lost, and the well known type resulting from inadequacy of the physiologic mechanisms for heat loss, have been stressed. The recently introduced "Sun Protection Factor" system for grading sunscreens has been briefly described. The treatment for poisonous snake bite emphasizes the minimal value of incision and suction for pit viper bites in the United States, their ineffectiveness for the bites of other poisonous snakes, the uselessness of other methods of nonhospital treatment except immobilization of the venom by wrapping and splinting the limb, and the need for hospitalizing the patient for antivenom therapy.

The nonhospital care for nontraumatic disease has changed little except for the availability of some improved drugs, particularly antibiotics, and improved understanding of some disorders such as traveller's diarrhea or giardiasis. Kirk Avent, an internist specializing in infectious diseases, a dedicated teacher, and a climber, is a second new contributor. He has rewritten the chapter on infections and reviewed the therapy of infectious disorders in other chapters.

Tom Hornbein, a contributor to the first two editions, did not take part in the third. His interest, support, and assistance are still deeply appreciated.

REFERENCES

1. Peters E, Editor: *Mountaineering: The Freedom of the Hills,* 4th ed, Seattle, The Mountaineers, 1982. (Quoted by permission of the editor and the publishers.)

Acknowledgments

FOR THE THIRD EDITION

Starting to work on the third edition of *Medicine for Mountaineering* has not been as difficult as starting on the second, although the analogy to rekindling an old love affair is still appropriate. New information in several fields, particularly high altitude disorders, made the need for a new edition more obvious. The availability of computer based word processors made the work much easier.

Suggestions for the third edition have been received from many individuals. All have been carefully considered; some have been of definite help; all have been appreciated. Many of the suggestions came from the contributors and are described in the Preface. My brother, Forrest Wilkerson, assisted with Appendix D, "Legal Considerations." Jo Allen Taylor has prepared the new illustrations for this edition; Rhonda Carnes entered the manuscript into the word processor. Staff members of The Mountaineers-Books — John Pollock originally, and Donna DeShazo and Ann Cleeland subsequently — have provided encouragement and indispensable assistance, sometimes just in the form of a sympathetic ear. Barbara Chasan has correctly positioned all of the punctuation, replaced many "which's" with "thats," and performed the Herculean task of copy editing with speed and grace.

Ed Peters and The Mountaineers-Books have allowed quotation from the fourth edition of *Mountaineering: The Freedom of the Hills.* William M. Lamars, Jr., M.D., Director of Hospice Calgary, has given permission to reproduce his Grief Cycle Chart which was presented at a symposium entitled "Death, Dying, and Bereavement" sponsored by the Swedish Cancer Society in 1982. Rob Taylor has graciously given permission for quotations from his book *The Breach: Kilimanjaro and the Conquest of Self.* Ray Smutek has generously allowed us to include quotations from his article "Good Morning, I'm Your Guest Victim for Today" which appeared in *Off Belay,* February 1978.

The continued love and support of my wife and children has made this endeavor possible and worthwhile.

Jim Wilkerson
Birmingham, Alabama
30 September 1984

FOR THE SECOND EDITION

Starting to work on the second edition of *Medicine for Mountaineering* has been much like trying to rekindle an old love affair. Recognition of new material to be added or inadequacies to correct has been rather easy, but developing the enthusiasm to attack the task and carry it through to completion has been surprisingly difficult. Contributors Herb Hultgren, Charles Houston, and Ben Eiseman have been principally responsible for initiating the second edition. John Pollock, of The Mountaineers, deserves credit for getting it finished. Without his encouragement and continuous gentle prodding the manuscript would still be half done.

Herb Hultgren; Dr. Burt Janis of the Division of Infectious Diseases, University of Utah College of Medicine; Dr. Warren Bowman of the Billings Clinic, Billings, Montana; Dr. Alen Barbour of the Stanford University Medical School; and Dr. Catherine MacInnes of Glenelg By Kyle, Highlands, Scotland have expended a considerable amount of time and effort to carefully go over the first edition and make many thoughtful suggestions and criticisms. Their interest and efforts have led to significant changes and improvements in the second edition and are acknowledged with gratitude. Dr. Paul Corbett of Merced has helped generously with ENT injuries and diseases. Herb Hultgren has invited the members of the Medical Committee of the American Alpine Club to review the first edition. Helpful comments have been received from Dr. Bruce Meyer, John Montgomery, Dr. Gil Roberts, Dr. Ben Ferris, and Dr. Harry McDade. Additional suggestions have been received from many other individuals, essentially all of which have contributed to the second edition and are certainly appreciated. My brother, Forrest C. Wilkerson, and his colleague Angela Roddey Holder have critically reviewed the appendix section "Legal Considerations."

Gerry Robertson, Medical Illustrator, Pacific Palisades, California, has produced the new or revised illustrations for the second edition with interest, understanding, and skill which have resulted in significant additions to the text. Peggy Ferber has contributed her considerable knowledge and ability to smoothing the rough edges of the manuscript, preparing it for the printer, and shepherding it through the processes of printing, proofreading and publication. To Barbara McBurney and Joan Boland must go a word of thanks for their assistance in typing the manuscript and the considerable correspondence which has been associated with this undertaking.

"The Journal of the American Medical Association" and Drs. Lawrence Corey and Michael A. W. Hattwick have granted permission to reproduce the algorithm for postexposure rabies prophylaxis from the article "Treatment of Persons Exposed to Rabies," J.A.M.A. *232*:272, 1975, which is acknowledged with pleasure and appreciation.

My wife has accepted my preoccupation with this second edition and the accompanying clutter and confusion without complaint. My children have given up their river trip and mountaineering outings for an entire summer so the work could progress without greater delay. To them I must express my gratitude and deepest affection.

J.W.

FOR THE FIRST EDITION

One of the major difficulties encountered in preparing this book has been the problem of describing diseases and their diagnosis and treatment in terms which could be readily understood by individuals who are not familiar with the vocabulary or basic principles of medicine. Although each of the contributors solved this problem in his own way, their chapters varied widely in approach, terminology, and the style of writing. These variations, which are to be expected in works by multiple authors, would not have seriously detracted from a book directed to a professional audience. However, this material is intended for individuals with a limited knowledge of the subject. Therefore, to provide the uniform approach and consistent style which were considered necessary to reduce confusion and misunderstanding to a minimum, the text has been extensively rewritten. The contributors have realized the need for such alterations and have consented to them in a manner which the editor is pleased to acknowledge and for which he is deeply appreciative.

Special recognition must also go to Harvey Manning, writer, outdoorsman, conservationst, and highly valued member of The Mountaineers. Without his conviction of the need for a book of its kind, this work would never have begun. Without his continued encouragement, stimulation, and support it would not have been completed. Without his editorial assistance and judgment it would never have acquired what literary merit it may have.

John Rossiter, Medical Illustrator for the University of Virginia Medical School, who made the earlier drawings, and Alan Cole, Medical Illustrator, Altadena, California, who completed this work after John's untimely and tragic death, have combined their considerable talents with an interest and understanding of the purpose of this book to produce illustrations which are both fitting and highly informative. To Marlene Kuffel, Helen Hunterman, and Joyce Braine must go a word of thanks for their generous assistance in typing the manuscript during its various stages of development.

Further appreciation is gratefully expressed to Dr. F. Dennette Adams and the William & Wilkins Company of Baltimore for permission to quote from *Cabot and Adams Physical Diagnosis, 14th Ed.*; to Dr. N. Howard-Jones, Director, Division of Editorial and Reference Services of the World Health Organization for permission to use the table of the treatment for rabies following varying types of exposure published by that organization; to the American College of Surgeons for permission to quote from *Early Care of Acute Soft Tissue Injuries*; to Harvey

Manning and The Mountaineers for permission to quote from *Mountaineering: The Freedom of the Hills*; to H. V. J. Kilness, Editor, and "Summit" for permisson to use illustrations from the article "Head Injuries" which appeared in Vol. 7, No. 5: 2-7, May 1961; to Dr. Julian Johnson and Year Book Medical Publishers, Inc., for permission to adapt for this book illustrations from *Surgery of the Chest, 3rd Ed.*; and to Walter L. Griffith, Director, Product Advertising and Promotion, and Parke, Davis & Company for providing photographs of their plastic inflatable splint, ReadiSplint, for use in preparing drawings of such splints.

Finally, to my wife and children, who have generously forgiven my frequent derelictions from the duties of a husband and father during the production of this book, I wish to express my heartfelt thanks and deepest affection.

J.W.

Introduction

The ability to rationally analyze a problem or situation and select and pursue a direct, logical course to a solution is a rare talent sometimes known as "common sense." No ability is more important in caring for individuals with medical disorders in mountaineering circumstances.

The functions of the body and the intricacies of its varied disorders are highly complex. Only those who are familiar with the principles of diagnosis and therapy can provide optimal medical care for the victims of injury or disease, particularly in remote situations. Knowledge of these principles, thoughtfully applied, has often been the difference between survival and death.

The members of mountaineering outings should know how to provide basic medical care and should be prepared to administer the treatment that is needed. The knowledge and medical equipment required depends upon the location and duration of the outing. Traumatic disorders — the injuries produced by physical forces such as falls or falling objects — are the most common in mountaineering, particularly on outings of only a few days. Signs and symptoms of nontraumatic disorders, such as infections or diseases of the heart or lungs, usually develop gradually over a period of several days and often do not become apparent during short trips. During longer trips, the slower onset may permit the victim to be evacuated under his own power before he is incapacitated. Additionally, climbers as a group tend to be young and healthy and are less susceptible to nontraumatic disorders.

Members of any mountaineering outing, regardless of its location or duration, should be capable of:

1. Caring for soft tissue injuries;
2. Anticipating and treating shock;
3. Recognizing and caring for fractures;
4. Diagnosing and treating head injuries;
5. Caring for and evacuating an unconscious individual;
6. Diagnosing and treating thoracic and abdominal injuries;
7. Recognizing and treating heat or cold injuries;
8. Recognizing and treating altitude disorders;
9. Carrying out cardiopulmonary resuscitation.

In addition, members of extended expeditions should develop:

1. The ability to take a simple medical history and perform a physical examination;
2. A familiarity with the techniques of patient care, including the administration of medications;
3. A knowledge of the diseases likely to be encountered on that particular expedition.

Every climber should have a thorough examination by a physician before beginning the climbing season. Mountaineering organizations should consider whether such examinations should be required before anyone participates in a climb. (Preexisting medical disorders that would be recognized during a physician's examination and treated are too complex for inclusion in a handbook such as this.) For prolonged expeditions into isolated areas, a prior medical examination is essential. Individuals with a peptic ulcer, gallstones, hernia, pregnancy, a history of intestinal obstruction following an abdominal operation, or chronic malaria with a large spleen should be advised of the risk in prolonged isolation where surgical help is not available.

SECTION ONE
GENERAL PRINCIPLES

CHAPTER ONE

Diagnosis

"Disease manifests itself by abnormal sensations and events (symptoms), and by changes in structure or function (signs). Symptoms, being subjective, must be described by the patient. Signs are objective and these the physician discovers by means of physical examination, laboratory studies, and special methods of investigation."[1]

This statement succinctly describes the means by which medical disorders are diagnosed. Traumatic injuries — those resulting from physical forces such as falls — are identified primarily by physical examination. The description of symptoms by the patient, the medical "history," plays a greater role in the recognition of nontraumatic diseases. The lack of facilities for laboratory studies or other investigations should not prevent the diagnosis of most illnesses occurring in wilderness circumstances. Most of the common diseases were being accurately diagnosed by history and physical examination long before most of the special investigative methods currently in use were available.

The diagnosis is usually the most difficult aspect of medical care for a patient with a nontraumatic disorder. Physicians commonly expend more effort identifying many diseases than actually treating them. In this chapter, outlines are provided to help individuals caring for a patient recognize the organs or tissues that are the sites of the disorder. Later chapters directed to disorders of specific organ systems contain more thorough discussions of diagnostic features, which should permit reasonably accurate identification of most common disorders. These guides should be consulted repeatedly and openly. "Mistakes are just as often caused by lack of thoroughness as by lack of knowledge."[1] Before a major expedition several members should practice taking medical histories — with the assistance of a physician, if possible.

Effectively examining the victim of a medical disorder is not as simple as following an outline, however. Tact, diplomacy, and a calm, understanding, and sympathetic manner are essential. The ability to appraise and understand the personality of the patient and to adopt an approach that instills confidence is vital. A seriously ill or injured person can not be expected to be cheerful and understanding or, on some occasions, even cooperative.

Interruptions during the examination should be avoided. For the victim of trauma, an initial rapid examination should identify major injuries that require emergency treatment such as the control of bleeding, establishing an open airway, or even splinting a fracture. Immediate evacuation from a position of imminent danger such as falling rock may be necessary, but a complete, unhurried, and uninterrupted examination should be carried out as soon as possible.

After the examination has been completed, the findings should be written out. While transcribing what he has found, the examiner can systematically consider the abnormalities he has discovered and utilize his knowledge of disease and the information that he is able to obtain from other sources to arrive at a diagnosis. Furthermore, he can periodically reconsider that diagnosis, particularly if new signs or symptoms appear or the response to treatment is not that which was expected. If the abnormalities are not written down, details are almost always forgotten or overlooked during later reconsideration.

THE MEDICAL HISTORY

The patient should be encouraged to describe his symptoms in his own words. Leading questions should be avoided as much as possible, although some direct inquiries are almost always necessary. A patient's failure to mention a symptom is no indication that it is not present.

Various features of illness point to specific diagnoses. The time or circumstances in which symptoms appear and their chronological sequence are often significant. The exact location of pain or discomfort, the time at which it began, whether the onset was gradual or sudden, the intensity or severity of the pain, and the quality of the pain — cramping, stabbing, burning, or others — should be ascertained. Whether symptoms are continuous or intermittent, how they are aggravated or relieved, how they are related to each other, and how they are affected by such factors as position, eating or defecation, or exertion and sleep must be determined. Nonpainful symptoms such as tiredness, weakness, dizziness, nausea — or their absence — may be highly significant.

An account of any past illnesses must always be obtained, even though in mountaineering circumstances the present illness is usually the most significant part of the history. If the patient's illness is a recurrence of a previous disease, awareness of that disorder can provide the key to its understanding. Additionally, preexisting disease such as diabetes or epilepsy must be brought to light so that necessary treatment can be continued. Even the victims of trauma can have such disorders and should be carefully questioned about their past medical history.

MEDICAL HISTORY

PAST HISTORY
Previous Illnesses: Bronchitis, asthma, pneumonia, pleurisy, tuberculosis, rheumatic fever; any other heart or lung disease; malaria,

diabetes, epilepsy, anemia; any other severe or chronic illnesses.

Operations: Date, nature of operation, complications.

Injuries: Date, nature of injury and residual disability; history of mountaineering related injuries, including cold injury, snow blindness, or altitude illness.

Medications: Any medications currently being taken or taken in the past; reason for medications.

Family History: Diseases that tend to run in the family, particularly heart, lung, kidney, or neurological disorders.

Exposure: Recent exposure to infection; recent residence in an area that was the site of an epidemic.

Immunizations: Initial immunizations, when administered, boosters.

Allergies: Allergy to food or similar substances, insect stings, or drugs, particularly penicillin and sulfa drugs.

REVIEW OF SYSTEMS (Including both present and past illnesses)

Head: Headache, dizziness, hallucinations, confusion, or fainting.

Eyes: Inflammation, pain, double vision, loss of vision.

Nose: Colds, sinus trouble, postnasal drip, bleeding, obstruction.

Teeth: General condition, abscesses, dentures.

Mouth: Pain, bleeding, sores, dryness.

Throat: Sore throat, tonsillitis, hoarseness, difficulty in swallowing or talking.

Ears: Pain, discharge, ringing or buzzing, hearing loss.

Neck: Stiffness, pain, swelling, or masses.

Heart and Lungs: Chest pain, palpitations, shortness of breath (greater than that expected or experienced by others with exercise or altitude), cough, amount and character of material that is coughed up, coughing up blood.

Gastrointestinal: Loss of appetite, nausea, vomiting, vomiting blood or "coffee ground" material, indigestion, gas, pain; constipation, use of laxatives, diarrhea, bloody or black (tarry) stools, pale or clay colored stools, hemorrhoids; jaundice.

Genitourinary: Increase or decrease in frequency of voiding, back pain, pain with voiding; passage of blood, gravel, or stones; sores, purulent discharge, venereal disease or sexual contact; menstrual abnormalities such as irregular periods, increased bleeding with periods, bleeding between periods, cramps.

Neuromuscular:	Fainting, unconsciousness from other causes, dizziness or vertigo, twitching, convulsions; muscle cramps, shooting pains, muscular or joint pains; anesthesia, tingling sensations, weakness, incoordination, or paralysis.
Skin:	Rashes, abscesses or boils.
General:	Fever, chills, weakness, easy fatigability, dizziness, weight loss.

THE PHYSICAL EXAMINATION

If a physical examination is to provide useful information, some previous experience on the part of the examiner is highly desirable, particularly for examining the chest and abdomen. For the inexperienced examiner, comparison of the patient with a normal individual may be helpful, but there is no substitute for prior tutelage by a physician.

A complete physical examination is an essential element of the evaluation of anyone with a medical disorder. The victim of trauma must be completely examined so no wounds are overlooked, particularly in the presence of an obvious injury. For the examination, the patient should be made comfortable and protected from wind and cold — so far as possible. The examiner's hands should be warm and he must be gentle. Any unnecessary roughness makes obtaining diagnostic information more difficult and can aggravate the patient's disorder.

To ensure that all areas of the body are examined, a definite routine should always be followed. The outline below is relatively complete and is adequate for both traumatic and nontraumatic disorders. The examination of some anatomical areas, particularly the chest and abdomen, is described in more detail in the chapters dealing with those areas.

PHYSICAL EXAMINATION

General (Vital Signs):	Pulse rate, respiratory rate, temperature, blood pressure, general appearance.
Skin:	Color, texture, rashes, abscesses or boils.
Head:	
Eyes:	Eyebrows and eyelids, eye movements, vision, size and equality of pupils, reaction of pupils to light, inflammation.
Nose:	Appearance, discharge, nature of discharge, bleeding.
Mouth:	Sores, bleeding, dryness.
Throat:	Inflammation, purulent exudates.
Ears:	Appearance, discharge, bleeding.

Neck:	Limitation of movement, enlarged lymph nodes.
Lungs:	Respiratory movements, breath sounds, voice sounds, bubbling.
Heart:	Pulse rate, regularity, blood pressure.
Abdomen:	General appearance, tenderness, rebound and referred pain, spasm of muscles, masses.
Genitalia:	Tenderness, masses.
Rectum:	Hemorrhoids, impacted feces, abscesses.
Back:	Tenderness, muscle spasm, limitation of movement.
Extremities:	Pain or tenderness, limitation of movement, deformities, unequal length, swelling, ulcers, soft tissue injuries, lymph node enlargement, sensitivity to pin prick and light touch, muscle spasm.

EXAMINING TRAUMA VICTIMS

The victims of traumatic injuries may have injuries that have produced conditions such as respiratory obstruction or severe bleeding that must be cared for immediately. After these emergencies have received attention, however, the rescuers must pause and essentially start over from the beginning. Frequently, the first action should be the organization of the rescue party, delegating some individuals to examine and treat the accident victims and assigning others the responsibility for preparing for evacuation, overnight bivouac, or whatever is most appropriate.

The persons assigned to each accident victim must start from the beginning with the medical history. They need to obtain an account of the accident and the time and circumstances in which it occurred. Frequently the nature of the accident provides major clues to the injuries that should be anticipated. If the victim is unconscious, any witnesses to the accident must be asked whether unconsciousness was the result or the cause of the accident. The examiner must determine whether the victim had any preexisting medical conditions that may have contributed to the accident or that may require additional treatment. All of this information must be recorded.

The victim's condition and the character and extent of his injuries must be determined. His pulse and respiratory rate (and blood pressure, if possible) should be measured — and recorded — immediately and every ten to fifteen minutes until they are clearly stable. These vital signs should be rechecked immediately after the patient is moved; an increase in pulse rate or fall in blood pressure at such times is often an early sign of shock.

Although a few injuries such as fractures of the legs may have to be cared for first, the victim must be completely and thoroughly examined. Concealed injuries must be carefully sought. Injuries of the back are most frequently overlooked, even in hospital emergency rooms. If the victim is lying on his stomach when first approached, his back should be examined before he is turned over. At some point, his back must be examined, even though fractures of the extremities or the vertebral column require that the examination be made with minimal movement of the patient.

A systematic routine must be learned and followed so that no areas of the body are overlooked. Chest injuries are unquestionably more threatening than hand injuries and deserve prior attention, but failure to recognize and care for a hand injury can result in a crippling deformity that leaves the victim permanently handicapped.

> "With a complete diagnosis, and an accurate evaluation of the general condition of the patient, the battle is half won. Many errors in care are due to incomplete diagnosis, to overlooking some serious injury while concentrating on the obvious. A systematic method of examination will obviate such errors."[2]

Examinations must be repeated, not only to monitor the condition of the patient, but also to ensure that all injuries have been found and treated. If the victim is unconscious at the time of the initial examination, he must be reexamined as soon as he regains consciousness.

THE MEDICAL RECORD

For disabling diseases or injuries in circumstances where a physician's help is more than a few hours away, a detailed written account of the medical history and the physical examination findings is an essential element in the patient's medical care. Memory alone can not be relied upon to determine whether a symptom was present or physical changes were detectable, even a few hours after the examination. Memory is not a dependable record of numerical data such as pulse and respiratory rates, temperature, and blood pressure. If any significant treatment, particularly drugs, has been administered, a written account of the doses and times they were given is essential.

For patients with nontraumatic illnesses in a remote situation, a written record allows the examiner to systematically review his findings while trying to arrive at an accurate diagnosis. Written records are much easier to use when consulting medical texts or when trying to obtain help by other means such as radio.

Written records of the vital signs (pulse, respiratory rate, blood pressure, and temperature) and other features of the patient's illness allow small changes in these signs to be detected. Such changes usually precede more obvious indications that the patient's condition is worsening and allow treatment to be instituted earlier, when it commonly is more effective. Small changes may also indicate a response to treatment and presage an improvement in the patient's overall condition, perhaps allowing a difficult emergency evacuation to be delayed until circumstances are more favorable.

In circumstances where evacuation of a patient is prolonged, written records allow more than one individual to share in the patient's care. Because all can determine what the patient's signs or symptoms were at any time in the course of his illness, all can recognize changes and take any steps that are needed. Written records are also needed for correctly administering medications so that doses are not omitted or duplicated.

If the patient is to be evacuated, written records are essential for the physician who is to care for him. In some circumstances, such as a helicopter rescue, the person caring for the patient may not be able to accompany him and provide a verbal record. If evacuation has required several days and more than one person has been involved in the patient's care, a written record is the physician's only source of accurate information about the patient's original condition, how that has changed, and the treatment that has been given — particularly the drugs that have been administered.

The value of written medical records is demonstrated by the way they are immediately begun when a patient enters a hospital emergency room or a physician's office. Such records are usually subpoenaed at the beginning of any medical malpractice action, and omissions or alterations have often been damaging to the physician's defense.

The outlines provided for the medical history and the physical examination are suitable outlines for the medical record. Obviously, all abnormalities should be recorded, but the absence of abnormalities is frequently of equal importance, particularly for nontraumatic disorders. If a specific statement that a sign or symptom was absent has not been made, a physician subsequently caring for the patient may be unable to determine whether that change was really absent or was simply not noticed.

For traumatic injuries, an account of the accident should be recorded at the earliest opportunity. All injuries should be carefully described. The absence of injuries, or any evidence of injury such as swelling or discoloration, in major areas of the body — chest, abdomen, head, arms, or legs — should also be noted. The vital signs should be recorded at intervals of thirty to sixty minutes for four to eight hours or as long as these signs are not stable. After stabilization, vital signs need to be recorded only about every four hours until the patient is well on his way to recovery. Any preexisting medical conditions should be described. The dosage, route, and time of administration of all medication must be accurately logged. Notes about any other treatment or changes in the patient's condition should also include the time.

The written record must be kept with the patient in an accessible location and not tucked away in a pack or similar inconvenient spot. Notations of changes in the patient's condition or of medications must be made immediately and not recorded from memory at a later time.

REFERENCES

1. Adams FD: *Cabot and Adams Physical Diagnosis,* 14th ed. Baltimore, The Williams & Wilkins Co., 1958. (Quoted by permission of the author and publishers.)
2. Kennedy RH in Committee on Trauma, American College of Surgeons: *Early Care of Acute Soft Tissue Injuries.* Chicago, 1957. (Quoted by permission of the publishers.)

CHAPTER TWO

Basic Medical Care and Evacuation

Most victims of major accidents or serious illness in the mountains are evacuated within hours or, at the most, one to two days. Occasionally, however, bad weather, difficult terrain, distance from a hospital or mechanical transportation, insufficient personnel for stretcher evacuation, or other problems may require that the patient be cared for in a remote wilderness situation. Persons with less severe disorders may not need evacuation, particularly if they are expected to recover enough to walk out or resume climbing within a relatively short time.

NURSING CARE

Anyone confined to bed (or sleeping bag) by illness or injury has certain basic needs that require attention, regardless of the nature of the illness. Ministering to these needs is most readily identifiable as "nursing care." The fundamental objective of this type of care is simple: to allow the body to heal itself.

Comfort and Understanding

Comfort and understanding — the essence of nursing — are needed by all, regardless of the nature or severity of their medical problems. Some have a greater need than others; many try to deny their need. Regardless of the situation, the medical supplies on hand, or the sophistication of available medical knowledge, interest and concern, sympathy and understanding can always be shown; comfort and reassurance can always be provided. All are essential.

Rest

Rest promotes healing during an illness or after an injury in several ways. External or emotional stress is reduced, and additional injury to damaged tissues is avoided. At high altitudes, rest can provide an opportunity for improved nutrition and the nutrients can be used for healing instead of muscular effort. A few patients with heart disease may need to be almost immobilized, but patients with other diseases, particularly disorders that do not involve the heart or lungs, do not need such confinement. Often, remaining in camp rather than hiking or climbing is all that is required to hasten recovery.

In the absence of any injury or disease involving the brain, medications promoting sleep may be given at altitudes below 10,000 feet (3,000 m). However, at higher elevations conventional sleeping medications should not be administered because they can lead to unnecessarily low blood oxygenation during sleep, which may aggravate symptoms of altitude sickness. Much of the sleeplessness and ir- regular breathing associated with high altitude can be relieved with acetazolamide. (See Chapter Twelve, "Medical Problems of High Altitude.")

For the victim of a painful injury, analgesia is necessary for restful sleep. Many patients are much more aware of pain at night when nothing is happening to divert their attention. For three or four days after a major injury, occasionally even longer, strong analgesics such as morphine or meperidine may be needed. (These drugs have so much sedative effect that additional sleeping medication is not needed and should not be given. Combining a sleeping medication with a ma- jor analgesic is hazardous.)

Warmth

Victims of illness or injury must be kept warm without overheating. At temperatures near or below freezing, a patient with a severe illness or injury may not be able to generate enough heat to maintain a normal body temperature, even in a sleeping bag and tent. For such patients, as well as some victims of exposure, external sources of heat may be necessary to restore and maintain normal body temperature. (See Chapter Thirteen, "Cold Injuries.")

Lower Altitude

Evacuation from altitudes above 15,000 feet (4,600 m) hastens healing and per- mits a more complete return to normal following traumatic injuries as well as other types of disease. Individuals with diseases of the lungs or heart should be taken as low as possible, preferably below 8,000 feet (2,400 m), and provided with supplemental oxygen if it is available.

Coughing

Patients who are immobilized with a severe injury or serious illness usually do not breathe deeply, particularly if breathing is painful. As a result of diminished respiratory activity, the lungs are not fully expanded and fluid and mucus tend to accumulate in the immobile segments. These collections are an ideal medium for bacterial growth and cause pneumonia unless they are evacuated. Such infections are the most common cause of death for elderly persons confined to bed with fractured hips or similar injuries.

To eliminate the fluids, expand the lungs, and reduce the danger of infection, patients must be encouraged — or even forced — to breathe deeply and to cough at frequent intervals. Coughing may be difficult and painful for a very ill patient or the victim of a chest or abdominal injury, but these patients are the most prone to develop pulmonary infections and most need to clear their lungs. The practice in most hospitals is to have the patient sit up, hold his sides, and cough deeply — not just clear his throat — at least once every two hours. A similar routine should be adopted under mountaineering circumstances, particularly at higher altitudes where any compromise in pulmonary function could be disastrous.

Elimination of fluids from the lungs can also be increased by postural drainage. If the patient's head and chest are kept slightly lower than the rest of his body, gravity helps get rid of the fluids. In a tent such positioning can best be achieved by elevating the abdomen, pelvis, and legs. After the patient has recovered to the extent that he is able to be up and walking around, forced coughing or postural drainage are usually no longer necessary.

Ambulation

Anyone confined to bed as a result of illness or injury should be encouraged to get up and walk around a little several times a day. Such exercise increases the circulation in the legs and plays an important role in the prevention of thrombophlebitis. (See Chapter Sixteen, "Diseases of the Respiratory System.") The only major exceptions to this rule in mountaineering circumstances are patients with injuries of the pelvis or lower extremities that prevent walking, and patients who have already developed thrombophlebitis and should remain as immobile as possible until the disorder has resolved.

Diet

Solid food is not as important during the acute stages of an illness as an adequate fluid intake. Unless an associated disorder dictates a particular type of diet, such as the bland diet for peptic ulcers, the patient should be permitted to eat whatever he desires. During convalescence more attention can be given to a nutritionally adequate diet that can contain extra amounts of protein.

Bowel Care

Difficulties with bowel evacuation are common in persons confined to bed. Repression of the urge to defecate, low food intake, and dehydration (resulting from a reduced fluid intake and increased fluid losses due to altitude, increased sweating, or other causes) all contribute to the problem. If not corrected, fecal impaction often results. (See Chapter Eighteen, "Gastrointestinal Diseases.") Even though stool volume is reduced in the absence of solid food in the diet, bowel movements should occur about every three to four days. The best way to ensure normal elimination is to make certain the fluid intake is adequate; roughage or fiber in the diet to increase stool bulk is also helpful. Laxatives or enemas should rarely be needed to prevent impaction in a bed ridden individual.

Convalescence

Although exercise should be encouraged during convalescence, strenuous activity prior to complete recovery may delay the return to normal health, particularly at high altitudes. In addition, an individual is more susceptible to other diseases or injuries during convalescence. To be certain that recovery is complete delaying a return to full activity for two or three extra days may be desirable.

FLUID BALANCE

An adequate fluid intake is always essential. A person can live for weeks without food, but only a few days without water. Fluid balance implies an equilibrium between losses (through the kidneys, skin, lungs, or other routes) and gains (from fluids and foods that have been ingested.) During an illness that increases fluid losses and makes fluid intake difficult or impossible, fluid balance can become critical. Dehydration resulting from massive diarrheal fluid loss was the cause of death for the hundreds of thousands who died in ravaging cholera epidemics of past centuries.

An adult male of average size normally loses one and one-half to two liters of water from his body each day. The "sensible loss" is excreted by the kidneys and ranges from one to two liters per day. The "insensible loss," of which he may be unaware, occurs through perspiration (even in cold climates) and evaporation from the lungs (to moisten air that is inhaled.) The daily volume of this loss is one-half to one liter in temperate climates and at low altitudes. Increased fluid losses occur in hot climates or with high fevers, when several liters of water may be lost daily through perspiration (which is no longer insensible), or at high altitudes, where up to four liters of fluid may be lost daily through the lungs.

Salt (sodium chloride), potassium, and bicarbonate are known collectively as electrolytes and are vital constituents of body fluids. As with water, a balance between intake and loss must be maintained. The daily salt requirement for an average adult is five grams. When large amounts of salt are lost through perspiration, needs may be as high as fifteen grams a day.

Normal kidneys are very sensitive to changes in the body's fluid balance and react immediately to conserve or eliminate water as circumstances may require. The urine volume provides a highly reliable indication of the balance between fluid intake and losses. A twenty-four hour volume of less than 500 cc of deeply colored urine is indicative of fluid depletion; a volume of 2,000 cc of very lightly colored urine is a sign of excessive fluid intake.

These water and electrolyte requirements represent the needs of a normal, healthy adult. Individuals with heart or kidney disease may be unable to get rid of excess salt or water and can have quite different requirements. The administration of normal quantities of electrolytes and water, particularly salt, to persons with one of these disorders can have serious consequences.

With a severe illness causing high fluid losses (such as dysentery or cholera) the volume of fluid lost as vomitus and watery stools should be measured — an unpleasant but necessary task — in order to stay abreast of a patient's fluid status. Insensible losses also must be estimated, taking into consideration fever, environmental temperature, and altitude. The volume of fluid ingested must also be measured. These measurements and estimates must be recorded as they are made so the patient's fluid needs can be calculated subsequently.

The twenty-four hour urine volume is a precise indicator of a patient's fluid balance but tends to reflect what has already happened rather than his current status. Measuring losses and gains as they occur provides a more immediate insight into the condition of a patient with a severe fluid losing disorder.

Dehydration at Altitude

Higher altitudes tend to produce dehydration, and this tendency becomes progressively greater as the elevation increases and the environment becomes colder. Probably most climbers are dehydrated to some extent above 18,000 feet (5,500 m). Some investigators have suggested that the depression, impaired judgment, and other psychological and intellectual changes that commonly occur at high altitudes and for which hypoxia has been blamed, may actually be the result of dehydration.

The principal cause of dehydration at high altitude is the increased fluid loss associated with more rapid and deeper breathing of cold air. Air is warmed to body temperature and is saturated with water as it passes through the upper air passages; it has a relative humidity of one hundred percent when it reaches the lungs. At higher altitudes a greater volume of air must be inspired to provide the oxygen that is needed, and a larger quantity of water is required to moisten the increased amount of air. Furthermore, cold air contains little moisture, and more water is required to humidify air that is initially cold than air that is warm. (The relative humidity might be quite high when the air is cold but can drop to below ten percent when the air is warmed to body temperature. Loss of heat through evaporation of water and warming cold air is a significant contributor to hypothermia at higher altitudes.)

In cold environments, some of the water that humidifies inspired air is regained during expiration by condensation in the upper air passages that have been cooled by the inspired air. However, mouth breathing during exercise or at other times bypasses the air passages where most condensation occurs and increases water loss. Many climbers are not careful about managing clothing to minimize sweating, particularly with the bulky clothing required to keep warm during periods of immobility at high altitude, and fluid loss from this source is not held to the lowest levels possible.

A decrease in fluid consumption probably contributes to dehydration at high elevations. Both the need to carry fuel and melt snow to obtain water for drinking or cooking, and the loss or dulling of the sensation of thirst that accompanies the loss of appetite, nausea, or even vomiting that occurs with acute mountain sickness, tend to reduce fluid intake.

Climbers must consciously force themselves to drink large volumes of fluid at high altitude. Thirst alone is not a reliable indicator of the need for water. Above 15,000 to 16,000 feet (4,600 to 4,900 m), fluid requirements often exceed four liters per day. The adequacy of fluid intake can best be judged by the urine color and volume. Darkly colored urine — orange snow flowers instead of light yellow — the absence of a need to void upon awakening from a night's sleep, or a twenty-four hour volume of less than one-half liter are indicators of significant dehydration.

Fluid Replacement

The easiest and most reliable method for replacing lost fluids is to drink them. Almost any nonalcoholic fluid is suitable, but since water contains no electrolytes, fruit juices, soft drinks, soups, and similar liquids should be encouraged. (Coffee, tea, and hot chocolate are not as satisfactory because they contain caffeine and related substances, which are diuretics and increase renal fluid loss.)

Seriously ill patients with very little appetite often refuse liquids as well as solid foods. However, they can often be persuaded to drink small quantities of fluids, just two or three sips, at frequent intervals such as every fifteen to twenty minutes. With tenacity, patience, and gentle encouragement such patients frequently can be coaxed into drinking several liters of fluid over a twenty-four hour period.

Some patients, most commonly those with protracted vomiting or who are unconscious, are unable to take fluids orally. If medical attention can be obtained within one or two days and fluid losses are not increased, the intervening fluid depletion is usually not too severe. However, longer periods without fluid, and disorders which increase fluid loss, can produce severe dehydration if fluids are not given intravenously.

Administering fluid intravenously should be attempted only by persons who are experienced and knowledgeable about such therapy. Fluids suitable for intravenous administration (which cannot be improvised) would only be carried by a large, well equipped expedition, although such fluids might by obtained by air drop. Such fluids are often left behind when expeditions are finished, and in some popular climbing areas a significant supply has accumulated. These fluids have come from many nations and their labels are printed in many languages, but the contents are usually listed in standard chemical symbols or in English.

The amount of fluids to be given intravenously must be determined each day. Fluids are required to replace both normal and abnormal losses. Two liters of five percent glucose and one-half liter of an electrolyte solution (preferably a balanced salt solution, but normal saline if only that is available) usually satisfy the body's daily needs when there is no abnormal loss. Fluids lost through vomiting, diarrhea, or excessive perspiration should be replaced with an electrolyte solution. Excessive fluid loss through the lungs due to altitude should be replaced by glucose since no electrolytes are lost with the moisture in expired air.

Most electrolyte solutions contain little potassium. Patients with poor kidney function cannot rid themselves of excessive potassium, which may rapidly accumulate to lethal levels. However, patients with normal renal function excrete potassium in the urine. As a result, blood potassium concentrations can fall to dangerously low levels during prolonged intravenous fluid therapy if the potassium is not replaced. Therefore, individuals receiving intravenous fluids for more than two to three days, or who have large abnormal losses from diarrhea, and who have a normal urine volume, should receive an extra 15 to 20 mEq of potassium per liter of electrolyte. (The occasions when such potassium supplements are available in mountaineering circumstances must be rare. When available, the supplements are usually supplied in a solution which can be added directly to the electrolyte solution.)

If a person with a healthy heart and normally functioning kidneys is provided with an adequate intake of water (as glucose) and electrolytes (balanced salt solution), the kidneys compensate for any imbalance that may exist. The inevitable inaccuracies inherent in measuring fluid intake and output are fully corrected. However, an individual with preexisting heart disease and a history of congestive heart failure, a person with severe kidney disease, or a patient with acute renal failure as a result of his disease or injury requires much more accurate therapy, which can only be provided with hospital facilities. For such patients, any error in administering fluids must be on the side of not giving enough.

CARE FOR TRAUMA VICTIMS

Traumatic injuries are produced by physical forces such as falls, avalanches, or the minor accidents of camp life and are by far the most common medical problems encountered by healthy, young climbers.

Emergencies

True medical emergencies in which a delay of a few minutes in providing care can significantly affect the outcome are rare. In mountaineering accidents the opportunity to provide such treatment may pass before anyone is able to get to the victim. Nonetheless, climbers must be familiar with the procedures for treating traumatic medical emergencies if they are to deal with them successfully on the rare occasions when they do occur. True emergencies do not allow time for referral to a textbook.

If immediate action is necessary to prevent loss of life following an accident, the order in which problems should receive attention is as follows:

1. RESPIRATION. An open airway must be established first; interference with breathing by chest wounds must also be quickly corrected. If needed, cardiopulmonary resuscitation should be started.
2. BLEEDING. After the patient is breathing or being resuscitated, bleeding should be controlled by direct pressure at bleeding sites, not by tourniquets or pressure points.
3. SHOCK. After cardiac and respiratory function has been established and bleeding stopped, attention should be directed to treating or preventing shock. Treatment given in anticipation of shock is more effective than treatment instituted after the presence of shock is apparent.

Although the order of the first two problems may appear reversed because control of severe bleeding should take only seconds but cardiopulmonary resuscitation can be prolonged, in reality they are not. Anyone whose heart has stopped does not bleed. Therefore, CPR must take first priority. Furthermore, anyone who has bled so extensively his heart has stopped can not be resuscitated. The combination of cardiac arrest and severe hemorrhage is essentially always lethal.

Other Injuries

All injuries should be treated as completely as possible before the patient is moved. Open wounds are always contaminated to some extent; further contamination should be avoided. Soft tissue injuries should be covered with voluminous dressings that compress the wounds to help control bleeding, immobilize the injured areas, minimize swelling, and control infection. Even when no fractures are present, extremities with severe injuries should be immobilized and should be elevated slightly to aid blood circulation. If the lower extremities are injured and evacuation requires the victim to walk or climb, frequent rest stops should be made during which he should lie down and elevate his feet. Splinting fractures before the victim is moved is particularly important. "Splint 'em where they lie" is a time proven adage.

The equipment necessary for the treatment of some injuries, such as injuries of the chest, is not available on most short outings and is almost never carried on an actual climb. However, this equipment should always be available in popular climbing areas and should be a part of the emergency gear of all mountain rescue organizations.

SPECIFIC ACCIDENTS

Avalanches

Most avalanche victims die from traumatic injuries produced by the impact of large blocks of hard packed snow or ice. A smaller number are suffocated under loose snow. The following outline can be followed in caring for avalanche victims immediately after they have been found:

1. Obviously lethal injuries should be sought. If present, attention can be directed to other victims and evacuation of the body can be delayed until the hazard of further avalanches has passed.
2. The victim should be assumed to have a broken neck if he is unconscious and no lethal injuries can be found. Appropriate support and prevention of movement must be continued as long as necessary.
3. An open airway must be established, chest injuries must be covered, and resuscitation must be initiated if the victim is not breathing. Movement of his neck must still be avoided, which is not a simple matter.
4. After the victim is breathing, his other wounds should be treated as rapidly as possible so he can be protected from cold injuries and moved out of the avalanche path at the earliest possible moment.

Lightning

Lightning kills more people than any other kind of natural disaster. In the United States between 150 and 300 persons die from such injuries every year; in 1943, 430 lightning deaths occurred. However, the number who die is less than one-third of those who are hit by lightning. Since only the more severely injured get reported, the true fatality rate is probably between ten and twenty percent. Most survivors have no significant residual disabilities.

Because the voltage in a bolt of lightning is so high (200 million to 2 billion volts of direct current), it tends to produce a "flashover" effect. When lightning strikes a person, it typically "flashes" over the outside of the body, particularly if the body is wet. Electricity does penetrate the body enough to disrupt the electrical functions of the brain and heart, but lightning injuries are not usually associated with the extensive burns resulting from electrical injuries of man made voltages (up to 200 thousand volts of alternating current, usually less than 30 thousand volts.) Instead, the current largely flows around the outside of the body, just like electricity tends to flow along the outside of a conductor. (The electrical energy can instantly vaporize the moisture on the body surface and blow away the person's clothing, which may explain some puzzling findings.)

The most significant effects of lightning are on the brain. The electricity does shock the heart, causing it to arrest, but the heart's intrinsic tendency to contract rhythmically causes it to resume beating, just as it often does after being shocked to stop ventricular fibrillation. However, the brain requires significantly longer to recover from the effects of the electrical current. Because the brain controls respiration, the victim often does not breathe. Although the heart has resumed beating, it can not function without oxygen, and subsequently goes into ventricular fibrillation, resulting in death.

Clearly the emergency treatment for a lightning victim consists of immediate, and sometimes prolonged, artificial respiration. (Cardiac resuscitation should be given also, if needed, but the heart most often resumes beating on its own.) Over seventy percent of the persons struck by lightning have enough disruption of brain function to lose consciousness. Recovery of enough function to resume breathing commonly takes as long as twenty to thirty minutes, and occasionally takes hours.

If more than one person has been struck by the lightning, which commonly occurs, attention should be directed first to the ones who are lying still, not breathing, and appear dead. Those who are groaning or rolling around, although unconscious, are breathing and do not require immediate attention.

After the victim is breathing on his own, he should be evacuated to a hospital, as other problems commonly occur. Occasionally and unpredictably, heart failure, which requires intensive care, develops several hours later, apparently as the result of electrical damage to the heart muscle. Most lightning victims lose their short term memory for two to five days and can never recall the circumstances of the accident. Emotional or psychiatric problems are also common, but they usually clear up with time and appropriate treatment. Various types of paralysis appear but are usually transient. The extremities may appear blue and pulseless, as if the arteries were obstructed. This change usually is the result of intense spasm of the muscles in the walls of the arteries, and it passes after a few hours. Over fifty percent of lightning victims have one or both eardrums ruptured, possibly as the result of incredibly loud (and nearby) thunder. Superficial burns are common and typically have a feathery or fernlike pattern but rarely are severe.

Delayed problems sometimes occur. Neurologic problems have developed three to twelve months after injury. Cataracts can appear as long as two years later.

EVACUATION

An effective mountain rescue requires a good stretcher and enough people to carry it without risking further injury to the patient or the rescuers. Basket stretchers are the best available in most areas. Leg dividers interfere with splinting broken legs and subsequent packaging of the victim and should be eliminated if they can be removed without destroying the structural integrity of the stretcher. Better stretchers have been developed but are rarely found in mountain rescue areas within the United States. The McInnes stretcher can be transported over the roughest terrain by only two people.

Few circumstances can justify rolling a patient with fractures of the legs, pelvis, back, or neck onto a makeshift stretcher and bouncing him along over a rough descent simply because a rigid support, such as a basket stretcher or a broad board, and enough people to carry it are not immediately available.

If bad weather makes evacuation urgent, it is rarely necessary to carry the victim very far below the tree line before obtaining the personnel and equipment needed to complete the evacuation in a manner which minimizes the risk of further injury. The rescue may be easier and the outcome better if equipment and supplies for an overnight stay are carried to the victim, and the evacuation is delayed until the following morning or even until the weathr improves.

"Four dozen" stretcher bearers are essential too. Transporting an injured climber over rugged terrain is physically demanding. Fewer than six ordinary individuals can not carry a basket stretcher containing an adult male very well. Even that many stretcher bearers tire rapidly and must be replaced every few hundred yards.

If the party is small, deciding who should go for help and who should stay with the injured may be a problem. If the group has signed out with a park ranger or similar official, the wisest course may be to wait until search efforts locate the entire party. In wooded areas a fire may be built to attract the attention of fire wardens and to provide warmth and comfort. Since at least one person must stay with an injured climber at all times, small parties obviously should always register before a climb.

The rules for safe mountaineering are the same after an accident as before. Further injuries or loss of life as the result of ignoring these rules simply because one accident has occurred can not be justified. One person must not go for help alone over terrain (such as a snow covered glacier) that he would not cross by himself under normal circumstances. The fundamental soundness of this policy was pointed out in a Pacific Northwest accident in which a climber died from hypothermia while attempting to go for help; the accident victim and a third uninjured climber who remained with him were subsequently rescued by a search party.

Helicopters

The use of helicopters for mountain rescues has not only greatly reduced the amount of time needed to get an accident victim to medical care but has reduced the number of required stretcher bearers to four or six. Most of these can be brought in by the helicopter, along with a stretcher and needed medical supplies.

Working effectively with helicopters requires some knowledge of their capabilities and limitations. Although landings have been made at altitudes above

20,000 feet (6,100 m) by turbine (jet) helicopters, most helicopters can not land or take off above 8,000 to 10,000 feet (2,400 to 3,000 m). The maximum altitude at which a helicopter can operate is determined by air density. Cold air is more dense and a helicopter can operate at higher altitudes at lower temperatures. Conversely, the altitude at which a helicopter can land or take off can be reduced by several thousand feet by high air temperatures.

Helicopters usually can not make absolutely vertical ascents or descents. Some space for an approach and departure is needed. The most level spot that is free of surrounding obstructions, particularly electrical or telephone wires which are difficult to see from the air, should be selected. The wind direction should be indicated to the helicopter pilot, preferably by smoke, which also indicates the wind speed, or with an easily seen article of clothing.

Helicopters are hazardous. The downward thrust from the main rotors can produce winds ranging from 60 to 120 miles per hour. Obviously a person helping to guide a helicopter to a landing should not be standing on the edge of a sheer drop. Eyes must be protected from flying dirt and debris. Personal equipment must be stored where it can not be blown away. Strong rotor winds can tumble full packs over the ground and over a cliff or into a crevasse. Burning embers from fires can be blown about, possibly causing injuries to climbers or starting fires in surrounding brush or forests.

The danger from the tail and main rotors would seem to be obvious, but a surprising number of people walk into spinning rotors every year. While the helicopter is on the ground the main rotors may be higher than a person's head, but a sudden gust of wind or slowing of their speed can bend them downward to an amazing extent. No one should stand beneath the tips of the rotors. Personnel should approach the helicopter in a crouched position, preferably from the front where they can be seen by the pilot.

CHAPTER THREE

Special Problems

Fever and chills are common signs of disease that occur with infections and many other illnesses. Shock, unconsciousness, and cardiorespiratory arrest are less common but also are associated with widely varying disorders. For convenience and brevity, each of these problems is discussed in this chapter instead of with the disorders with which they might occur.

FEVER

Fever is an elevation of the body temperature and most commonly is a sign of infection. However, many noninfectious disorders and some normal conditions are associated with temperature elevations. A mild fever frequently follows traumatic injuries; sunstroke causes a very high fever.

Although human body temperatures average about 98.6° F (37° C) when measured orally, they range from a low of about 96.5° F (35.8° C) to as high as 100° F (37.8° C) in completely normal individuals. Furthermore, a person's temperature usually varies 1.25° F to 3.75° F (0.7° to 2.1° C) during each twenty-four hour period, usually reaching its lowest level between 3:00 and 5:00 A.M. and its highest in the late afternoon or early evening. Women's body temperatures vary with their menstrual cycles, rising about 1.0° F (0.5° C) at the time of ovulation and remaining elevated until menstruation begins. During vigorous exercise a completely healthy person's temperature can climb as high as 104° F (40° C) because he is generating heat faster than it can be lost.

A person usually should not be considered to have a fever until his temperature at rest exceeds 100° F (37.8° C) orally or 101° F (38.5° C) rectally. Lower values are within the range of normal. Furthermore, a significant illness or infection usually produces a definite fever. In a cold environment, however, hypothermia can mask a high fever by reducing the body's temperature to normal or even sub-normal levels.

Oral temperatures are easier to measure, but suffer the disadvantage of being affected by recently consumed food or beverages, smoking, or mouth breathing and talking. Therefore, oral temperatures should not be taken for at least ten minutes after eating or smoking, and the patient should preferably have been sitting or lying quietly. Rectal temperatures are more reliable and usually are about one degree Fahrenheit (one-half degree Centigrade) higher than the oral temperature. If rectal measurements are necessary, a rectal thermometer is preferable. It should be lubricated, gently inserted about one and one-half inches into the rectum, and left for three minutes.

If the patient is delirious or thrashing about, he must be watched carefully and perhaps even restrained to prevent his breaking the thermometer and injuring himself, regardless of where the temperature is measured.

As long as an illness persists, the temperature and pulse rate should be measured and recorded in a permanent form every four hours (although a soundly sleeping patient rarely needs to be awakened just to have his temperature taken). Fevers sometimes follow specific patterns that are diagnostically helpful. The temperature may go up and stay up, gradually coming down at the termination of the illness; alternately, the temperature may spike to high levels and then fall to normal or below normal every day or every second or third day. A continuous record is essential if such patterns are to be recognized.

A moderate fever, although it may make the patient uncomfortable, does not produce any lasting harmful effects. In contrast, temperatures above 106° F (41 °C) orally can cause irreversible damage if not immediately lowered. In hot or temperate climates such high fevers should be reduced by removing most or all of the patient's clothing and covering his body and extremities with cool (tepid), wet cloths, which should be replaced as they become warm. The patient can be fanned to increase evaporation and cooling. A patient with a life threatening fever in an environment of ice and snow may only require removal of a portion of his clothing.

These measures should be continued until the temperature is below 103° F (39.5°C). Aspirin may be given orally if the patient is fully conscious or rectally if he is stuporous or comatose. The patient's temperature must be watched very carefully for eight to twelve hours after it has dropped because high fevers frequently recur quite rapidly.

Although his fever must be lowered, the patient must also be protected from environmental extremes of heat or cold such as bright sunlight or snow and ice. After cooling he should be redressed in clothing similar to that being worn by everyone else. He must not be closed up in a sleeping bag, which traps the heat and can cause his temperature to go up again, unless sleeping bags are necessary for everyone else to keep warm.

CHILLS

A patient with a chill feels cold and shivers uncontrollably; he also feels miserable. These symptoms are produced by small showers of bacteria or viruses entering the blood stream. Frequently a chill is the first sign of an infection. In comparison with the chills commonly resulting from exposure to cold or sunburn, chills caused by infections are much more severe and produce violent, uncontrollable shaking of the entire body. The teeth chatter, the lips and nails are purple, the skin is pale and cold, and the victim feels miserable. (In years past, a chill could be diagnosed when a patient was shaking hard enough to make his hospital bed rattle.) The cold feeling persists in spite of blankets and heating pads until the chill has run its course, usually five to fifteen minutes.

A chill is usually followed in a short time by a fever that may reach high levels. The only treatment consists of caring for the underlying infection. Pneumonia, meningitis, and "strep throat" are frequently introduced with a single shaking chill. Malaria, infections of the liver and bile ducts or kidneys, and generalized bacterial infections are characterized by recurrent chills.

SHOCK

Shock is not a disease entity but a sign of disease produced by an illness or injury. The most common cause is a sudden reduction in the volume of the blood, typically as a result of hemorrhage. All of the constituents of blood — red blood cells and serum — are lost when bleeding occurs. However, the blood volume can also be reduced by disorders in which only the fluid portion of the blood is lost. Large volumes of serum pour into the damaged tissues following a severe burn. Dehydration resulting from fluid loss caused by severe vomiting or diarrhea, as typically occurs with cholera, can cause a reduction in blood volume that is lethal if uncorrected.

When the blood volume is reduced, regardless of the cause, the arteries in the skin and muscles constrict, tending to direct the available blood to the vital organs. At the same time, the heart begins pumping at an increased rate in order to circulate the remaining blood faster and enable a smaller volume of blood to carry the required oxygen to the tissues. When these mechanisms can no longer compensate for the reduction in blood volume, the blood pressure falls and shock results. If untreated, severe shock eventually becomes irreversible in spite of therapy and the victim dies.

Shock also occurs in other disorders in which there is no obvious reduction in blood volume. Severe infections or heart attacks are often associated with shock. A period of shock of varying duration is characteristic of the terminal stages of any fatal disease. The mechanisms by which shock is produced in these conditions are poorly understood and efforts at treatment, other than therapy directed toward the underlying disease, are frequently unrewarding.

Diagnosis

The severity of shock following hemorrhage depends upon the volume of blood lost and how fast it is lost. The symptoms of shock are usually more severe when bleeding is rapid than when blood loss is more gradual, even though the total amounts lost are identical. Estimating the volume of blood loss is not easy, and most individuals tend to overestimate. A small amount of blood can cover an amazingly large area.

A person 6 feet (180 cm) tall and weighing 175 pounds (80 kg) who is normally hydrated has a blood volume of about 6,000 cc. A person 5 feet 2 inches (155 cm) tall and weighing 110 pounds (50 kg) has a blood volume of about 4,000 cc. Individuals of different sizes have roughly proportional blood volumes.

Mild shock results from loss of ten to twenty percent of the blood volume. The patient appears pale and his skin feels cool, first over the extremities and later over the trunk. As shock becomes more severe, the patient often complains of feeling cold and he is often thirsty. A rapid pulse and reduced blood pressure may be present. However, the absence of these signs does not indicate shock is not present since they may appear rather late, particularly in previously healthy young adults.

Moderate shock results from loss of twenty to forty percent of the blood volume. The signs characteristic of mild shock are present and may become more severe. The pulse is typically fast and weak or "thready." In addition, blood flow to the kidneys is reduced as the available blood is shunted to the heart and brain, and the urinary output declines. A urinary volume of less than 30 cc per hour is a late indication of moderate shock. In contrast to the dark, concentrated urine observed with dehydration, the urine is usually a light color.

Severe shock results from loss of more than forty percent of the blood volume and is characterized by signs of reduced blood flow to the brain and heart. Reduced cerebral blood flow initially produces restlessness and agitation, which is followed by confusion, stupor, and eventually coma and death. Diminished blood flow to the heart can produce abnormalities of the cardiac rhythm.

Treatment

Treatment for shock is much more effective if begun before the typical signs appear, but such anticipation may require considerable perspicacity. Shock would obviously be expected after a severe hemorrhage. However, some fractures, particularly those involving the spine, pelvis, or thigh, and many injuries to the internal organs, are associated with severe bleeding that produces no external evidence of hemorrhage. Shock also should be anticipated in some other disorders, particularly those such as severe diarrhea, which result in severe fluid loss.

Successful treatment of shock depends largely upon treating the cause. However, several measures should be taken regardless of the underlying disorder. Treatment must be started as early as possible. Following any injury, the first step after controlling bleeding and ensuring adequate respiration should be treating shock.

The victim should be lying down with his head at the same level or lower than the rest of his body and his feet elevated ten to twelve inches (twenty-five to thirty centimeters). This position allows the considerable volume of venous blood normally present in the legs to drain back into the body, making that blood available for circulation to more vital tissues. In severe shock, the lower position of the head may aid circulation to the brain.

The patient's body temperature must be maintained. Blankets or sleeping bags are not adequate in severe shock because the victim can not produce enough heat to warm himself. Hot water bottles or heated stones are needed, particularly in a cold environment. Warmth should be supplied at once, not after the patient's body temperature has begun to fall.

Any impairment of respiration must be corrected; oxygen should be administered if it is available.

Pain, movement, or unpleasant emotional stimuli such as fear or the sight of blood often increase the severity of shock. If severe pain is present (a patient in moderate or severe shock usually does not feel much pain), the patient does not have a head injury or other contraindication to such medication, and evacuation is going to be prolonged, morphine or meperidine can be administered.

Circulation to the skin and muscles of the extremities is impaired in shock, and drugs injected at those sites may not be absorbed. Badly needed analgesics can be injected intravenously, but multiple small doses should be injected slowly (sixty to ninety seconds for each injection) instead of the single larger dose usually given intramuscularly. Alternatively, injections could be given into the pectoral muscles of the chest where circulatory impairment is less severe. Subsequent injections must be only half as large and should be given at six hour intervals as long as shock is evident. Larger, more frequent injections could lead to a severe overdose. If circulation to the injection site is poor and the drugs are not absorbed, when the patient recovers from shock and the circulation is restored, all of the injected medication could be absorbed at once.

Morphine also helps to allay anxiety. With or without its use, the victim should be given all possible comfort and reassurance to minimize the effects of fear and emotional turmoil. (See Chapter Four, "Psychological Responses to Accidents.")

The victim may have to be moved immediately from the path of falling rock or a potential avalanche, and he can be carried a short distance to a helicopter without harm. However, moving the victim greater distances, particularly evacuation by stretcher, should not be attempted until all injuries have been treated, shock has been controlled as well as possible, and the patient appears to be in a stable condition.

Low blood volume from hemorrhage or other causes can be temporarily corrected to a considerable extent by the intravenous administration of a balanced salt solution. Blood plasma or plasma expanders may be somewhat more effective but also are associated with potentially harmful side effects and should only be given by a physician or an individual trained in their use. The red blood cells necessary for carrying oxygen are not replaced by these fluids, and such therapy does have limitations. Whole blood is the optimum replacement for blood loss, but preservation and cross-matching are impossible outside of a hospital with an appropriately equipped laboratory.

Intravenous fluids should be given in anticipation of shock, particularly with injuries such as extensive burns or major fractures when the development of shock appears to be a certainty. (Finding a vein suitable for inserting a needle through which intravenous fluids can be administered is usually quite difficult once shock has appeared.) Fluids should be administered in amounts that approximate the volume of lost blood. However, blood loss is usually difficult to estimate accurately, particularly with injuries where most of the loss is hidden from view.

A previously healthy adult with no indication of prior heart disease is rarely harmed by under or over replacement of fluids by as much as one or even two liters. For such individuals, as much as three to four liters of fluids may be administered fairly rapidly until the heart rate begins to slow and the patient appears to be responding to treatment. Thereafter, fluids should be given at a much slower rate, and no more than four liters should be given within the first eight hour period. If blood loss is so great that more fluids are needed, the administration of a balanced salt solution alone probably would not be adequate treatment. However, burn patients may need larger volumes and should receive them whenever they are available. (See Chapter Eight, "Burns.")

If the victim does have heart disease, any error in fluid administration must be on the side of under replacement. Excess fluids could lead to the unneeded complication of heart failure in such individuals.

The adequacy of treatment following hemorrhage can be determined by measuring the pulse rate, the blood pressure, and the urinary output. Pulse and blood pressure should return to levels close to normal within a few minutes to a few hours after replacement of the lost blood volume. A low urinary output and increasing pulse rate indicate the need for reinstituting therapy. All data regarding pulse rate, blood pressure, urinary output, and all therapy that has been administered must be carefully recorded so the patient's course can be accurately followed and a physician can know the patient's status more precisely.

The treatment of shock associated with nontraumatic disorders is less clear cut, and the results are often less satisfactory. Patients in shock from peritonitis or similar disorders may benefit from one or two liters of balanced salt solution per day, but more should not be given. A victim of a heart attack who has sustained no blood loss must not be given fluids as they increase the work load on his already damaged heart.

UNCONSCIOUSNESS

An unconscious patient requires special attention to four general needs: respiration, fluid requirements, protection from the environment, and specific treatment for the cause of his unconscious state. The nature of the last two requirements depends upon the circumstances in which the victim is found; fluid requirements are discussed under fluid balance in Chapter One, "Diagnosis."

If unconsciousness is the result of trauma, the victim must also be treated as if he had a broken neck. Fifteen percent of all injuries to the head that result in prolonged unconsciousness also cause cervical fractures.

The victim of a disorder so severe that breathing ceases can rarely be kept alive by manual artificial respiration for more than a few hours (see resuscitation). Therefore, the only specific care for unconscious patients in mountaineering circumstances is the maintenance of an open airway to permit unimpeded respiration.

Medications for sleep or pain are completely unnecessary, would further depress brain function, and must not be administered.

The care of an unconscious patient is simple, but vitally important. Skilled treatment of other injuries or heroic rescue efforts may be completely wasted by five minutes of neglect. No matter how precarious the situation, no rescue efforts can be justified until means for keeping the air passages clear during the entire evacuation have been established. It should be obvious that an injured climber must be left in an exposed and dangerous situation if rescue attempts would cause certain death due to airway obstruction.

AIRWAY MAINTENANCE

The mouth and nose, throat, larynx (voice box), trachea, and bronchi form the passages through which air moves into the lungs and are known collectively as the airway. The mouth, throat, and tongue are constructed so that the base of the tongue moves backward and closes off the opening to the trachea during swallowing to prevent food or fluid entering the lungs. Partial obstruction of the larynx by the tongue during sleep results in snoring. However, the larynx is only partially blocked during natural sleep because the muscles that hold the tongue and structures of the throat are not totally relaxed. In contrast, disorders resulting in unconsciousness can produce complete relaxation of these muscles, permitting the tongue to totally obstruct the passage of air into the lungs.

The easiest way to prevent such airway obstruction is to tilt the unconscious victim's head back by placing one hand on the back of his neck and lifting while pushing down on his forehead or pulling his chin forward with the other hand. When the head is in this position, the tongue is pulled forward and can not fall back far enough to produce obstruction. If the patient has no injuries that might

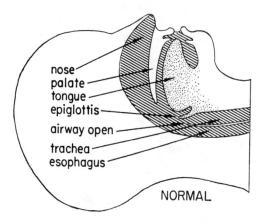

Figure 1. Structures of the mouth, throat, and airway in a normal, conscious individual.

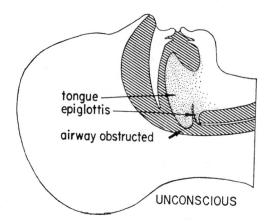

Figure 2. Position of the tongue and epiglottis in an unconscious patient.

be aggravated by turning him, particularly a broken neck or back, he may be placed on his side with his head facing downward. In this position his tongue tends to fall forward instead of backward and does not block the throat. However, the head also should be extended to provide additional help in keeping the airway open.

The adequacy of the airway is very easily checked. If the victim is breathing quietly, the airway is open. Snoring or noisy breathing, labored respirations, or the absence of respiratory movements indicate partial or complete airway obstruction.

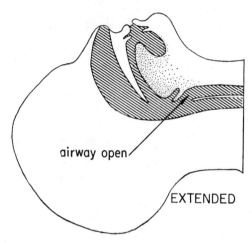

Figure 3. Position of the tongue and epiglottis in an unconscious patient with the head and neck extended to relieve airway obstruction.

If a broken neck is suspected, the airway can be opened by placing the fingers at the angles of the victim's jaws and pulling forward. Alternately, a finger or thumb can be hooked behind the teeth of the lower jaw and the jaw pulled forward. The neck should not be moved.

Disorders that produce unconsciousness are also frequently associated with vomiting. The vomitus may be aspirated, completely obstructing the air passages or producing a severe, often lethal pneumonia. To prevent such accidents the victim's head must be lower than his chest and turned to the side whenever he is vomiting or appears likely to vomit. If there is no reason not to do so, he can be placed on his side to help keep his airway open and prevent aspiration. (Unconscious persons must never be given food, fluids, or medications by mouth.)

If the victim does not recover consciousness within a few hours and evacuation requires a long stretcher carry over rough terrain during which the maintenance of an open airway in this manner would be impossible, a more permanent plastic airway or tracheostomy is necessary. Many first aid kits contain plastic airways (oropharyngeal airways) which are flattened curved tubes that fit over the base of the tongue, allowing air to enter the larynx. (If the patient starts to regain consciousness, the tube causes him to gag and cough and can be removed.)

Another method of keeping the airway open is to insert a large safety pin through the meaty part of the tongue and hold the tongue forward by taping the

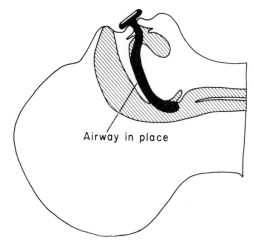

Figure 4. Oropharyngeal airway in place in an unconscious patient.

pin to the chin or anchoring it in a similar manner. Although this technique sounds and appears brutal, it is simple, highly effective, and produces no permanent damage.

In rare circumstances a permanent artificial airway (tracheostomy) may be required.

Tracheostomy

A tracheostomy is an opening into the trachea that allows the patient to breathe when the upper air passages are obstructed. Although tracheostomies are commonly performed in hospitals, the occasions when one would be needed by a victim of a mountaineering accident or illness are very rare. Probably the most common need for a tracheostomy in mountaineering situations would be to maintain an open airway during evacuation of an unconscious person, but other means for maintaining the airways of such patients are available. Accident victims with severe facial fractures may be unable to breathe through their nose or mouth due to the deformity and swelling accompanying their injuries. A crushing blow to the larynx commonly produces airway obstruction.

A tracheostomy is simply a hole in the trachea, and any acceptable technique for creating the hole and keeping it open works quite well. The site for the tracheostomy must be selected carefully to minimize subsequent scarring and deformity, and to avoid damage to other structures in the neck, particularly large blood vessels which can produce a massive hemorrhage. (The location of the opening has little to do with how well the tracheostomy functions except that it obviously must be below an obstructing injury.) Most hospital tracheostomies are placed just above the sternum at the base of the neck. This site must not be used by inexperienced individuals for tracheostomies because the thyroid and the common carotid arteries (two of the body's largest) may be encountered. Instead, an opening should be made in the cricothyroid membrane. The thyroid cartilage forms the Adam's apple. The cricoid cartilage is the large cartilagenous ring just below the thyroid cartilage. The cricothyroid membrane connects these two structures. (A physician's help in identifying this structure should be obtained before such knowledge is needed to care for a patient.)

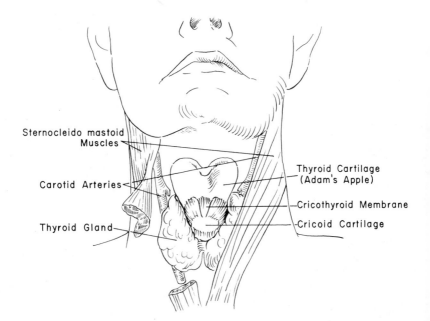

Figure 5. Location of cricothyroid membrane and carotid arteries.

The patient should be lying on a flat surface, if possible, with his head extended backward to stretch the structures in the neck. The skin of the neck should be cleaned with soap and water and an antiseptic applied if time is available. The space between the thyroid and cricoid cartilages should be precisely identified and an opening made with some type of sharp instrument. (A variety of devices specifically for performing crycothyroidostomies are commercially available, but the techniques for using them obviously must be learned before the moment they are needed. An eight to ten gauge needle is suitable for this purpose and easy to use; a fifteen gauge needle is large enough to provide an adequate airway for most individuals if nothing larger is available. However, a climber who had one of these devices available could just as easily have carried a plastic airway.) A one-quarter inch skin incision can be made in the midline of the neck over the cricothyroid cartilage with a scalpel or similar sharp blade, but is not essential. Then the needle or other device should be inserted into the trachea. Air can be heard moving in and out immediately.

The opening in the trachea collapses unless something is inserted to keep it open. Commercially available devices have a tube for this purpose. If a large needle is used to perform the tracheostomy, the needle can be left in place to provide an opening. The needle, or whatever device is used, must be anchored to keep it from falling out or from being jammed into the back wall of the trachea and obstructed.

The needle or tube should generally be left in place until the victim is under a physician's care. If, during a prolonged evacuation, an unconscious patient should recover enough to not need the tracheostomy, the needle or tubing can be plugged (so that it can be easily opened again) or removed. The wound almost always closes and heals with no further attention.

FOOD ASPIRATION ("CAFE CORONARY")

A cause of respiratory obstruction that has been recognized with increasing frequency and has received much publicity in recent years is the aspiration of food, most commonly meat. Prior to the development of the Heimlich maneuver, a procedure that usually dislodges the food and was named for its originator, approximately 4,000 people are estimated to have died each year from this type of accident in just the United States. Surprisingly large food fragments can be impacted in the larynx. Whole radishes and similar sized pieces of poorly chewed food are typically found. The food plugs the larynx and obstructs the passage of air, usually completely. Since no air can move through the larynx, the individual can not speak, cough, or breathe.

While eating, the victim suddenly indicates that he is choking, usually rises out of his chair, and after a brief struggle collapses. Since the food is jammed into his larynx, he can not speak! A signal has been devised for the victim to indicate that he is choking; it consists of thrusting the "V" between the thumb and first finger of the hand against the throat.

Attempts to dislodge the food with a finger (or a special device developed for that purpose) inserted through the mouth are rarely successful and may only force the food farther down. Pounding the victim on the back also is usually fruitless. Such measures may be tried, but no more than a few seconds should be spent in this way. Airway obstruction by aspirated food is a true emergency and only three or four minutes are available to correct the problem.

The Heimlich maneuver consists of thrusting a hand or fist into the upper abdomen in such a way that the diaphragm is suddenly forced upward. The abrupt pressure on the diaphragm forces air out of the lungs at high speed and usually pops the obstructing food out of the larynx. In fact, the food is commonly ejected completely out of the victim's mouth. This maneuver is so effective it can be used to evacuate aspirated pills or similar objects that do not completely obstruct the airway. Some have stated the maneuver can effectively expel water from the airways of drowning victims, but such claims have been questioned.

The victim can be stood up if he is still conscious. Without delay, the rescuer's arms should be extended around him, and one fist placed in the top of the "V" formed by the ribs just below the sternum. The knuckle of the thumb of that hand should be against the victim. The second hand should be placed on top of the first, and both should be pulled inward and upward as sharply as possible. Several attempts may be required to expel the food.

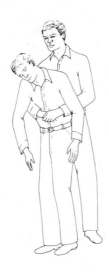

Figure 6. Position for Heimlich maneuver with victim standing.

When performing the maneuver in this manner, as little pressure should be placed on the ribs as possible. (Some is unavoidable.) Squeezing the ribs does not expel the food; thrusting against the diaphragm does. Squeezing the ribs has led to fractures, in a few cases multiple fractures.

If the patient is unconscious or obese, he should be placed on his back on the flattest surface that can be found. After straddling the victim (*not* kneeling beside him), both hands, one on top of the other, should be placed on the upper abdomen just below the sternum, and pressed down briskly to force the diaphragm upward and dislodge the food.

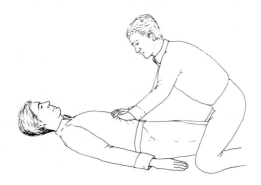

Figure 7. Position for Heimlich maneuver with victim lying down.

If the Heimlich maneuver is not successful after a number of tries, a tracheostomy must be performed. It should be done as quickly as possible. Artificial respiration through the tracheostomy may be necessary for a short time if the victim has stopped breathing. However, most failures have not been failures of the Heimlich maneuver but failures to apply it in time to prevent permanent brain damage.

RESUSCITATION

Occasions for effective resuscitation of the victims of disease or trauma in mountaineering circumstances are rare. However, victims of lightning and drowning can definitely be revived by resuscitative measures. In fact, resuscitation, sometimes for hours, should be attempted for all lightning victims and for all cold water drowning victims who have been submerged for an hour or less.

Avalanche victims can occasionally be successfully resuscitated. Even a person knocked unconscious in a relatively minor accident may temporarily stop breathing and require artificial respiration. Furthermore, even though a patient is breathing on his own, he may benefit from artificial respiration if he is breathing inadequately.

Resuscitation is usually not effective if an underlying disorder that has caused breathing to stop or the heartbeat to cease is not corrected or significantly improved. Diseases affecting the lungs (such as pneumonia or high altitude pulmonary edema), severe infections, extensive trauma (particularly severe head, chest, or abdominal injuries), and severe shock of almost any origin are disorders for which cardiopulmonary resuscitation is not effective, particularly in wilderness situations.

Resuscitative measures take time and energy; an unsuccessful attempt at resuscitation extracts a heavy emotional toll. Such expenditures may be critical for the survival of other members of the party in a threatening situation.

Attempts to resuscitate anyone who has been more than fifteen minutes without breathing or a heartbeat, *and has a normal body temperature,* are futile. At normal temperature, the brain can survive only about five minutes without oxygen before suffering permanent damage. After this period, deterioration is rapid and by ten to twelve minutes death is inevitable. (Much longer periods without breathing, even as long as an hour, are survivable if the body has been cooled, particularly if the cooling has been rapid, as occurs with cold water immersion.)

Resuscitative techniques must be practiced beforehand if efforts to apply them are to have a reasonable chance for success.

Artificial Respiration

Whenever an individual who appears to require resuscitation is encountered, he first should be checked to see if he can be aroused. If the victim is truly comatose, he should be placed on a firm, flat surface and the rescuer should place his face close to the victim's mouth to listen and feel for air moving through the nose or mouth. If breathing is impaired or absent, the respiratory passages must be cleared of any obstruction. The fingers should be inserted into the victim's mouth and throat and any foreign matter or vomitus removed. (Efforts to breathe by avalanche or drowning victims often cause them to gulp in snow or other material.)

If the victim has not been subjected to trauma that could have broken his neck, his head should be tilted backwards by placing one hand under the neck and lifting upward while pushing down with the other hand on the forehead. This maneuver places tension on the tongue and structures in the throat so that the airway is not obstructed. In some cases relieving such obstruction is all that is necessary for the patient to resume breathing.

If artificial respiration is necessary, it should be started with the least possible delay using the mouth-to-mouth technique. The hand behind the neck holds the head forward while the hand on the forehead pushes downward and the thumb and forefinger pinch shut the nostrils. (In an alternate method, the fingers of both hands are placed behind the angles of the jaw, pulling the jaw forward while the thumbs close off the nose. This technique should be used if the victim is thought to have a broken neck.) Rarely the victim's jaw is so tightly clenched that it cannot be opened. The head must still be tilted backward to keep the airway open and artificial respiration given through the nose.

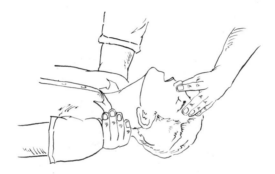

Figure 8. Positioning of the head and neck for mouth-to-mouth artificial respiration.

The rescuer should inhale, place his mouth over the victim's open mouth, and exhale with enough force to cause the victim's chest to rise. Then he should remove his mouth and inhale again while the victim's lungs empty. Upon initiating artificial respiration, the rescuer should give the victim four quick breaths without allowing time for the victim's lungs to empty. This maneuver distends the lungs, which may have been partially collapsed, and provides for more effective air exchange. Artificial respiration should be carried out at a rate of approximately twelve to fourteen breaths per minute and should be synchronized with any respiratory efforts being made by the victim.

If artificial respiration is effective, air can be heard moving in and out of the victim's upper air passages. Usually the victim's chest can be seen to rise and fall also. If such evidence of successful artificial respiration is not present, the airway must be examined for obstruction. Foreign matter must be removed and the head must be tipped backward as far as it will go with the jaw pulled well forward.

During mouth-to-mouth artificial respiration the stomach may become distended with air forced through the esophagus instead of into the lungs. This air should be removed to prevent the distended stomach from impinging on the diaphragm and interfering with respiratory movements. In children, the stomach may even rupture. Moderate pressure on the upper abdomen with the palm of the hand usually forces the air back out through the esophagus in a large belch. This maneuver may have be to repeated periodically. The victim must be watched carefully because vomiting commonly follows the belch.

The mouth-to-mouth method of artificial respiration is so far superior to any other method it should be used exclusively. It is almost impossible not to perform artificial respiration correctly and effectively by this technique if the precautions described are observed.

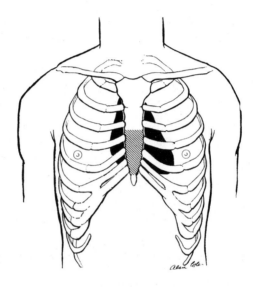

Figure 9. Area of the chest to which pressure is applied during external cardiac massage.

Cardiac Resuscitation

Following the first four quick breaths at the initiation of artificial respiration, the rescuer should determine whether the victim's heart is beating by checking the carotid pulse. The examiner can find this pulse by placing his fingers on the thyroid cartilage (Adam's apple) and moving them to either side into the groove between this cartilage and the prominent muscle that runs from the base of the ear to the center portion of the upper chest (sternocleidomastoid muscle). If no pulse can be felt, cardiac resuscitation should be instituted.

The normal heart pumps blood by contracting, which forces the blood out into the arteries. Cardiac massage accomplishes the same thing by compressing the chest from the outside. By pressing on the lower part of the sternum, the pressure in the chest is raised to a level sufficient to force the blood out of the heart. Blood circulation can be effectively maintained by this technique for many hours.

The rescuer should kneel beside the victim and place the heel of one hand on the lower end of the victim's sternum at a point two finger widths above the tip. (The hand must not be on the tip of the sternum as this may fracture and puncture the liver, resulting in severe hemorrhage. The fingers must be lifted from the chest wall so that only the heel of the hand is in contact with the sternum in order to reduce the probability of fracturing ribs.) The second hand should be placed on top of the first, and the arms should be kept straight so that force can be exerted by shifting the rescuer's weight onto his arms. The use of muscular force alone for cardiac massage is too tiring to be carried out for more than a few minutes. Enough pressure should be exerted to depress the sternum one or two inches. The pressure should be released immediately and the maneuver repeated about sixty times a minute. The cycle should consist of approximately equal periods of time

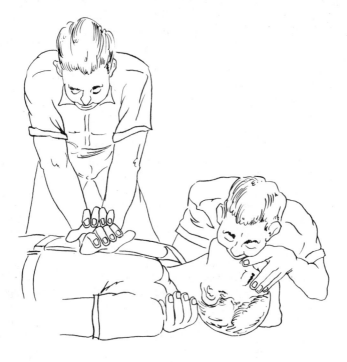

Figure 10. Administration of external cardiac massage and mouth-to-mouth artificial respiration.

during which pressure is being applied and pressure is not being applied. The effectiveness of the massage can be checked by feeling for the pulse at the victim's neck or groin.

Pressure on the chest by cardiac massage does not move enough air into the victim's lungs to keep him alive. Therefore, mouth-to-mouth artificial respiration must be given simultaneously. If a second rescuer is on hand, he can give artificial respiration at a rate of one breath for every five cardiac compressions. The artificial respiration must be timed so it is given during the interval when the pressure is not being applied to the chest. The two rescuers should alternate periodically between cardiac massage and artificial respiration to avoid tiring either to the point of becoming ineffective. The switch should be made without interrupting the pattern of cardiac massage.

If only one rescuer is present, he must give both cardiac massage and artificial respiration. The technique generally recommended is to give fifteen compressions of the heart at a rate of approximately eighty per minute and then two quick breaths of artificial respiration. Repetition of the cycle at this rate provides approximately sixty cardiac compressions a minute.

Other Considerations

The victim should be checked at approximately one to two minute intervals to determine whether spontaneous cardiac function has returned. After the victim has responded to resuscitation, he must be watched closely in case a relapse occurs. A prolonged period of unconsciousness usually follows even though he is breathing on his own. The airway must be kept open. If the victim is vomiting, he should be placed with his head lower than his chest and turned on his side. Shock must be anticipated and treated appropriately. The victim should be evacuated as fast as possible.

One of the most difficult questions concerning resuscitation is when to give up. The final decision in every case must be based on consideration of the circumstances in which the accident has occurred, the extent of the victim's injuries, the treatment required and administered, the persons available for care of the victim, and the possibility of obtaining medical assistance within a short time. Artificial respiration should be kept up for anyone whose heart is still beating. On the other hand, anyone requiring cardiac massage who also has a normal body temperature has a much poorer prognosis. If spontaneous heart action has not resumed and if the pupils of the eyes are widely dilated and do not contract when exposed to light after thirty minutes of massage, the victim is beyond further help. In contrast, resuscitative attempts for victims of hypothermia should not be abandoned — in most instances — until the victim has been rewarmed to a body core temperature above 92° F (33° C).

For most patients, cardiopulmonary resuscitation fails. Usually the injury or disease is too severe to begin with, or resuscitation is initiated too late. However, rescuers are often reluctant not to make the effort, even if prospects for success appear very remote. The few individuals saved may make the efforts expended on others more than just worthwhile, but the physical and emotional costs of unsuccessful attempts may be quite high.

CHAPTER FOUR

Psychological Responses to Accidents

Emotional responses to traumatic accidents should be expected in both accident victims and their rescuers. Most reactions are normal and tend to be consistent. However, anyone involved in an accident can benefit from attention to his psychologic needs. For some individuals, attention to their emotional needs during a rescue can be just as vital as medical care if they are to return to a functioning role in society.

The emotional responses provoked by an accident are similar to the reactions that follow loss of a loved one and are known as bereavement or grief. Since many more persons have experienced grief than have been involved in major accidents, the emotional reactions to trauma have been compared with grief reactions to make them easier to understand. This comparison provides two additional benefits: it illustrates the normality of psychologic reactions to accidents, which may seem abnormal to individuals who have not experienced such phenomena, and it describes grief reactions, which can be expected among accident survivors who have witnessed the death of close friends.

GRIEF REACTIONS

Grief is the emotional and behavioral train of reactions set in motion by the loss or separation from a loved one. Due to his emotional involvement with the lost person the survivor experiences a period of mourning or grief, which can be lengthy and painful. If his grief is properly worked through, however, the survivor reconciles himself to the loss and resumes his life with renewed vitality; sometimes with even greater commitment. Grief, like other emotional states, is more easily and profitably experienced when shared with others who are trusted.

Grief evolves through several stages and, like "being in love," the boundary between what is normal and what is abnormal is often blurred. Bereaved persons commonly display widely ranging attitudes, beliefs, and behavior that smack of irrationality. The first stage of their emotional response has been labeled the protest phase and is initially characterized by stunned shock and denial. ("He can't be dead!") Anger commonly follows and may be illogically directed at the person or circumstance that appears to have caused the loss, at the victim for having gotten into the unfortunate situation, or inwardly at the grieving survivor himself for not having been present to help, for not having prevented the loss, or even for surviving. The bereaved frequently manifest external signs of emotional pain, such as crying, weakness, loss of appetite or even nausea, or sleep disturbances. Survivors may search for their loved ones or mementos of their loved ones.

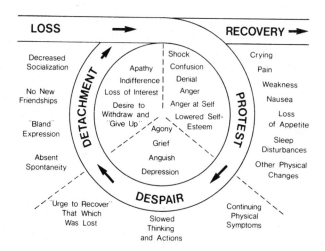

Figure 11. Diagram of reaction cycle associated with grief. (From William M. Lamers, Jr., M.D. Used by permission.)

After days or weeks, bereaved individuals typically move into a second stage dominated by despair, internally experiencing anguish, grief, and depression, and externally displaying such signs as slowness of thought, physical symptoms similar to those of the protest phase, and further searching for loved ones and remembrances of them. After weeks or months, they move slowly into the third or detachment stage, during which they lose interest in life and want to withdraw and give up. Externally they appear bland, lack spontaneity, are devoid of social energy, and behave like robots or "zombies."

Normally the cycle of protest, despair, and detachment takes six to eighteen months. The bereaved finally work through their loss, say their final good-byes, and move on to reorganize their lives and personalities, emotionally renewed by reconciliation with their loss. The success with which the bereaved can resolve his grief is proportional to his capacity to face the sense of hopelessness and helplessness evoked by the finality of death, whether the death of others or himself.

Sometimes grief can not be handled successfully. When the relationship with the deceased has been charged with an ambivalent mixture of love and hate and the hostile feelings have been denied, a bereaved person may be tortured with guilt. The grief process may go on indefinitely with great emotional cost to the survivor. An inability to mourn can be manifested emotionally by reactions such as depression, emotional numbness or anesthesia, hypochondria, addiction to drugs including alcohol, or other "acting out" behavior by which emotions are discharged through impulsive actions. Physical manifestations include hysterical reactions such as weakness or paralysis, and psychosomatic disorders involving the skin, stomach and intestines, or other body systems. The survivor may place himself in the same illness or accident producing situation that led to the death of the deceased or may mimic the medical or traumatic conditions of the deceased.

The basic remedies for grief are time and opportunities for verbal and nonverbal expression of memories and feelings about the deceased, death, and the survivor's relationship with the deceased. If depression is prolonged and pathologic, a therapist's help may be needed to work through the blocks to normal mourning.

NORMAL RESPONSES BY ACCIDENT VICTIMS

The normal emotional state of mountaineering and wilderness accident victims, or the victims of any sudden, unpredictable, and overwhelming crisis, is similar to an acute grief state. For a trauma victim, the overwhelming emotion results from experiencing the possibility of death and fearing for his life. An accompanying sense of powerlessness or helplessness, of having lost control over his survival, adds to the impact. The victim is aware of seeking to escape and of being weak, vulnerable, and helpless. His self esteem and sense of competence have been assaulted, and he sees himself as unable to keep out of harm's way or as having acted with poor judgment.

Five "phases of disaster" for accidents have been identified:

1. Preimpact (threat);
2. Warning;
3. Impact;
4. Recoil;
5. Postimpact.

The preimpact or threat phase occurs months or years before the incident and is characterized by a failure to take appropriate measures to minimize the possibility of an accident. The warning phase takes place immediately before the incident and usually consists of ignoring obvious hazards such as avalanche paths. Since both of these phases take place before the accident, rescuers are not involved.

Impact Phase

The impact phase refers to the time during which the incident occurs. It can last for seconds to hours during an accident such as an avalanche or a fall, or for months to years during and after a war.

One-eighth to one-fourth of the people involved in an accident react effectively. They are often excited and "too busy to worry." About three-fourths of the victims are stunned and bewildered. They show no emotion, are inactive or indecisive, and are usually docile, although they may be totally unresponsive or behave in an automatic, robotlike manner. They may have physiologic manifestations of fear such as sweating, palpitations, tunnel vision, or a dry mouth. This type of reaction is known as "psychologic shock" but should not be considered an abnormal reaction. A final one-eighth to one-fourth of accident victims react with grossly inappropriate behavior such as paralyzing anxiety, hysteria, or psychotic reactions.

Recoil Phase

The recoil or fourth phase of disaster occurs hours to weeks after the incident, depending upon the individual and the nature of the incident. The primary stress of the accident has passed, but the accident victim is subjected to secondary stresses such as the prospect of being immobilized and isolated without food or shelter, the prospect of being totally dependent upon someone he does not know for rescue, or the more distant prospect of not being able to go back to work.

Reactions during the recoil phase occur in three stages which are similar to the stages of the grief reaction. The first stage is one of protest or denial. The victim may not be able to deny that a problem exists but refuses to admit the magnitude of the problem. The problem is understood intellectually but not emotionally, and the victim is blase and unconcerned.

During the second stage, recall normally returns (to ninety percent of accident victims), and the victim becomes aware of the problem but regards it as overwhelming and unbearable. Strong emotions are manifested by tightening of muscles, sweating, restlessness, difficulty in speaking, sadness and weeping, irritability and anger, or passive dependency and childlike behavior. Some victims develop a "zombielike" stare — the "1,000 mile stare." The victim may need to tell and retell the experience.

During the third stage, the victim begins to return to normal, accepts his problems, and makes efforts to solve them. He is more hopeful and confident, and emotions from the second stage are less intense.

Helping with Emotional Responses in Impact and Recoil Phases

Accident victims, uninjured members of the party, and rescuers must cope with the reactions of both the impact (third) phase and the recoil (fourth) phase at the scene of the accident or during evacuation. Psychologic assistance provided at that time can greatly diminish the emotional aftereffects. Rescue leaders and their crew members must be prepared to provide as much psychologic help as possible with constructive, understanding listening.

At the time of the accident and for several hours afterward, some victims are stunned, confused, and paralyzed with anxiety. Others are vigilant and cool. Some victims are emotionally expressive, displaying anxiety, anger, sobbing, a sense of relief, or a tendency to blame others. Others are very controlled, exhibit little distress, and appear very composed. Both types of symptoms reflect denial and emotional exhaustion or "shock." Both reactions are normal, but the victims need acceptance and assurance of the normality of their responses. They may be vulnerable to damaged self esteem if they perceive their behavior as inadequate or abnormal.

A person's self esteem and sense of mastery are also based on his judgment of how well he responds to problem situations. Success heightens self esteem; failure lowers it. Therefore, involving the victim in the rescue, encouraging him to take part in any way possible, either to help himself, other victims, or members of the rescue party, can be critical for the victim's morale and subsequent mental health. Rescue leaders must be aware of this need and do all they can to ensure it is met.

The victim may say "this will hit me later." He should be reassured (or informed) that indeed it will hit him later and that his emotional responses may take time and talking out.

Postimpact Phase

The final phase of a disaster, the postimpact phase, usually takes place six to twelve months after the incident and may last a life time. The source of stress is the personal and social aftereffects of the incident. The normal reaction, after recovery from the accident, is to return to normal activities. A sense of well-being returns, and the victim is able to make decisions and act on them. He successfully works through grief he may have encountered. Many survivors develop altered attitudes toward life and death and display a definite philosophic mellowing and growth.

Abnormal reactions occasionally occur and have been labeled the "delayed stress syndrome." The characteristics of this disorder are posttraumatic neurosis, psychosomatic illness, increased physical illness, depression, accident proneness, accidental death, or suicide. Professional counselling is often needed to work out the problems of this syndrome. However, proper emotional support during rescue can significantly reduce the severity of such disorders or prevent them altogether.

ABNORMAL RESPONSES TO ACCIDENTS

Abnormal psychologic reactions to trauma may affect four functional areas:
1. Orientation to time, place, and person;

2. Observable motor and physical acts;
3. Verbal behavior;
4. Emotional or affective expression.

Since typical abnormal behavior patterns are rather easily recognized, they are outlined without further discussion.

Orientation
   Mild derangement (adequately aware of time, place, events, and person):
      a. Dazed, confused;
      b. Minor difficulty understanding what is being said;
      c. Minor difficulty thinking clearly or concentrating;
      d. Slow or delayed reactions.
   Severe derangement (confused about time, place, events, and person, but may gradually respond to information and reassurance [unlike patients with brain trauma, which must be considered]):
      a. Forgetful of own name and names of associates;
      b. Unclear about date — year or month;
      c. Unable to state clearly his location;
      d. Unable to recall clearly events of the previous twenty-four hours;
      e. Regresses to an earlier period of life;
      f. Complains about memory gaps of thirty minutes or more;
      g. Confused about who he is or what he does;
      h. Appears unaware of what is happening around him.

Motor Behavior
   Mild:
      a. Wringing hands or clenching fists; stiff and rigid appearance; continuously sad expression;
      b. Some restlessness; mild agitation and excitement;
      c. Difficulty falling asleep or keeping down food;
      d. Rushing about trying to do many things at once, but accomplishing little;
      e. Feelings of fatigue inconsistent with previous and concurrent activity;
      f. Halting or rapid speech that is out of character; difficulty getting words out.
   Severe:
      a. Agitated movements; inability to sleep or rest quietly;
      b. Grimacing or posturing of recent onset;
      c. Markedly reduced activity; sits and stares; remains immobile for hours;
      e. Mutilation of self or objects for no reason;
      f. Repeated ritualistic acts of no functional significance; attempts to prevent the acts create resistance and excessive emotion;

g. Excessive use of drugs or alcohol;
h. Inability to carry out simple functions such as eating, dressing, organizing equipment.

Verbal Behavior
Mild:
a. Verbalizes hopelessness: "It's no use," "I can't go on;"
b. States he cannot make a decision; doubts his ability to recover;
c. Overly concerned with small things and neglectful of more pressing, major problems;
d. Denies any problems; overconfident; claims he can do everything without help;
e. Blames the problems on others; has difficulty making plans or discussing future actions.
Severe:
a. Hallucinations, auditory or visual, unverifiable by others;
b. Verbalizes fear of losing his mind; claims the world seems unrecognizable and unreal; claims his body feels unreal and completely different;
c. Preoccupied with an event or idea to the exclusion of anything else;
d. Unrealistic claim that an agency, object, group, or spirit is out to harm him and others such as his family or friends;
e. Expresses inability to make a decision to carry out familiar activities;
f. Expresses a real fear of killing or harming himself or others; far exceeds simple statement of anger or hopelessness.

Emotional Expression
Mild derangement (significantly different from most victims but largely appropriate to situation):
a. Frequent uncontrolled tearing and weeping; rehashing of traumatic events;
b. Blunted expression of feelings; apathetic; seemingly withdrawn emotionally and unable to react with feeling to what is happening;
c. Unusual laughter and gaiety;
d. Overly irritable; quick to get angry over trivia.
Severe derangement (markedly unusual affect or emotion):
a. Excessively flat emotionally; virtually no expression of feeling;
b Excessive emotional expression; inappropriate joy, anger, fear, or sadness for situation.

TRAUMA OR DISEASE SIMULATING
PSYCHOLOGIC ABNORMALITIES

A number of physical, organic disorders can produce abnormal behavior that simulates abnormal psychologic reactions. Most of these disorders produce a change in the availability of oxygen to the brain by altering the blood supply, but some produce metabolic derangements. Hypoxia is most common in mountaineering circumstances and can result not only from altitude but from pneumonia, chest injuries, shock, and other disorders. Hypothermia typically produces progressive changes ranging from fatigue with forgetfulness and slow thought processes, through loss of coordination and greater mental dullness, to irrationality, and finally coma. Hyperthermia (increased body temperature) can cause headache, irritability, agitation, and mental dullness before progressing to stupor and coma. Hypoglycemia (low blood glucose or sugar) leads to restlessness, irritability, lethargy, poor judgment, agitation, disorientation, and finally coma. Severe hypoglycemia is almost always a complication of diabetes, but milder glucose depletion occurs in normal individuals who are exhausted and have not maintained an adequate food intake. Dehydration can produce similar abnormalities.

Head injuries may result in immediate or delayed changes which include disorientation (most typically); drowsiness, apathy, and irritability; forgetfulness and wandering off; bizarre behavior, including homicidal or suicidal mania; and abnormal, heavy breathing, convulsions, and finally unconsciousness. Specific signs such as unequal pupils or abnormal reflexes may be present. Severe infections of the nervous system can produce such signs, as can pneumonia or severe generalized infections. Intoxication by drugs, including alcohol, or drug withdrawal, particularly alcohol, tranquilizers, and barbiturates, can have similar effects.

Generally speaking, in association with these disorders, personality changes such as silliness, irritability, agitation, belligerence, and lethargy occur first and are followed by loss of cognitive functions, which progresses from mild mental dullness through disorientation to time, place, and person (in spite of frequent reminders), loss of calculating ability and specialized knowledge, to loss of judgment and memory. Eventually, obvious confusion with anxiety or hallucinations supervenes and may be associated with incoordination, which produces staggering and slurred speech. As the condition worsens, tremors can appear, followed by convulsions and unconsciousness progressing to deep coma and eventual death.

If sedation is essential for the evacuation of a person whose behavior is uncontrollable, a tranquilizer is preferable. Barbiturates or narcotics complicate the neurologic abnormalities, depress respiration, and should be avoided.

PROVIDING PSYCHOLOGIC AID
FOR ACCIDENT VICTIMS

Listening effectively and creatively is the essence of psychologic care. The counselor must look directly at the person who is speaking, giving his complete attention, and asking questions or paraphrasing the victim's statements to make certain he fully understands what is being said. The victim must be allowed to express his feelings openly and freely; the counselor must understand that such expression is the major purpose of the conversation. The counselor's functions do not include judging what the victim should feel, and he certainly must not convey any such opinion to the victim.

While listening, the rescuer must be thinking about how he can help the victim preserve his dignity. He particularly must evaluate the victim's capacity for taking part in the rescue operation, because participation is so essential for restoring and preserving self esteem and a sense of mastery and control, and for minimizing psychic trauma, guilt reactions, and delayed stress reactions. (The victim obviously must not be allowed to jeopardize the rescue effort or increase the number and extent of casualties. His need for continuing observation, reassurance, and support or restraint must be determined.)

Some goals, particularly psychologic goals, a rescue leader should strive for are:

1. To create acceptance of the victim's feelings as normal reactions to stress;
2. To reduce feelings of guilt by not assessing blame for the accident; to reduce feelings of inadequacy by involving the victims in their own rescue in whatever ways are possible;
3. To restore a feeling of well-being with rest, food and water, warmth, attention to injuries, and comfort and support through listening and touching;
4. To give realistic, honest answers balanced with judicious omissions when advisable;
5. To reduce panic and rage; to remove the most disruptive individuals from the scene; to allow ventilation of feelings and to accept them; to stress the need for help from the victim, particularly for any special abilities he may have;
6. To restore a sense of hope and of belonging through quiet, firm, and knowledgeable leadership with clearly understood goals and sensitivity to the need of victims and rescuers;
7. To provide physical guidance or restraint when necessary, analgesia when indicated;
8. To be aware of the special needs due to the victim's sex when a victim is immobilized and dependent (as in a litter) and assign a person of the same gender to be in constant contact with the victim — the "head person" who always remains by the victim's head during the evacuation;
9. To maintain awareness that supposedly unconscious victims often hear some of what is said around them.

Some attitudes or actions rescue leaders must try to avoid are:

1. Callousness or flippancy; the "M*A*S*H" syndrome;
2. Lying to provide unrealistic optimism and reassurance;
3. Talking around the victim without talking to him;
4. Authoritarian style; telling victim how to feel or imposing ideas on victim; not really listening;
5. Expecting victim to function at top level too quickly;
6. Expecting too little of victim, damaging his chances to salvage self esteem;
7. "Chicken soup" style; oversolicitousness, which interferes with victim's recovery of self esteem;
8. "Democratic" leader(less)ship; floundering by committee, with no definitive leader, goals, plans for achieving them, or communication within the party, including rescuers and victims.

CASE STUDY ONE

Some helpful insights into the psychology of accident victims and recommendations for rescuers have been made by Ray Smutek in his account of his own mountaineering accident and rescue. When describing his fall, he recalls "accelerated mental activity, the detached over-view of the situation, the recollection of past events. Most amazing was the absence of pain, coupled with a very acute awareness of the damage being done."[1]

He observes that potentially the most dangerous stage of an accident is immediately afterwards, "not necessarily to the victim. . . . I think the natural tendency in a situation like this is to rush to the victim, perhaps unbelayed. Action! Do something! Don't just stand there!" But Smutek continues, "this is not the time to rush; few situations require that immediate an action. There is only one thing that you should do immediately and that is to think."

He describes directing his immediate rescue and first aid to the extent that he was conscious and able to state what his injuries were and what he was capable of doing. Further in the article he says that the long wait for rescue "psychologically was the worst part of the entire episode. There was nothing to do but worry." He was very happy to have the company of a fellow climber and thinks everyone in a similar situation should have an "official comforter."

When rescue did come, some of the rescuers were "over their heads," and Smutek states, "nothing is more devastating to a person's morale than an obviously incompetent rescuer." Finally, he reports that administration of a pain killer muddled his mind and increased his anxiety because he could not understand the procedures to which he was being subjected. He feels that rescuers should use pain medication on a highly selective basis, particularly if that medication may interfere with a victim's need to feel in control and be aware of what is going on. These feelings clearly reflect the victim's need to maintain a sense of efficacy. On the other hand, some people are not used to being in control and may be more comfortable being medicated or being told that everything is being cared for.

CASE STUDY TWO

In *The Breach: Kilimanjaro and the Conquest of Self,* Rob Taylor traces the various phases of his devastating accident on Kilimanjaro, his almost miraculous rescue, his prolonged recovery, and his reactions to them. Following a fall in which he suffered a severe compound fracture of his lower leg, a subsequent descent on his own down a perilously steep snow slope, and, finally, a solitary, exposed, life threatening bivouac lasting several days, his thoughts and behavior were strikingly well organized. His self control becomes more understandable when he says, "unrestrained emotions and unbridled feelings in the end, after the fact, are fine, but during the crisis they are illusory defenses."[2]

Nonetheless, on the mountain Taylor experienced grief over the loss symbolized by the injury to his leg. He also felt anguish over the days of waiting for the unknown, but was preparing for and accepting the worst. He writes of "the need to re-live the event" during his recovery and of becoming "daily more aware of the positive aspects of the pilgrimage. . . and [of a] renewal of a reverence and deep appreciation of the gift of life." Finally, he speaks of a heightened sense of self definition, of altering his concept of death, and of coming to realize that he "must make the most of each encounter, each meeting" as a result of his experience.

Taylor recommends to rescuers the therapeutic use of concern, small talk, encouragement, and infectious optimism.

PSYCHOLOGIC RESPONSES OF RESCUERS

Rescuers have psychologic or emotional reactions to accidents, contrary to popular belief and their television image, and their reactions can create problems. Such problems, which have been labelled "rescue trauma," are well known to many rescuers, but few have talked about them with their colleagues, probably from fear of appearing unmanly or even unbalanced.

Dissociation

To perform well, even heroically, saving lives or minimizing the effects of trauma requires a high level of objectivity in spite of the emotional assault by the sights and sounds of the victims and their injuries, the survivors, or the onlookers at the accident scene. To maintain their objectivity, most rescuers dissociate or "split" their intellect from their emotions and deny the emotional magnitude of the events surrounding them. This defensive dissociation, or "splitting," is effective but can not be kept up indefinitely. Eventually the "mental circuits" become overloaded and rescuers begin to develop symptoms of decompensation. The term "rescue trauma threshold" has been coined for "the point at which the intensity of traumatic rescue work begins to overwhelm a person's psychological defenses."[3]

When the overloaded person begins to break down, he develops signs and symptoms similar to accident victims. He may become withdrawn and appear dazed, apathetic, forgetful, or tired. He may become outwardly expressive and be irritable, irrational, destructive, or violent. Or he may shut off his feelings and become less able to experience intimacy with his family and friends. Some rescuers become increasingly reliant on alcohol or drugs.

Overload may come on suddenly after a major disaster that produces many casualties with mutilating injuries, or it may come on insidiously from the accumulated stress of a series of less distressing accidents. Additionally, a rescuer's susceptibility to overload, his rescue trauma threshold, may change from day to day as the result of factors entirely unrelated to the rescue itself, such as poor health, family problems, or insufficient sleep.

Sources of Stress

The causes of rescue stress are many and interrelated but can be separated into two categories: overt and covert stressors. Overt stressors are those immediately related to the accident scene, the victims, and the rescuers. The senses may be assailed by the sights or smells at the scene. Injuries can be bloody and mutilating. The victim may be dead or die in route. Rescue equipment may be inadequate and personnel insufficient, so more effort is demanded of fewer people. Victims of mountaineering accidents frequently must be evacuated by long "carries" over difficult, trailless terrain, often at night. Many hours of gruelling, exhausting labor are required. (Rescues require an average of twelve hours in the White Mountains of New England; they require days in more remote areas when helicopters are not available.)

Covert stressors include the rescuer's body, which may be weakened by fatigue or illness, and his mind, which may be preoccupied with legal, financial, or family problems. Another source of stress is the attitude of rescuers toward the rescue and their abilities. At the start of a rescue operation, rescuers may have high expectations of success, only to be disappointed by the victim's death, their fallibility or their coworkers', and by lack of appreciation for their work, including inaccurate, critical, or even censorious reports in the media.

Another stressor reported by an experienced professional is the enforced inactivity a portion of a rescue team experiences after arriving at an accident scene. Only a few are needed to administer medical treatment; the rest must wait. While waiting, their energy and enthusiasm ebb; some sink so low that they need to be "psyched up" to carry out the victim. The stress of this "middle period" is often overlooked and appears to result from a feeling of not being needed, from the "settling in" of fatigue, and sometimes from newness of the rescue experience.

Normal Reactions to Stress

Reactions to stress may be immediate or delayed. Immediate reactions among rescuers at the accident site — which are normal — include anxiety and apprehension, doubts about their abilities, or hopelessness and despair, which are often mixed with denial or "splitting." Some rescuers experience cognitive difficulties, forgetting where they put things and finding decisions hard to make. "Rescuers in all types of incidents report nausea, a pounding sensation in their hearts, muscle tremors, cramps, profuse sweating, chills, headaches, and muffled hearing." These symptoms tend to dissipate within one to three days, but if the underlying emotions are not recognized as normal and allowed to surface within a reasonable period of time, they eventually work their way into the rescuer's daily life and can cripple him emotionally, cognitively, and physically.

Delayed stress reactions appear hours to weeks after an accident and may be directed either inward or outward. Inward reactions include depression, apathy, or feelings of guilt for not helping or for further injuring the victim. Rescuers may experience nightmares, insomnia, or occasional visual flashbacks, and physical signs such as headaches, loss of appetite, or nausea. Outward reactions typically include irritability, explosiveness, and, in some cases, anger with others who contributed to the stress of the incident, particularly with the press for inaccurate or distorted reporting. Like the immediate stress reactions, these delayed reactions are entirely normal.

Preventing Adverse Stress Reactions

Rescuers, whether they are occasional amateurs or career professionals, must be emotionally prepared for the worst casualties, including the dead, dying, and mutilated, and for the worst situations, such as watching helplessly while someone dies because he is inaccessible, equipment is inadequate, or he just does not respond to the best possible medical care — which occasionally does occur. In preparing for the worst, rescuers also must be aware of their limitations and must balance their expectations with reality. Rescuers must be prepared to serve under leaders who do not have time for explanations or who are not aware of the needs of their crew members. They must expect recognition and thanks from others to be sparse and criticism abundant. Rescuers also should not be surprised when, to paraphrase one Northwest climber's description of mountaineering, rescue work turns out to be ninety percent drudgery and boredom and ten percent sheer terror.

Despite training and experience, situations occur with which the rescuer can not deal due to personal sensitivities or involvement. Such problems include injuries to family or friends, injuries to children, or specific kinds of injuries and mutilation. The rescuer's sensitivity must be respected by himself and his leader and associates. If he is clearly having trouble, the leader should reassign him quickly and tactfully to some other responsibility.

Similarly, rescuers must be aware of the virtual inevitability and normality of developing signs of stress overload, in spite of training and extensive experience, and the acceptability and necessity for sharing those accumulated emotions with others. However, awareness of these phenomena is not enough. To ensure the emotional health of rescuers, preventive or therapeutic measures are essential.

1. Within twenty-four hours after a rescue, the team members need to engage in strenuous aerobic exercise to relieve tension and achieve greater muscular relaxation.

2. Within twenty-four to forty-eight hours after completion of a rescue, a mandatory "debriefing" of an hour or more for the entire team should be focused on expressing and sharing each participant's emotional reactions to the rescue. No one's performance or technique should be criticized, nor should plans for the future be made. Instead, the participants should share their humanity and support each other. Support is needed specifically for the pain, sadness, terror, guilt, or feelings of helplessness experienced by each in differing ways. These emotions must be expressed and accepted without shame or embarrassment.

   Although some groups can manage this process quite well by themselves, such exercises frequently are more effective when guided by someone not directly involved in the rescue, particularly someone with experience in stress management. Working through or completely resolving the stress may require more than one meeting, but all meetings should be conducted as close to the event as possible, preferably within three days. Delays of a week or more increase the risk of converting early, tenuous emotional reactions into more entrenched and chronic disorders. The stress debriefing should be conducted without any alcohol. To maximize the benefits, the minds of all must be fully functional.

3. After debriefing, rescuers need to eat and rest well, rounding out the recovery of the entire organism.

4. Finally, after physical and emotional recovery has been assured, the rescue team should critique the rescue objectively, learn from successes as well as mistakes, and plan for the future.

CASE STUDY THREE

A professional rescuer who is also a climber has been willing to share his thoughts about an experience on a recent Himalayan trek. On the hike in, a member who was a close friend of the rescuer became seriously ill and clearly had to be evacuated. The group leader decided to split the party, most continuing to their objective, while the rescuer and two physicians stayed behind with the victim. After the main party had moved on, the victim's condition deteriorated catastrophically, and over a period of days the three rescuers worked virtually to the point of exhaustion to save him.

During this ordeal, the rescuer became aware of several strong feelings. He found that rescuing a close friend aggravated normal feelings of inadequacy and guilt, particularly guilt for not having more forcefully cautioned the victim before he became so ill. He also felt guilty for not having resisted more vigorously the decision to split the party, which left the victim with a support team barely able to provide for his care. In retrospect, the rescuer realized that he had deferred to the leader despite his own considerable judgment and experience due to a difference in credentials. (The leader was a physician.) During and after the subsequent vigil, the subject began to question his confidence in the leader, in his associates, in himself, and even in some categories of people (doctors and nurses) who were members of the rescue group. His confidence was further eroded following reuniting of the party when "significant" people "acted like nothing had happened."

The rescuer kept these feelings hidden for some time, not realizing that others were experiencing the same emotions. Only months later, when he made an off-hand comment that he was considering dropping out of the group, did he have an opportunity to share his pain and begin to reconstruct relationships. Since then he has been free to make a variety of recommendations, particularly that the emotional residue of stressful situations be discharged through mandatory debriefings.

He also observed that even though external support from a rescuer's associates is helpful, in the long run the benefits fade unless the rescuer himself recognizes the value of his efforts and learns from his mistakes, rather than wallowing in destructive self criticism. To grow, everyone must accept responsibility for his actions, both good and bad.

POSTTRAUMATIC STRESS DISORDER

Should the rescuer not be allowed to work through his normal reactions, he risks developing a more severe abnormality known as the "posttraumatic stress disorder." This condition has been repeatedly described during the past century and has been given widely varying names, depending on its origin. These labels include accident neurosis, shell shock, traumatic neurosis, combat fatigue, combat exhaustion, post-Vietnam syndrome, and neurasthenia. The term "post-traumatic stress disorder" has been used to unite these conditions under one label.

The features of the posttraumatic stress disorder are:

1. The victim has undergone a recognizable stressful experience that would evoke significant symptoms of distress in almost everyone.
2. The victim re-experiences the trauma in one or more of the following ways:
    a. Recurrent and intrusive recollections of the event;
    b. Recurrent dreams of the event;
    c. Sudden acting or feeling as if the traumatic event were reoccurring due to the stimulus of an environment or thought associated with the event.
3. The victim has a numbed responsiveness to or reduced involvement with the external world, beginning some time after the trauma, manifested by one or more of the following:
    a. Markedly diminished interest in one or more significant activities;
    b. Feeling of detachment or estrangement from others;
    c. Constricted affect.
4. The victim usually has two or more of the following symptoms that were not present before the trauma:
    a. Hyperalertness or exaggerated "startle" response;
    b. Sleep disturbances;
    c. Guilt about surviving when others have not, or about behavior required for survival;
    d. Memory impairment or difficulty concentrating;
    e. Avoidance of activities that arouse recollections of the traumatic event;
    f. Intensification of symptoms by exposure to events that symbolize or resemble the traumatic event.

Three subtypes of the posttraumatic stress disorder have been identified:

Acute. Symptoms appear within six months of the trauma and last less than six months;
Chronic. Symptoms appear within six months and last longer than six months;
Delayed. Symptoms appear six months or more after the trauma.

Diagnostic studies during the past half century suggest that with sufficient unrelieved stress, anyone would develop the post-traumatic stress disorder. Vietnam veterans who developed this disorder shared five characteristics:

1. A positive attitude toward the war before engaging in combat;
2. A high level of combat exposure;

3. Immediate separation from the military service upon returning to the United States;
4. A negative perception of family helpfulness upon returning home;
5. A feeling that forces beyond their control were directing the course of their lives.

The correlative experiences for wilderness rescuers would be:

1. Unrealistic expectations;
2. A high level of exposure to hazardous terrain or weather;
3. Infrequent opportunities to share emotional experiences; frequent "suffering in silence;"
4. Frequent lack of support or appreciation;
5. Feeling that uncontrollable factors such as weather, timing, inadequate personnel or equipment, communication failures, or accidents involving members of the rescue group have determined the outcome of the rescue.

Treatment for the posttraumatic stress syndrome is the province of professional therapists. However, the earlier the disorder is recognized, the faster and more successful is the outcome of therapy. Recognizing stressful events and taking measures to relieve the emotional pressures they engender, or recognizing the symptoms of this disorder are certainly within the province of rescuers, climbers, or simply friends.

SELECTION OF RESCUERS

Enthusiasm alone is not an adequate qualification for wilderness rescuers. Members of rescue teams should be chosen on the basis of at least the following criteria:

PHYSICAL CONDITION
Cardiorespiratory endurance from regular exercise;
Strength, upper and lower body;
Good health with no significant medical problems, acute or chronic.

TECHNICAL EXPERTISE
Medical knowledge, particularly about the care for trauma victims;
Familiarity with search and rescue procedures;
Knowledge of evacuation techniques;
Experience with hostile or difficult environments such as mountains, white water, underwater (scuba).

GENDER

The "head" or communication and support person should be the same gender as the victim.

PERSONALITY

Reasonable, not excitable or impulsive;

Capable of following own initiative;

Capable and cooperative in following others;

Attentive to details of procedure and equipment;

Endowed with a sense of humor;

Empathetic, capable of feeling for another's plight without being overwhelmed;

Optimistic, although prepared for the worst;

Able to minimize or shelve worry or fear and yet be able to accept those feelings as normal;

Not prone to harbor anger.

PSYCHOLOGIC REACTIONS TO DEAD BODIES

When faced with the dead bodies of intimates or strangers, many people experience emotional difficulties. In *The Hour of Our Death,* Aries states that people have long resisted believing that death deprives the body of all life. He says, "belief in the sensibility of the cadaver has the support of the people, and what we would call folklore. . . though scientists consider such to be superstition."[4] Many believe that the body still hears, feels, and remembers after death, a belief reinforced by recent descriptions of out-of-body, life-after-death experiences. They treat the dead gently for fear of hurting them or, in some cases, for fear of angering them.

Other reactions to dead bodies include anxious discomfort, horror and panic, fear of the unknown or of one's own death, and fear of contamination. A few people react with intellectual or morbid fascination and curiosity. Defensive behavior such as indifference, joking, hostility, or detachment are more commonly encountered.

In nursing and medical students the fear of dying and the death of others decreases with increasing academic preparation and experience. However, the fear of their own death and dying remains the same or increases as they near the age where their death is more likely.

Professional rescuers encounter death so commonly on the streets or highways that they lose their feeling of being uncomfortable when near a body, at least when near the body of someone they do not know. For amateur rescuers who do not have so many encounters with death, two methods for reducing the emotional shock of the experience have been suggested: desensitization through gradual, nontraumatic exposure to death; or coming to terms with their own death by experiencing it in fantasy, discovering what is really essential for them to have accomplished during their lives, and taking steps to leave as little unfinished as possible. The value of anticipatory grief as a buffer for sudden and serious loss has been demonstrated.

Finally, many individuals have come to accept death as another stage of life, but that crosses into the purview of religion.

ACKNOWLEDGMENT

The author wishes to express appreciation to Roger Zimmerman, Ph.D., and William Moss, EMT, for their professional expertise.

REFERENCES

1. Lamers W: Death, dying, and bereavement. Symposium, Stockholm, Sweden, 20 June 1982. (Reproduced by permission.)
2. Smutek R: Good Morning, I'm Your Guest Victim for Today. *Off Belay* February 1978. (Quoted by permission of the author and publisher.)
3. Taylor R. *The Breach: Kilimanjaro and the Conquest of Self.* New York, Coward, McCann, and Geoghegan, 1981. (Quoted by permission of the author and publisher.)
4. Nydam RJ. Rescue trauma threshold. *Emergency* February 1983; 35-45.
5. Aries P: *The Hour of Our Death.* New York, Alfred Knopf, 1981.

ADDITIONAL READING

1. Mitchell MS, Jeffrey T: Recovery from rescue. *Response!* 1982; 7:10.
2. Missouri Department of Mental Health: *Mental Health and Disaster Relief: Leaders Manual.* St Louis, Missouri, 1974.

CHAPTER FIVE

Preventive Measures

In wilderness areas, illness is usually coupled with inaccessibility. The advantages of preventing such mishaps are obvious. Loss of life, permanent disability, or even the failure of an outing, trek, or expedition to reach its goal are high prices to pay for disabilities that could be avoided. In many underdeveloped countries, including Nepal, cholera is a constant threat, and polio immunization is not practiced; malaria is a problem throughout the tropics and subtropics; tetanus has a worldwide distribution and is usually catastrophic in a remote situation. All can be prevented.

This chapter is directed to the problems of infectious diseases and their prevention by immunizations and sanitation, particularly water disinfection. These precautions are of obvious significance for the expeditionary mountaineer for whom exposure to unusual infections usually represents the greatest hazard in travelling to and from the mountains. The risk of infection in many foreign cities, even in the "best" hotels, and the almost total lack of sanitary measures in areas traversed during approach marches make extensive precautions essential. However, many aspects of preventive medicine are important for mountaineering in countries where sanitary practices are reputedly more sophisticated. (Drugs for the prevention of malaria, and other methods for avoiding infections, are discussed in Chapter Twenty-three, "Infections.")

IMMUNIZATIONS

Immunization is the easiest and most reliable method for preventing infections. Unfortunately, only a few totally effective immunizations are available. However, those that are only partially effective can significantly reduce the likelihood of infection and lessen the impact should the infection occur. For expeditions, all members should perhaps be required to obtain immunization against the diseases likely to be encountered for which such protection is available. (The immunologic principles upon which immunizations are based are discussed in Chapter Twenty-four, "Allergies.")

General Considerations

When travelling, an International Certificate of Vaccination is a convenient means for keeping a record of all immunizations and is required for entrance into some countries.

As vaccines are improved and more experience is gained with their use, recommendations for immunization change. Sometimes changing political situations also cause countries to change their immunization requirements for entry. The Centers for Disease Control annually publishes a bulletin describing in detail which immunizations or other preventive measures are advisable for travel in any specific area, as well as the latest legal requirements for entry. This bulletin, "Health Information for International Travel," can be purchased from the Superintendent of Documents, U.S. Government Printing Office, Washington, D.C. 20402. Additionally, most local health departments have a copy which can be consulted, sometimes by telephone.

The International Association for Medical Assistance to Travellers (IAMAT) is a volunteer, nongovernmental organization of hospitals, health care centers, and physicians throughout the world who have pledged to provide travellers with physicians who speak their language and who meet IAMAT's standards, which are generally consistent with U.S. standards. Membership in IAMAT and a directory of its affiliated institutions in over 115 countries, including most of the countries containing major mountain ranges, is free. The address of the U.S. affiliate is IAMAT, 736 Center Street, Lewiston, N.Y. 14092. Also free from that organization is its *World Immunization Chart* which lists the potential risk for over a dozen diseases, country by country, in a quick reference format.

Scheduling Immunizations

Mountaineering expeditions do not take place without months of planning and preparation. Scheduling immunizations is a critical part of such preparations and must not be put off until the last minute.

Viral vaccines, including hepatitis B, and tetanus and diphtheria toxoid can be given six months or more before departure. The benefits from such immunizations persist for years. Bacterial immunizations, such as typhoid fever and cholera, are not as enduring and should be given much closer to the date of departure. The last immunization probably should be administered two to three weeks before leaving. Pooled immune globulin, which would be given to help prevent hepatitis A and non-A, non-B hepatitis, should be given as close to departure as possible — almost while walking onto the aircraft.

The repeated injections for some immunizations such as typhoid fever or hepatitis B must be administered four weeks or more apart. Live virus vaccines such as yellow fever and oral polio vaccine must be given at the same time or one month apart. Immune globulin should not be given for three months before and for at least two weeks after any live viral vaccine to avoid neutralizing that vaccine.

SPECIFIC IMMUNIZATIONS

Smallpox

Smallpox has been eliminated worldwide by a vigorous vaccination campaign carried out by the World Health Organization, an outstanding medical triumph. The last reported case of smallpox outside of a laboratory was in Somalia in 1977. Most countries have eliminated their requirements for recent smallpox vaccination for entry. The vaccine is now considered more hazardous than the risk of contracting the infection and should not be administered.

Rubella

Rubella (German measles) is one of the most widely documented causes of birth defects. The Centers for Disease Control recommends that everyone, not just women, be vaccinated unless he has been previously vaccinated or has laboratory evidence of immunity. A single injection of live rubella virus vaccine provides lasting immunity.

Measles

Measles can be a severe disease, particularly in adults. In 1981, thirteen percent of the cases reported in the U.S. were contracted in other countries. Individuals who have not had a documented vaccination or a physician diagnosed infection, or who do not have laboratory evidence of immunity, should receive measles vaccine, whether or not they plan to travel.

Poliomyelitis

Poliomyelitis is now almost entirely preventable by immunization. Trivalent oral live virus vaccine provides much longer effective immunity than the inactivated virus (Salk) vaccine. The oral vaccine should be taken even though prior inactivated virus immunization has been carried out. A booster should be obtained in preparation for a trip to an underdeveloped country. Some countries, like Nepal, can not afford routine polio immunization and infection by those viruses is widespread.

Tetanus

The organisms producing tetanus are widespread, and infections can result from trivial wounds. Because the treatment for tetanus is not very effective, the mortality rate is so high, and immunization provides such reliable protection, no excuse for inadequate immunologic protection against this disease can be found. The initial series of tetanus toxoid immunizations is two injections four to eight weeks apart. A third inoculation should be obtained six to twelve months later. A booster should be obtained at least every ten years thereafter. However, if a booster has not been received within five years, one should be obtained before departing on a mountaineering outing (or following a contaminated wound in any circumstance).

Typhoid

Initial typhoid immunization is achieved by two injections four weeks apart. A booster suffices within three years of initial immunization, although yearly inoculation is desirable in areas where the disease is known to be present. Typhoid immunization is estimated to be only about seventy percent effective in preventing typhoid infection, but it does significantly reduce the severity of infections that do occur. Such immunization is recommended, sometimes strongly, for travellers outside of major cities in underdeveloped countries, which would include almost all climbers in those areas.

Cholera

Cholera immunization is required for entry into some countries by travellers from areas where the infection is widespread. Immunizations are only about sixty to eighty percent effective for a period of about six months. Protection is maximal when injections are obtained shortly before going to the endemic area. The initial inoculation should be followed by a second injection one month later. Boosters must be obtained every six months.

Yellow Fever

Yellow fever is endemic in the equatorial regions of Africa and South and Central America. The possibility of a resurgence in the Caribbean has appeared as the carrier mosquito, *Aedes aegypti,* has developed resistance to insecticides. Yellow fever has never been recognized in Asia, and officials fear its introduction there would result in disastrous epidemics. For that reason, yellow fever immunization is required to travel in many Asian countries, particularly for persons arriving from countries where yellow fever is endemic. A single inoculation provides effective immunization; boosters are needed only every ten years. Immunizations must be obtained from a World Health Organization Yellow Fever Vaccination Center. The location of the nearest center can be obtained from the local health department.

HEPATITIS

Hepatitis is caused by a number of completely different viruses, two of which have been isolated and characterized: hepatitis A and hepatitis B. A third type of hepatitis has been labelled non-A,non-B hepatitis because it is not caused by either of these viruses. Currently available evidence indicates that non-A,non-B hepatitis is caused by two different viral agents, but more may be involved. Prevention of all types of hepatitis is essential because no specific medical treatment is available for any of them.

Hepatitis A

Hepatitis A is produced by a simple RNA virus that is most commonly transmitted by fecal contamination of water. This virus is responsible for most epidemics of acute hepatitis within institutions, such as those for the mentally retarded, and for hepatitis resulting from eating shellfish from contaminated water.

Hepatitis A almost always produces a brief illness from which the patient completely recovers in a few days to a few weeks. (The details of this illness are discussed in Chapter Eighteen, "Gastrointestinal Diseases.") Actually, more than ninety percent of the infections are "subclinical"; the victim does not realize he has been sick, or he only feels bad with no symptoms suggestive of liver disease. On a mountaineering expedition, such infections would often produce enough disability to be disruptive.

The Hepatitis A virus has been successfully grown in culture and a vaccine is being developed, although it is not available at the present time (1984). When this vaccine becomes available, it should be taken by almost everyone. Due to the sophisticated water sanitation facilities prevalent within most developed countries, many of the residents in those countries have never come in contact with the Hepatitis A virus. Since this infection tends to be more severe in older persons, its prevention by vaccination is advisable.

Until a vaccine becomes available, the only immunoprophylaxis available for hepatitis A is pooled immune globulin. Although the protection provided by this agent is incomplete and transient, it is probably advisable for back country travel in underdeveloped countries. The administration schedule has already been discussed. However, diligent water disinfection is probably at least equally effective for preventing this infection; without this precaution, immune globulin may be inadequate.

Hepatitis B

Hepatitis B is caused by a large, complex DNA virus that is quite different from the virus producing hepatitis A. Hepatitis B is primarily transmitted by body fluids, although it can be transmitted by contaminated water or food. This infection was transmitted by needles used for injections prior to the initiation of rigorous sterilization procedures and the introduction of disposable needles and syringes. It was also transmitted by blood transfusions prior to the development of methods for detecting its presence in blood. Currently, in developed countries it is most commonly transmitted by sexual contact; among residents of underdeveloped countries it is transmitted most commonly by mothers to their fetuses or newborns or by young children who play together.

Hepatitis B is a much more dangerous infection than hepatitis A because hepatitis B can progress to a chronic form. Within the U.S. and similar developed countries, approximately ten percent of the individuals with acute hepatitis B develop chronic hepatitis. About three percent develop progressive hepatitis, and half of these progress to cirrhosis. The fourth most common cause of death in the thirty-five to sixty year old age group (usually life's most productive years) in the U.S. is cirrhosis, and approximately half of the cases are attributed to chronic hepatitis. Most of the remainder are the result of chronic alcoholism, but even in those patients chronic hepatitis may be in part responsible. (Chronic hepatitis B is one of the world's most prevalent diseases. It is estimated to affect approximately five percent of the world population, or about 200 million individuals. Furthermore, hepatitis B is directly related to the development of hepatocellular carcinoma, a malignant tumor originating within the liver, which is the most common of all malignant tumors on a worldwide basis.)

Fortunately, a safe, effective vaccine is available for hepatitis B. The vaccine clearly provides protection against infection for most of its recipients. Additionally, the vaccine is prepared from only the surface coat of the hepatitis virus, not the entire organism, and can not transmit hepatitis. Even though the vaccine has been prepared from the serum of male homosexuals, who have a high incidence of the acquired immunodeficiency syndrome (AIDS), no instances in which that disorder has been transmitted by the vaccine have been identified.

Hepatitis B vaccination should be obtained by everyone travelling into back country areas of underdeveloped countries, although individuals who have previously come into contact with this virus and developed natural immunity do not need to be vaccinated. Such subclinical infections are common and can be detected with a simple blood test which is cheaper than the vaccine. At the present time the vaccine is relatively expensive (compared to other vaccines — it costs about one-half as much as one day in an average hospital), but less costly vaccines have been developed and should be available soon.

Non-A,Non-B Hepatitis

Although these infections are rather common, the viral agents causing them have not been isolated. Non-A,non-B hepatitis is currently the most common cause of hepatitis transmitted by blood transfusions, although only about five to ten percent of such infections are transmitted in that manner. Of the remaining infections, about half are transmitted by intravenous drug abuse and half are transmitted by "travel to underdeveloped countries." The latter group is probably the result of contaminated food or water.

Non-A,non-B hepatitis progresses to chronic hepatitis more frequently than hepatitis B. Estimates of the incidence of chronic non-A,non-B hepatitis following acute infections have ranged from fifteen to ninety percent, although the lower rate appears more accurate. Cirrhosis also develops more frequently following non-A, non-B hepatitis. (This infection has no demonstrable association with hepatocellular carcinoma.)

Since the organisms responsible for non-A,non-B hepatitis have not been isolated, no vaccines are available. Pooled immune globulin is probably as effective for the prevention of these infections as it is for hepatitis A. However, that protection is incomplete and transient.

The most compelling reason for compulsive water and food disinfection while travelling in an underdeveloped country is to avoid non-A,non-B hepatitis. Giardiasis and tourista are unpleasant infections, but neither commonly lasts more than a week. Chronic hepatitis can last for the rest of the victim's life, which typically is significantly shortened.

SANITATION

Informed sanitation practices play a vital role in preventing infections. Many residents of underdeveloped countries do not follow even the most rudimentary sanitation procedures, such as washing their hands after using the toilet. Even when they become accustomed to such practices, they do not understand the reasons for them and consider them idiosyncrasies of foreigners. When local inhabitants are employed as cooks or in similar roles, hand washing, disinfection of water for drinking, cooking, or even washing dishes, and sanitary preparation of food must be vigorously and constantly enforced to prevent a lapse into old habits.

Locally obtained food must be regarded with the same skepticism as the water supply. Diseases carried by food include the bacillary dysenteries, amebiasis, and a variety of parasites. The only food that can be regarded as safe from contamination is that which has been thoroughly cooked *under supervision*. Fruits must be picked above ground level, cleaned, and peeled by the eater. All other foods must be assumed to be dangerous, particularly previously peeled fruits, custards, cakes, bread, cold meats, cheeses, and other dairy products. Milk is a potential source of tuberculosis. Bottled carbonated drinks are generally safe, but any ice that might be added often is not.

Sites for garbage disposal and latrines should be downstream, downhill, and downwind. Such sites should be as far as possible from streams. However, such considerations must also be balanced against convenience. Placing latrines too far from camp leads to underutilization, which can make the camp unpleasant and unsafe. Local inhabitants often must be instructed to use latrines. Nepal suffers an epidemic of cholera at the beginning of each rainy season because the rain washes human feces from the streets into the streams that serve as the water supply.

WATER DISINFECTION

A water disinfection system for wilderness use must be simple and reliable in addition to being lightweight and small. Boiling water is time consuming and inconvenient, and the additional time required to compensate for lower boiling temperatures at higher altitudes apparently has not been determined. Micropore filtration effectively removes bacteria and parasites, but the water still must be chemically treated to destroy viruses (which produce infections such as hepatitis). For chemical disinfection, only chlorine or iodine containing compounds are sufficiently simple and inexpensive to be used routinely.

Although chlorine is used in most municipal water systems, available chlorine compounds are too unstable to be relied upon for wilderness water disinfection. The disinfectant action of chlorine is relatively slow and pH sensitive, and in water containing organic residues, chlorine combines with ammonia ions and amino acids to form chloramines, making disinfection unpredictable.

IODINE AS A WATER DISINFECTANT

Diatomic iodine (I_2) consistently and reliably disinfects water containing as many as one million bacteria per milliliter, a concentration approximately ten times greater than would be expected in grossly polluted water. It also destroys viruses, parasites, and parasitic cysts. Additionally, iodine is faster acting than chlorine, resists inactivation by organic compounds, is active over a wide pH range, and is available in stable preparations. Even in moderately turbid water with moderate amounts of organic color, at 23 °C (73 ° F) and an iodine concentration of 8 mg/L (8 parts per million), a contact time of ten minutes eradicates bacteria, viruses, parasites, and parasitic cysts and provides a considerable margin of safety. (Such high iodine concentrations are needed primarily to destroy parasitic cysts. A concentration of 0.5 mg/L is adequate if parasites are not a problem.)

Another advantage of iodine is its visibility. Water containing 8 mg/L of iodine has a definite brown color.

Precautions

Several precautions must be taken when iodine is used for water disinfection. In cold water (0° to 5° C [32° to 41° F]) the chemical activity of iodine is slower, just as all chemical reactions are slower at lower temperatures. Contact time must be increased to twenty minutes to insure complete disinfection. Cloudy, heavily contaminated water requires more iodine to compensate for binding of the disinfectant by organic compounds. Doubling the iodine concentration to 16 mg/L is sufficient.

Artificial flavorings can be added to disinfected water to mask the iodine taste, but these additives usually contain ascorbic acid which reacts with the iodine, impairing its antimicrobial activity. Such flavoring must not be added to iodine treated water before enough time has elapsed for the microorganisms to have been destroyed.

Acute Iodine Toxicity

Iodine is not highly toxic. In fact, the third edition of Goodman and Gilman's textbook of pharmacology states "That iodine is highly toxic, however, is a popular fallacy."[1] The generally accepted lethal dose is 2 to 3 gm, but survival after ingestion of 10 gm has been reported. Iodine is a strong gastrointestinal irritant and causes immediate vomiting, which eliminates most of the iodine. That remaining in the gastrointestinal tract is largely neutralized by the intestinal contents. (The immediate treatment for iodine poisoning is administration of starchy food.)

Accidental iodine poisoning is rare. Almost all fatalities are suicidal, but successful suicide is uncommon if the victim receives medical care. No deaths occurred among 327 patients attended at the Boston City Hospital between 1915 and 1936 following attempted suicide with iodine.[2]

Chronic Iodine Toxicity

Ingested iodine is absorbed as iodide, and an average adult requires 150 to 200 micrograms a day.[3,4] Daily consumption of one to two liters of water disinfected with 8 mg/L of iodine would provide thirty to eighty times that amount, but such quantities would not affect most individuals with normal thyroid function. Almost all patients who have developed iodide goiter after consuming excess iodide have consumed far larger amounts for six months to more than five years.[3] (The recommended dose of the expectorant potassium iodide for asthmatics ranges from 1.2 to 8.0 gm daily [0.9 to 6.0 gm of iodine].) [3,4]

Iodine can cause large fetal goiters that produce lethal respiratory obstruction at birth. However, the mothers of infants with iodide goiters are almost all asthmatics who have consumed a gram or more of iodine daily for many months or years.[3]

Inmates of three Florida prisons have consumed water disinfected with 0.5 to 1.0 mg/L of iodine for fifteen years. No detrimental effects on the general health or thyroid function of previously normal persons have been detected with careful medical and biochemical monitoring. Of 101 infants born to inmates who had been in prison for 122 to 270 days, none had detectable thyroid enlargement.[5]

These studies indicate that individuals, including pregnant women, with normal thyroid function can consume water disinfected with 8mg/L of iodine for several months with no ill effects. Most individuals can safely drink water disinfected in this manner for much longer periods, but a system that incorporates a filter to remove parasitic cysts and adds only 0.5 to 1.0 mg/L of iodine would eliminate the risk of iodide goiter.

Although iodine is used to treat thyrotoxicosis, iodine can produce that syndrome in rare individuals with thyroid abnormalities, usually those with large, iodine deficiency goiters (Jodbasedow phenomenon).[3][4] All four individuals with hyperthyroidism encountered in the Florida prisons became more symptomatic while consuming iodinated water.[5] Persons with known thyroid dysfunction or goiter should avoid or be careful when using iodine for water disinfection, perhaps drinking water containing that quantity of iodine at home under the supervision of their physician before using it in a wilderness situation. The rare individuals allergic to iodine (usually manifested by a chronic skin rash) should not use iodine for water disinfection.

SPECIFIC IODINE DISINFECTANT PREPARATIONS

Tetraglycine Hydroperiodide

Tablets containing tetraglycine hydroperiodide are widely sold under trade names such as Globaline and Potable-Aqua. One *fresh* tablet dissolved in a liter of water provides an iodine concentration of 8 mg/L. The major advantage of tetraglycine hydroperiodide tablets is their convenience. A small bottle of fifty tablets can be carried easily. Sealed bottles can be stored for months with little loss of iodine.

The principal disadvantage of tetraglycine hydroperiodide is its tendency to disassociate after exposure to air. In studies to document their stability, tetraglycine hydroperiodide tablets that were placed in a single layer in an open dish at 140° F (60° C) lost forty percent of their iodine in seven days.[6] At room temperature and one hundred percent humidity, the tablets lost thirty-three percent of their iodine in four days.

Tetraglycine hydroperiodide tablets individually packaged in metal foil are supplied to members of the U.S. Army but apparently have not been made available to others.

Tincture of Iodine

Tincture of iodine has been widely recommended for water disinfection. Its major disadvantages are its taste and its iodide component. Some writers consider the taste imparted by tincture of iodine to be much stronger than other preparations containing equivalent quantities of iodine. The U.S. Pharmacopoeia (USP) standard tincture of iodine solution is 2 percent iodine and 2.4 percent sodium iodide in fifty percent ethanol. The iodide has no disinfectant activity and unnecessarily increases total iodine consumption.

Ticture of iodine is readily available and resists freezing. It can be used to disinfectant skin, but aqueous solutions are just as effective for that purpose and do not sting. Addition of 0.4 cc of a two percent solution to a liter of water provides an iodine concentration of 8 mg/L. An accurate dropper should be used to dispense a precise volume. Although a two percent solution is the USP standard, solutions of different concentrations are also sold as "tincture."

Iodine tincture is rarely sold by pharmacies in quantities larger than one ounce, but larger volumes are available from chemical suppliers. A quantity sufficient for the water disinfection needs of a major expedition would be bulky and heavy; the tincture must be stored in glass bottles, which can break.

Resin Bound Iodine

Quaternary ammonium anion exchange resins combined with iodine are recently developed water disinfectants. As water is filtered through the resin, microorganisms come in contact with the iodine and are destroyed, but iodine is released into the water in such small quantities that the resulting concentration is less than 2 mg/L, which is too little to taste or see. The most widely distributed device employing this method of disinfection is a cup originally known as the Mini Water Purifier, later renamed the Walbro Water Purifier, and more recently renamed again the Water Tech Travelmate Water Purifier.

Although convenient, this system has several disadvantages. The most significant is the absence of any indicator that the resin has been exhausted. The filter releases so little iodine into the water that no visible color is produced. The Water Tech Purifier is claimed to have the capacity for disinfecting 100 gallons of water, but few users would keep the records needed to know when that quantity has been filtered. Another disadvantage is the time required for filtration — ten to twelve minutes for a liter of water.

Faster systems have already been developed. If an indicator of iodine exhaustion can be devised, such devices should be very effective and useful for water disinfection.

Saturated Aqueous Iodine Solution (Kahn-Visscher)

In 1975 Kahn and Visscher described a procedure for disinfecting water with a saturated aqueous solution of iodine. Iodine crystals (2 to 8 gm, USP grade, resublimed) are placed in a 30 cc (1 oz) clear glass bottle with a paper lined bakelite cap. The bottle is filled with water and shaken vigorously for thirty to sixty seconds to produce a saturated solution. After the crystals have settled, one half of the supernatant (15 cc) is poured into one liter of water to be disinfected. If the water in the 30 cc bottle has a temperature of 68 ° F (20 ° C), which can be achieved by carrying it in a shirt pocket, the iodine concentration in the disinfected water will be about 9 mg/L.

The Kahn-Visscher method has two distinct advantages: compactness and reliability. If 4 gm of iodine are placed in the 30 cc bottle initially, it can disinfect approximately 500 liters of water. If crystals can be seen in the bottom of the bottle, enough iodine for disinfection is known to be present.

This technique for water disinfection has been denounced, even in inflammatory terms such as "it can kill you," because in decanting the supernatant, iodine crystals can be poured into the water to be consumed. The significance of this hazard is questionable. Iodine is so weakly toxic that three or four crystals would not be expected to produce any symptoms. When this procedure is used for water disinfection small flakes of iodine are commonly ingested but do not produce any detectable ill effects. The risk can be reduced by pouring the saturated iodine solution into an intermediate container before adding it to the water to be disinfected. Suitable filters are not available.

Sublimation of iodine has also been identified as a major disadvantage of the Kahn-Visscher technique, but sublimation is minimal under water, and toxic effects from the vapors of the quantities of iodine used for this type of water disinfection have not been documented.

Crystalline iodine has been found ineffective for eradicating giardial cysts at low temperatures, largely due to difficulty in consistently obtaining a saturated solution. However, other iodine based techniques did eradicate giardial cysts in these studies. The most active antimicrobial component of all of the iodine containing disinfectants is diatomic iodine, and this form of iodine is released by all.

One real problem with the Kahn-Visscher system for water disinfection is the tendency of the glass bottles to break, particularly as the result of freezing (which can be avoided by leaving an air space in the bottle when it is not being carried). Unfortunately, glass is the only satisfactory container for iodine solutions.

The Kahn-Visscher disinfection method is widely used because it is convenient and reliable. For informed adults who are aware of the hazards, particularly for members of prolonged expeditions or urban residents in underdeveloped countries, experience indicates the method is safe, although children must not be entrusted with a potentially lethal quantity of iodine. For weekend outings other methods of water disinfection are more readily available. Crystalline iodine is not sold in drugstores or camping supply outlets and must be purchased from chemical supply companies.

Alcoholic Iodine Solutions

Another iodine preparation that has been used but not widely publicized is a concentrated alcoholic solution of iodine. Iodine is much more soluble in ethanol than in water, and concentrated solutions can be easily prepared. If a solution contains 8 gm of iodine in 100 cc of ninety-five percent ethanol, only 0.1 cc needs to be added to each liter of water to be disinfected. An accurately calibrated dropper or similar device is needed to measure out such small quantities, but 100 cc of the solution contain enough iodine to disinfect 1,000 liters of water. Such solutions are reliable because loss of iodine does not occur. Smaller quantities, which would not contain a lethal quantity of iodine, could be used safely around children.

Alcohol evaporates slowly and the solution will become more concentrated with time. Therefore, any remaining solution should probably be discarded after each climbing season. The solution should be relatively inexpensive but somewhat inconvenient to prepare. Individuals need to order the iodine from chemical supply houses and have to find a way to weigh out 8 gm accurately. They also might have difficulty obtaining ethanol without paying alcoholic beverage taxes.

Table One. A Comparison of Iodine Preparations for Water Disinfection

Method	Advantages	Disadvantages
1. Tetraglycine Hydroperiodide	1. Convenient	1. Undetectable Loss of Iodine After Bottle Has Been Opened
2. Tincture of Iodine	1. Reliable 2. Available 3. Resistant to Freezing	1. Strong Taste 2. Extra Iodide 3. Bulky (Expedition Quantities) 4. Glass Container
3. Resin Bound Iodine	1. No Iodine Taste	1. No Indicator of Iodine Status After Prolonged Use 2. Tedious
4. Crystalline Iodine (Kahn-Visscher)	1. Reliable 2. Compact	1. Possibility of Decanting Iodine Crystals 2. Not Readily Available 3. Glass Container
5. Concentrated Alcoholic Iodine Solutions	1. Reliable 2. Compact 3. Resistant to Freezing	1. Not Readily Available 2. Requires Accurate Measuring Device 3. Glass Container

Lugol's (Iodine-Potassium Iodide) Solution

Iodine-iodide solutions are not ideal sources of iodine for water disinfection. The iodide has no disinfectant activity and increases the total iodine intake. Therefore, such solutions are less suitable for extended outings. Additionally, the concentrations vary. Although the USP standard is five percent iodine and ten percent potassium iodide, one percent, two percent, five percent, and eight percent solutions have been authoritatively identified as "Lugol's." Concentrated solutions require precise metering devices. Like all iodine solutions, Lugol's must be kept in glass containers, which can break. In view of these problems, other iodine sources appear preferable.

Povidone-Iodine Solutions

A ten percent solution of povidone-iodine, an organic iodine complex sold as Betadine and other trade names, has been recommended for water disinfection in a widely publicized letter to a medical journal. However, a 1:1,000 solution of povidone-iodine, which would be expected to yield a free iodine concentration of 10 mg/L, has been found to have severely limited antibacterial activity. Until the effectiveness of povidone-iodine for water disinfection has been established, these agents should not be used for this purpose.

REFERENCES

1. Goodman LS, Gilman A: *The Pharmacological Basis of Therapeutics,* 3rd ed. New York, The Macmillan Co., 1965:1033.
2. Moore M: The ingestion of iodine as a method of attempted suicide. *New Eng J Med* 1938;219:383.
3. Wolff J: Iodide goiter and the pharmacologic effects of excess iodide. *Amer J Med* 1969;47:101.
4. Gilman AG, Goodman LS, Gilman A: *Goodman and Gilman's The Pharmacological Basis of Therapeutics,* 6th ed. New York, Macmillan Publishing Co., 1980:972, 1412.
5. Thomas WC Jr, Malagodi MH, Oates TW, McCourt JP: Effects of an iodinated water supply. *Trans Amer Clin Clim Assoc* 1978;90:153.
6. Morris JC, Chang SL, Fair GM, Conant GH Jr: Disinfection of drinking water under field conditions. *Ind Eng Chem Ind Ed* 1953;45:1013.

SECTION TWO
TRAUMATIC INJURIES

CHAPTER SIX

Soft Tissue Injuries

Lacerations, abrasions, bruises, and blisters are the most common injuries occurring in the mountains. They are called "soft tissue" injuries to distinguish them from injuries to bones and ligaments.

The treatment of soft tissue injuries has four objectives: (1) control of bleeding, (2) control of infection, (3) promotion of healing, and (4) preservation of function in the injured part.

CONTROL OF BLEEDING

Direct pressure is the only effective means for controlling bleeding from a soft tissue wound in the field. The severed vessels must be collapsed, obstructing the flow of blood and permitting clots to form. Furthermore, the pressure must be applied directly over the wound. Pressure points are not worth considering. Tourniquets are dangerous and are essentially never needed or even justifiable. To apply a tourniquet for the time required to evacuate a climber is to sacrifice the limb below that point.

Bleeding from most superficial wounds is from capillaries, the small vessels that connect arteries to veins. The pressure in capillaries is so low that simply elevating the injured part or holding a dressing on the wound for about five minutes allows the blood to clot and plug these vessels.

Deeper lacerations may cut veins, which can lose larger amounts of blood than do capillaries. Occasionally, even superficial lacerations injure one of the veins visible beneath the skin of the arms and legs and produce profuse bleeding. But venous bleeding can also be stopped by elevation and compression because veins have thin walls and the pressure within them is low.

Arteries have much thicker, rubbery walls and lacerations rarely cut them. However, arterial blood is under much higher pressure, and blood loss can be much harder to control when these vessels are damaged. Therefore, every major wound must be inspected for arterial bleeding. The only reliable way to identify arterial bleeding is to look for blood spurting from the wound with each heartbeat. Depending upon the color of the blood to determine its source is unreliable.

Bleeding from almost all soft tissue injuries can be controlled by placing several sterile compresses directly over the wound and pressing firmly for about four to six minutes. Rarely, bleeding persists, even after pressure has been applied for fifteen to twenty minutes, particularly when an artery has been cut. On such occasions the wound should be packed with sterile gauze and wrapped snugly with a continuous bandage. This bandage must only be tight enough to control bleeding and must not obstruct circulation to the rest of the limb, an ever present danger with any bandage that completely surrounds a limb. Absent pulses, bluish discoloration of skin or nails, tingling sensations, or pain indicate that the blood supply to the tissues beyond the bandage is inadequate.

Since swelling at the site of the wound can greatly increase the pressure beneath a circumferential bandage, the limb beyond the bandage must be carefully examined for circulatory impairment at the time the bandage is applied, every thirty to sixty minutes for several hours, and every two to three hours thereafter. If the bandage becomes too tight it must be loosened; after bleeding is controlled the bandage should be removed.

Even after severe bleeding has been stopped, movement may cause it to recur. To avoid further blood loss, severely injured limbs should be splinted before the patient is evacuated. In expedition circumstances, delaying evacuation for two to three days to allow the clots within severed vessels to become more firmly anchored may be desirable.

CONTROL OF INFECTION

Wound infection results from contamination, and all open wounds are contaminated to some extent. Preventing infection by minimizing contamination and eliminating conditions that promote bacterial growth is far preferable to treating an established infection.

Wound Cleansing

After bleeding has been controlled, further contamination of soft tissue injuries must be avoided. First, the person caring for the patient must wash his hands thoroughly, preferably with an antibacterial agent such as pHisoHex or one of the povidone-iodine preparations such as Betadine. Sterile gloves, if available, should be used, but only after the hands have been scrubbed. Next, the skin around the wound should be vigorously cleaned, preferably by scrubbing with the same antibacterial agent. Washing dirt, dried blood, or other contaminants into the wound must be avoided.

Finally, the wound itself must be cleaned. Although cleansing must be thorough, further damage to the tissues must be avoided. The wound should be rinsed rather than scrubbed. The water must be uncontaminated or disinfected. A weak solution of a mild soap or an antibacterial agent can be used. Any foreign material, even if uncontaminated, or any dead tissue including blood clots left in the wound virtually ensures infection. Therefore, wound cleansing must be complete. Sterile forceps should be used to remove any debris that cannot be rinsed away. Small tags of tissue may be snipped off with sterile scissors.

For puncture wounds, bleeding to help remove bacteria and debris should be encouraged. The depths of such wounds are not reached by air, and anaerobic bacteria, including those that cause tetanus and gas gangrene, can produce virulent infections.

Antiseptics

Antiseptics have surprisingly little value in the control of wound infections. Antiseptics can not compensate for negligent wound cleansing and, for wounds that are thoroughly cleaned, provide little additional bacterial control. However, the informed use of the proper antiseptics is prudent, particularly for animal bites or heavily contaminated wounds.

Antiseptics for use in a wound must be able to kill bacteria without injuring the tissues. Minimizing tissue damage is important because no agent can kill all of the bacteria, and injured tissue provides an excellent medium for the growth of the remaining organisms. Only two readily available antiseptics meet these qualifications: a 1:750 aqueous solution of benzalkonium chloride (Zephiran) and a ten percent solution of povidone-iodine, an organic iodine complex sold under the trade names Betadine, Pharmadine, Povidine, and others. Povidone-iodine has two advantages over benzalkonium chloride: it's ideal for scrubbing hands (and is routinely used by surgeons) or the skin around a wound, and it can be packaged in polyethylene bottles rather than glass.

Either agent can be used undiluted for cleansing skin prior to needle punctures. Zephiran should be diluted four to one (by adding three times its volume of water) prior to use in a wound; povidone iodine can be diluted much more (ten to one or twenty to one.) The wound should be flooded with either solution.

The more widely known antiseptics — alcohol, tincture of iodine, or the mercurial preparations — injure the tissues and should not be placed directly in an open wound.

Wound Closure

In the wilderness, soft tissue wounds *never* need to be sutured.

If a wound is left open, the purulent material exuding from infected areas drains out onto the dressings. This purulent material cannot escape from a sutured wound and is extruded into the surrounding tissues, spreading the infection. Eventually the infection spreads into the blood and is carried to other parts of the body. Much of the involved tissue is destroyed and is later replaced by a nonfunctioning scar.

In hospitals, soft tissue wounds are sutured to promote healing and minimize scarring. However, the antiseptic conditions available in hospitals cannot be duplicated in the wilderness, and the damage done by an infection in a sutured wound would greatly prolong healing and lead to far greater scarring and deformity. Furthermore, if an unsutured wound is not infected, the edges tend to fall together, healing is rapid, and scarring is minimal.

If desired, clean, minor wounds that appear to present little risk of infection can be held together with "butterflies" or tape that has been sterilized by flaming. Such devices can easily be removed and the wound opened and drained should infection develop. Wounds that are too large to close with tape should never be closed by anyone but a surgeon who knows how to obliterate the spaces beneath the skin surface and avoid further damage by the sutures, including excessive tension on the tissues.

The danger of introducing infection, and the far greater destruction of tissue that results from infection in a wound that has been sutured, far outweigh any benefits that might be obtained from early closure.

Diagnosing Infections

If infection occurs in spite of preventive measures, early detection minimizes tissue damage and the threat to the patient's general health. The dressing over any wound except a burn should be changed daily until healing is clearly underway in order to watch for signs of infection. The patient's general condition should also be monitored, including measuring his temperature three to four times each day.

The signs of infection found around the wound itself are primarily the signs of inflammation — pain, redness, swelling, heat, and limitation of motion. These signs can be found with every wound but are much more severe in the presence of infection. Pain from soft tissue injuries usually begins to subside by the second or third day after injury. Persistence of severe pain beyond this period, or an increase in pain, suggests infection. Redness is usually limited to the margins of the wound. More extensive discoloration, particularly the presence of streaks extending upwards along a limb, indicates infection. Severe swelling around a wound, particularly a wound such as a simple cut with which swelling would not be expected, is a sign of infection, as is a detectable increase in the skin temperature. Swelling and pain combine to limit voluntary and involuntary motion, which is more obvious in the presence of infection.

The signs of a generalized infection also can be present with localized infections. An oral temperature of 100° to 101° F (37.8° to 38.3° C) can be expected for one or two days after a severe injury. A temperature elevation after a minor injury, a higher temperature, or an elevation persisting for a longer time is suggestive of infection.

Located throughout the body are accumulations of lymphoid tissue called lymph nodes. Bacteria and the products of tissue destruction from an infection are trapped in these nodes, which become enlarged and tender. Tissue destruction occurs with any injury and the regional lymph nodes become slightly enlarged, but in the presence of infection the nodes become more enlarged and painful. Additionally, the lymph nodes in more than one area often are enlarged and tender with an infection.

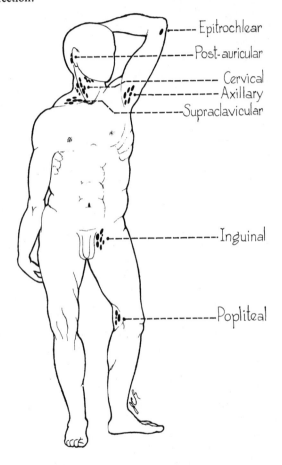

Figure 12. Location of the major collections of lymph nodes.

The diagnosis of a wound infection is confirmed by the finding of purulent material — "pus" — in the wound or on the dressings. The discharge may be cream colored, green, or even pink or reddish in color depending upon the infecting organism. Occasionally the discharge may be clear and straw colored. A foul odor is usually present. Rarely, an infected wound produces a very scanty discharge, and a diagnosis of infection is not necessarily wrong just because little purulent drainage is present.

The skin edges of an infected wound are sometimes sealed by coagulated serum, and exudate from the infection can not escape onto the dressings. If other signs of infection are present, the coagulum can be softened by soaking the wound in warm, disinfected water. Then the edges of the wound should be spread apart and the wound gently probed with a pair of sterile forceps. If an infection is present, pus usually pours out when the wound is opened. If no infection is present, opening the wound usually does little harm except for the discomfort, which is nominal when compared with the damage that could result from an undiscovered infection.

Treatment of Wound Infections

Treatment for an infected wound consists of drainage and antibiotic therapy. The wound should be opened by prying apart its edges with a pair of sterile forceps. Since pus within an infected wound tends to collect in pockets, the deeper parts of the wound must be probed and all such pockets drained. If one is found, others should be expected. After drainage, gauze should be placed in the wound to keep it open. The gauze, preferably vaseline impregnated, should be changed whenever the wound is dressed. The edges of the wound should not be allowed to reseal as long as any evidence of infection is present.

Infected wounds covered by a crust of coagulated serum and pus, particularly on the extremities, benefit from soaking in warm water. Moisture softens the crust and permits more thorough drainage. Heat causes the blood vessels to dilate, increasing the flow of blood to the tissues, which promotes healing and eradication of the infection. For small infected wounds on the extremities — or for large wounds if the patient cannot be evacuated — the dressing should be removed and the wound immersed in warm, sterile water for periods of twenty to thirty minutes three to four times a day. An antiseptic such as povidone-iodine should be added to the water. Afterward, the skin should be carefully dried and a fresh dressing applied.

Antibiotics should not be given routinely to patients with soft tissue injuries because the probability of infection is generally low, antibiotics have only a limited ability to prevent soft tissue infections, and the risk of allergic reactions and other adverse side effects is significant. However, for severe soft tissue injuries or badly contaminated wounds, antibiotics should be administered prophylactically before signs of infection appear. In a remote situation, antibiotics should also be given to patients with major wound infections with the understanding that the major benefit would be to inhibit spread of the infection and not to eradicate the infection within the wound.

If antibiotics are administered as a preventive measure, they should be given in large dosages for only two days; such a brief course of antibiotics does not allow the emergence of resistant bacterial strains. If a significant, established soft tissue infection is being treated, however, high doses of antibiotics should be given for at least five days, or until all signs of infection are gone. If the patient is not allergic to penicillin, he should be given a penicillinase resistant penicillin or a cephalosporin. If he is allergic to penicillin, erythromycin or some other antibiotic must be used.

BANDAGING

A bandage is usually composed of three layers, each with different functions.

Inner Layer

The inner layer of a bandage is a thin layer of a special material such as vaseline impregnated gauze or Telfa, which does not stick to the wound and allows the bandage to be changed relatively painlessly and without aggravating the injury. Obviously, this material must be sterile.

Dressings

The middle portion of a bandage is referred to as dressings and has five different functions:

1. Prevent infection or limit infection to organisms already present;
2. Absorb all drainage from the wound, which must not be allowed to contaminate clothing or other wounds;
3. Keep the skin adjacent to the wound dry to prevent maceration and infection;
4. Apply pressure on the underlying wound to aid in the control of bleeding or swelling;
5. Protect the wound from further trauma during evacuation.

In order to perform these functions, dressings must be sterile and bulky. Although special dressing materials are available, simple gauze pads that have been opened out and crumpled to increase their bulk work almost as well, and are easier to transport into wilderness areas.

Dressings that have been contaminated by purulent drainage should be handled with forceps or similar instruments which can be sterilized. Such dressings should never be touched with the fingers and should be disposed of by burning. If more than one wound or more than one accident victim must be cared for, attention to the infected wounds should be put off until last, and the attendant must scrub his hands thoroughly after dressing each wound to prevent the spread of infection.

Outer Wrapping

The outer portion of the bandage also has more than one function:

1. Hold the dressings securely in place;
2. Keep the dressings from getting wet by water or perspiration, which would inevitably carry along bacteria;
3. Apply pressure to help control bleeding and swelling;
4. Splint and immobilize parts of the body such as the hand.

Materials that have some elasticity are easier to use and stay in place better than plain gauze. Such materials also compress the wound slightly, but an elastic bandage is more satisfactory if significant compression is needed. If the wound must be kept dry, it should be covered with waterproof tape. However, moisture accumulates beneath waterproof tape, lifting the tape from the skin surface. If protection from wetting is not needed, porous tape should be used to hold the bandage in place. When the bandage is changed, the tape should be clipped off at the skin edges and new tape placed on top of the old to avoid the skin irritation that results from repeatedly stripping off the tape.

SPECIFIC INJURIES

Lacerations

Lacerations are cutting or tearing injuries and may be clean and straight or quite ragged. Such wounds commonly bleed. Infections are also a threat, particularly when small tags of dead tissue are present in ragged wounds. Blood vessels, nerves, or tendons may be damaged, but attempts to repair such structures in the field would almost always cause further damage and increase the risk of infection. The patient should be evacuated so that restoration of the damaged structures can be accomplished in more ideal surroundings.

Puncture Wounds

A puncture wound with only a small opening may extend deeply into underlying tissues. Hidden structures may be damaged and infection is always a threat. Bleeding to wash out dirt and bacteria should be encouraged. Foreign bodies should be removed if they are superficial and can be extracted without probing. A small piece of gauze should be inserted into the opening of the wound to prevent its being sealed and to permit the exudate from any infection to drain to the outside. In remote areas, antibiotic therapy is probably a justifiable precaution.

The greatest danger from such wounds is tetanus, which should be prevented with tetanus toxoid inoculations well before any outing is even contemplated.

Abrasions

Abrasions are scraping injuries produced by forceful contact with a rough surface. Severe bleeding is rare with such injuries and the objectives of treatment are to control infection and promote healing.

Before bandaging, large fragments of foreign material should be removed from the wound with sterile forceps, but removing numerous small embedded particles usually aggravates the injury and does more harm than good. Many such particles are extruded during healing; the rest should be removed under more propitious circumstances.

The wound should be covered with a layer of nonadherent material such as gauze impregnated with petroleum jelly, over which should be placed a bulky dressing to absorb drainage and cushion against further trauma. During dressing changes, the inner layer should not be removed until it spontaneously separates from the wound surface. Similarly, crusts that form during healing should not be removed.

Infection of abrasions is characterized by a purulent exudate, but since the entire wound is open and usually superficial, drainage occurs spontaneously. Dressings should be changed frequently and should be thick enough to retain the exudate.

Avulsions and Skin Flaps

Forces roughly parallel to the skin surface tend to lift or tear out chunks of tissue. If the tissue is completely torn away, the injury is considered an avulsion. A limb may be completely severed or avulsed, but few survive mountaineering accidents in which such powerful forces are generated. If the skin along one side remains intact, a skin flap is created. Small skin flaps are rather common, but occasionally larger flaps are produced.

If the full thickness of the skin is avulsed, the injury should be bandaged like an abrasion. As a general rule, wounds of this type that are more than one inch in diameter require skin grafting, so the patient eventually will have to be evacuated and hospitalized. Large avulsions are incapacitating.

If a thick flap of tissue with fat or muscle attached to the undersurface has been produced, the patient usually requires evacuation. Such injuries heal poorly and tend to become infected. The wound should be thoroughly cleaned and the tissue flap replaced in its original position. If the tissue flap is large, a strip of gauze should be placed along the lip of the wound so that the edges do not seal and purulent exudate can escape if the wound becomes infected. The wound should be bandaged with a bulky compression dressing, and the entire limb should be splinted. The flap, which must not be allowed to move or shift its position, is in essence a skin graft. If the wound is to heal, the flap must remain stationary while new blood vessels grow into the tissues.

The patient must be closely watched for signs of infection, and any wound infection that does occur must be promptly drained. Antibiotic therapy should be started at the time of the injury.

In expedition situations, evacuation may not be necessary if the wound appears to be healing satisfactorily without infection. The tissue flap is much less likely to be moved inadvertently while the patient is lying in a tent than when he is walking or being carried over rough terrain. However, such wounds do not usually heal without infection, and evacuation may be much more difficult for a patient with both a severe injury and a severe infection. (When such wounds are treated in a hospital, the fat, muscle, or other tissue on the undersurface of the flap — which is the tissue that typically dies or becomes infected — is usually trimmed away, and only the skin is preserved.)

If the flap does not survive, it first acquires a dusky appearance and then becomes progressively darker until it eventually is totally black. Uninfected flaps are dry and hard; infected flaps are usually moist, foul smelling, and soft. Surgical excision is typically required.

Small skin flaps with little or no fat on the undersurface are an entirely different matter. The wounds must be cleaned and the flaps held securely in position by bulky bandages just as larger flaps are, but such wounds often heal with no complications or severe infection. The skin flaps commonly do not "take" or attach to the underlying tissue, but they protect the delicate new skin that grows in from the sides and allow it to cover the wound. By the time the wound is covered, the flap usually has dried up and fallen off. The new skin may need to be protected for a few days, but no further therapy is required.

Contusions

Contusions, or bruises, are crushing injuries that cause bleeding into the damaged tissues. Usually the subcutaneous tissue and muscle are injured without a break in the overlying skin. Most contusions are minor, almost insignificant injuries, but rarely the damage can be great enough to severely incapacitate the victim.

The ideal treatment for a severe contusion is immediate rest until bleeding has ceased. However, such treatment may be impractical — even life threatening — in some mountaineering circumstances. Cessation of bleeding usually requires six to eight hours, by which time the injured muscles can be so stiff and painful that the victim is unable to walk. Therefore, the victim of a severe contusion in a remote area may need to walk out, or at least back to his camp, while he is still able to do so. After the muscles have become stiff and painful, three or four days may be required for them to start to relax, and weeks may be required for the injury to heal.

If circumstances do not require immediate evacuation, the injured area should be elevated. Cooling by wrapping the injured area with wet towels or clothing — not by applying snow or ice directly against the injury — causes the blood vessels in the area to constrict, may reduce the bleeding into the tissues, and tends to reduce pain. (Cooling can hasten the appearance of disabling muscle pain and stiffness and should not be used for lower extremity injuries if the victim must be able to walk.) If extensive swelling develops, the extremity may be wrapped with an elastic bandage or similar dressing that applies mild pressure. The wrapping should encompass the entire limb from the finger tips or toes to well above the area of injury and must not occlude the circulation.

After twelve to eighteen hours, movement of the injured area may be resumed, if tolerated, in order to speed resorption of the blood. Heat in the form of hot packs, a hot water bottle, or even warmed stones may also accelerate blood resorption and tends to relieve some of the muscle pain.

Stiffness persisting for more than two to three weeks in a muscle that has been severely bruised may herald the onset of calcium deposition in the injured tissues. Rarely, this process can continue until the entire clot has been transformed into bone — about twelve to eighteen months. The amount of muscle damage varies and is sometimes significant, so the condition should be recognized and treated to minimize disability. Diagnosis requires x-ray demonstration of the calcium deposits.

Wounds of the Hands and Feet

Wounds of the hands or feet are of special importance because these structures are so anatomically complex. All wounds in these areas must be thoroughly cleaned, but no tissue should be trimmed away unless it is unmistakably dead. If these members are enclosed in a large bandage, the fingers or toes must be separated by gauze to prevent maceration of the skin from the continuous dampness produced by perspiration. Such bandages should splint the hand in the

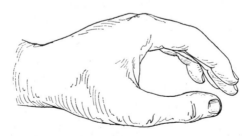

Figure 13. "Position of function" of the hand.

"position of function," which is the position the hand takes when holding a pencil. The color and sensation in the fingertips must be checked every thirty minutes for two to three hours, and every three to four hours thereafter, to ensure the bandage is not too tight and has not compromised the blood circulation. For severe injuries, antibiotic therapy should be instituted at the time of injury and evacuation begun immediately.

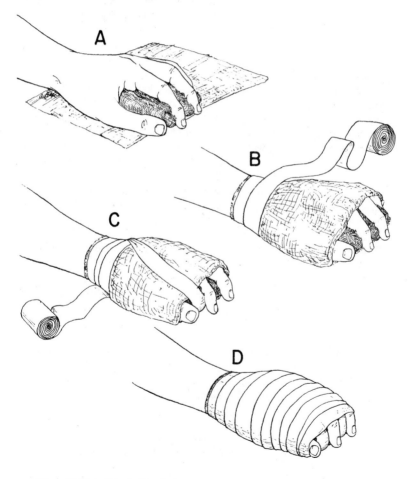

Figure 14. Technique for bandaging the hand in the "position of function."

Neck Injuries

Injuries of the neck require special attention because large blood vessels and the respiratory passages are located there. The danger from injury to these structures is so great that deep or extensive wounds in this location should not be treated in the same manner as soft tissue wounds elsewhere. No effort should be made to wash out the wound or remove foreign bodies or blood clots. The wound should be covered with a bandage that does *not* encircle the neck, and the victim should be evacuated immediately. (Superficial wounds that do not involve vital structures do not require special treatment.)

During evacuation respiratory obstruction must be avoided. Cervical fractures, head wounds, or chest wounds associated with the injury must receive appropriate care.

Blisters

Blisters are caused by friction that pulls the skin back and forth over the underlying tissues. Eventually a cleft or tear develops in the midportion of the epidermis, the most superficial portion of the skin, and fluid collects in this cleft.

For a blister to develop, the epidermis must be thick and tough enough to resist destruction by the friction, which otherwise would produce an abrasion. Also, the skin and subcutaneous tissues must be bound to the underlying bone to some extent, or the friction would just move the skin and no shear stresses would develop. Finally, the skin must be somewhat moist so that the object producing the blister adheres slightly to the skin surface rather than sliding back and forth. Only the last condition can be modified to help prevent blisters, but the first two conditions explain why blisters usually form at only a few specific sites such as the heels.

The most common cause of blisters is new or ill fitting boots. A common mistake is to wear boots that are too loose in the instep, which allows the foot to slide forward when going downhill, producing "downhill blisters," usually on the toes or front part of the foot. 'Uphill blisters" are most common over the heel or the Achilles tendon at the back of the ankle.

Blisters can be avoided by wearing boots that fit properly, breaking them in slowly, protecting areas that are prone to blister with adhesive tape or moleskin, and minimizing friction between the skin and boot. Friction can be reduced in at least two ways: keeping the foot dry with powder to reduce adherence between the boot and skin, and wearing a thick outer sock and a thin inner sock made of nylon or a similar material, which allows most of the slippage to take place between the two socks.

Once a blister has formed, further injury to the area should be prevented by covering it with tape or moleskin. The blister itself first should be covered with gauze or felt so the roof is not torn off when the tape is removed. Healing is faster, pain is diminished, and the risk of infection is greatly reduced when the blister roof is preserved. Often the blister fluid must be drained two or three times within the first twenty-four hours after the blister has formed to allow the roof to become adherent to the base.

If the roof of the blister has been torn away, the injury should be treated just like an abrasion — covered with a nonadherent inner layer and protected with a thicker outer layer. The feet should be kept clean to help prevent infection.

CHAPTER SEVEN

Fractures and Related Injuries

Mountaineering accidents usually involve the impact of a body with a solid surface such as rock, snow, or ice when one or both are moving at a considerable speed. Broken bones are a common result. The care for accident victims with fractures presents challenging problems requiring an understanding of the nature and possible complications of bone injuries.

Although all fractures share the common feature of broken bones, their severity varies widely. The two bone ends resulting from a simple fracture may be driven into each other (impacted), resulting in a fracture that is rather stable, produces little or no deformity, and causes little damage to the surrounding tissues. In contrast, fractures can be so extensive that the limb feels as if no bones at all were present. With such wounds, damage to the surrounding tissues is usually severe and further injury may occur during efforts to splint the fracture, even penetration of the skin.

The variability of fractures is reflected in the terms applied to different types of bone injuries. Fractures in which there is a single, clean break are called "simple." If the bone is shattered into one or more fragments, the fracture is labelled "comminuted." When the surrounding skin is intact, the risk of infection is small and the fractures are called "closed." If the skin has been penetrated or significantly injured in any way, not just by the ends of the broken bone, the risk of infection is far greater and the fracture is called "open" or "compound."

Almost all bone or joint injuries are of major significance, particularly in mountaineering situations, where just the immobilization resulting from a fracture can be life threatening. If other structures are damaged, permanent disability or even death can result. Disruption of major blood vessels can produce severe hemorrhage; vascular obstruction can cause gangrene of the extremity; breaks in the skin can lead to severe bone and soft tissue infections; damage to nerves may result in a paralyzed, useless extremity.

DIAGNOSIS

The principal signs of a fracture are:

1. Pain and tenderness;
2. Swelling and discoloration;
3. Deformity.

A fracture is often distressingly painful, and the pain is aggravated by any movement or manipulation. The fracture site is usually exquisitely sensitive. Typically, swelling and discoloration appear rapidly around the fracture. Both may extend for a considerable distance a day or two later. However, all of these signs, although suggestive of a fracture, are not diagnostic and may occur with sprains or occasionally with simple contusions.

Obvious deformity is diagnostic of a fracture; grating of the ends of the broken bones as they rub together is also diagnostic. One or both ends of the bone can occasionally be seen in open fractures. A less obvious but definite sign of a fracture or dislocation is shortening of the extremity in which the fracture is located. With fractures of the thigh or hip, the affected leg is usually one to two inches shorter than the uninjured leg due to overriding of the bone ends. (In a few individuals such shortening may have been present previously as the result of an old injury.)

Loss of function of the injured extremity is a suggestive but unreliable sign of a fracture. Some injuries are so painful that function is lost without an actual fracture having occurred. Loss of function can also occur as an emotional response to an injury without a fracture. Conversely, and more significantly, function may persist, particularly with fractures in the feet and hands or fractures in which the bone ends are impacted. If the patient is permitted to continue using the injured extremity, damage to the bone and surrounding tissues may be greatly increased.

Making certain that a fracture exists is not essential. Manipulation of the bones to test for the presence of a fracture almost inevitably produces further injury and in most circumstances is not justifiable. If a fracture is suspected, its existence should be assumed until x-ray examination proves otherwise. Occasions commonly arise, particularly with ankle injuries, in which an extremity is severely injured but does not appear to be fractured. In a remote area, evacuation can be delayed for several days until the character of the injury becomes obvious. If a fracture is present but the site has been kept immobilized and slightly elevated, such a delay rarely has any adverse effect on the final outcome. If no fracture is present, the victim may be able to walk out, or occasionally even continue climbing.

TREATMENT

Immobilization

The treatment for any fracture is immobilization; additional measures are necessary for open fractures and fractures associated with profuse bleeding. Immobilization prevents further damage to surrounding tissues by the bone ends, reduces pain, and decreases the risk of shock. However, the alignment of bone fragments necessary for healing can not be obtained in the field and should not be attempted.

Immobilization of a fracture in an outdoor setting is occasionally a challenge because material for splints is difficult to obtain. However, rope or nylon webbing are usually available in mountaineering circumstances, and many climbers carry triangular bandages. Any material that stabilizes the fracture can be used. A folded newspaper is particularly effective for fractures of the forearm and wrist. Brush, a pillow, a sleeping bag, or even a heavy piece of clothing can be satisfactory. A well prepared expedition probably should carry inflatable plastic splints. These splints are lightweight, easy to apply, and help control hemorrhage by applying pressure over the leg when the splint is inflated. (The air pressure in the splint may need to be temporarily lowered every one to two hours to ensure the blood supply to the skin is not impaired.) Standard splints are readily available in most downhill ski areas. Cross country skis make excellent splints; two make a sled. Bony prominences, especially at the wrist, elbow, ankle, and knee must be padded to prevent discomfort and permanent nerve damage from the pressure of splints made of hard materials such as wood.

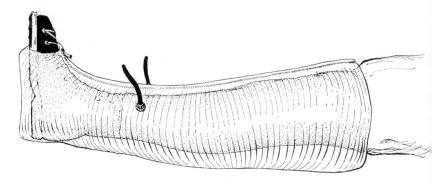

Figure 15. Inflatable splint for fractures of the lower leg and ankle.

For a fracture to be effectively immobilized, both the joint above and the joint below must be immobilized. For a fracture of the forearm, the wrist and elbow should be included in the splint. If the bone in the thigh is broken, both knee and hip motion must be controlled. In addition, as can be seen by examining an outstretched leg (the position in which the splint is usually applied), the knee can be moved by rotating the ankle. Thus, stabilization of the foot is also necessary to provide immobilization of the thigh or hip.

Straightening an extremity may be necessary in order to apply a splint, relieve blood vessel obstruction, or to pack the patient in a basket stretcher. However, such manipulation is usually painful and can cause further damage. Blood vessels or nerves can be injured; retraction of the contaminated ends of bone fragments protruding through the skin can pull in dirt and debris, leading to severe infection; the blood supply to the bone can be impaired, prolonging healing or even causing death of the damaged bone.

No attempt to straighten a fractured arm or leg should be made until strong traction can be applied by pulling on the end of the limb while someone holds the upper portion of the limb or the body. Restoration to the normal position should be attempted only when the fracture surfaces are separated by the pull and any necessary rotation can be performed gently and easily. The maneuvers can be carried out more readily immediately after the fracture has occurred. Later, muscle spasm and swelling restrict motion and increase deformity.

If the bone ends protrude through a break in the skin, they should be thoroughly cleansed with disinfected water and as much foreign material removed as possible before any attempt to straighten the extremity is made. (Traction almost always causes the bone ends to retract beneath the skin, and any foreign material carried with them greatly increases the severity of the subsequent infection.) If possible, open fractures are best splinted without reduction.

Another indication for manipulation is loss of the limb's blood supply beyond the fracture site. A patient with this complication usually has severe pain, numbness, and coldness in the affected limb, which typically is cyanotic or pale and swollen. If the bone ends are only pressing against the artery or vein, restoration to normal position may relieve the obstruction. However, if the vessel is actually torn, such manipulations are usually not helpful. Loss of sensation may also result from injury to a nerve, and unskilled manipulation can increase the damage that has already occurred.

Bleeding

Hemorrhage occurs with all fractures. The sharp, jagged ends of some broken bones cause extensive destruction of the surrounding muscle and other soft tissues, resulting in profuse blood loss. The hemorrhage can be entirely internal, and can be so voluminous that shock or even death results, even though there is little or no visible evidence of bleeding at the site of injury. Severe bleeding usually occurs following fractures of the pelvis or the thighs. Anyone caring for an accident victim with either of these injuries, or multiple fractures of any bones, must be aware of the threat of shock and should administer treatment in anticipation of its appearance.

Open Fractures

The danger of infection makes open or compound fractures much more serious problems than closed fractures. Osteomyelitis, an infection of bone, often produces extensive bone destruction, usually hinders or completely prevents healing of fractures, and frequently leads to permanent, crippling deformities — even amputation. The infection is often difficult to eradicate, even with antibiotic therapy, and occasionally persists for years, producing widespread debilitating effects.

Any fracture is considered to be open if the skin is broken, regardless of whether the skin was damaged by the jagged bone ends or in any other way. A fracture produced by a penetrating injury, such as a gunshot wound, is considered open because the skin is no longer able to keep bacteria away from the injured bone.

An open fracture should be treated like any contaminated soft tissue injury. All dirt and foreign material must be carefully and completely washed away. The wound should be left unsutured and covered with a bulky bandage. The patient should be evacuated as rapidly as possible. If evacuation can be completed in a few hours, antibiotics should not be administered unless they can be given intravenously. If evacuation is delayed, high doses of intravenous or oral antibiotics should be given. A cephalosporin is the drug of first choice; a penicillinase resistant penicillin or erythromycin are reasonable second choices.

Control of Pain

Pain resulting from a fracture is greatly reduced by immobilization. If the fractured extremity is splinted very shortly after the injury, no medications are usually needed during splinting. Later, a strong analgesic such as morphine may be required to relieve the pain of the inevitable jolts encountered during evacuation over rough ground.

Morphine should be injected intramuscularly every four hours as needed. However, absorption of the drug from the injection site is reduced if the victim is in shock. Repeated or large doses can lead to an overdose when normal circulation is restored. Accident victims often do not need medications for pain when they are in shock. If such patients do require analgesia, morphine should be injected intravenously in small amounts (one or two milligrams every fifteen minutes) until any necessary manipulation has been completed or the pain has been reduced to a level at which the patient is no longer thrashing about.

TRANSPORTATION

Treatment for fractures and all other injuries must be completed before the victim is moved unless his location is imminently dangerous due to hazards such as an avalanche, falling rock, or an electrical storm. Bleeding must be arrested, shock brought under control, all fractures splinted, and any other injuries attended before the subject is transported. After obvious injuries have been treated, but before evacuation is begun, the patient must be thoroughly and slowly examined to ensure that no additional injuries have been overlooked in the (unavoidably) hasty initial evaluation. Deliberate attention must be directed to the victim's back, which is often forgotten and neglected. If not treated, such injuries could be seriously aggravated during evacuation.

Individuals with fractures of the upper extremities, collar bone, or ribs and some persons with head injuries can walk under their own power. These patients must be closely attended since weakness and instability can result from the injury or from drugs given for pain. Subjects with fractures of the lower extremities, pelvis, or vertebral column and the victims of severe head injuries must always be carefully supported or carried. Considerable ingenuity, resourcefulness, and sheer determination are sometimes required to successfully evacuate individuals with these injuries, particularly in bad weather.

SPECIFIC FRACTURES OF THE UPPER EXTREMITIES

Hand and Fingers

The hand and fingers can be immobilized by bandaging the hand with a wad of material held in the palm. A rolled up pair of socks fits the hand well and serves nicely for this purpose. If the fracture involves the portion of the hand adjacent to

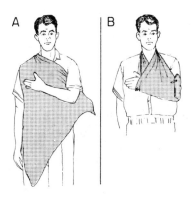

Figure 16. Application of a forearm sling.

the wrist, a splint should be applied to the entire hand and forearm to prevent motion of the wrist. Splints of this type are more comfortable when placed along the palm and the underside of the forearm. A forearm sling should be used to keep the hand elevated.

Forearm
Most wrist and all forearm fractures require inclusion of the hand and elbow in the splint. After splinting, the injured arm should be suspended in two slings as described for fractures of the upper arm.

Elbow, Upper Arm, and Shoulder
Immobilization of fractures of the elbow, upper arm, and shoulder is best achieved with two slings. The first is tied behind the neck and supports the elbow, forearm, and hand. The second is tied around the chest and holds the upper arm against the body, which serves as a splint. Should numbness of the little and ring fingers develop, padding of the elbow to prevent pressure on the nerves located there may be necessary. If only one triangular bandage is available, rope, nylon webbing, or some other material can be substituted for one of the slings. Rope can replace the chest sling if the fracture involves the elbow or forearm. If the upper arm or shoulder is injured, the forearm can be supported by a carefully padded rope extending around the neck and tied to the wrist.

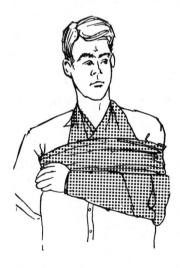

Figure 17. Forearm sling with an upper arm binder.

Collar Bone

Fractures of the collar bone (clavicle) are less uncomfortable if the individual holds his shoulders back. The shoulders can be splinted in this position by alternately passing a bandage or rope over the shoulder and under the armpit on opposite sides, forming a figure eight. The bandage should be applied over the victim's clothing, and the shoulders and armpits must be heavily padded. The coils should be applied while the shoulders are thrown back and should be just tight enough for the victim to be able to relieve pressure on his armpit by holding his shoulders back.

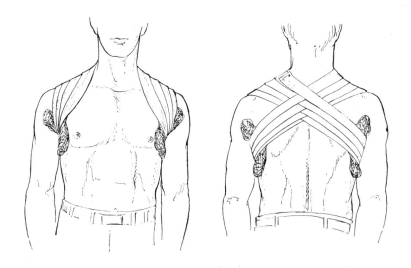

Figure 18. Figure-eight bandage for splinting a fractured collar bone.

SPECIFIC FRACTURES OF THE LOWER EXTREMITIES

Foot and Toes

Injuries of the toes and foot are best splinted by a well fitting boot. Since the boot is usually in place at the time of injury, fractures below the ankle are uncommon among climbers or skiers. Some fractures of the small bones of the foot result from accidents that seem insignificant at the time and are associated with relatively little pain. However, if pain persists for several weeks, the victim should consult a physician.

Crippling fractures of the heel bone (calcaneus) can result if a person falls some distance and lands on his feet. Pain usually prevents bearing weight on the fractured heel during evacuation.

Ankle

Fractures of the ankle are more common than fractures of the foot, and require immobilization by splints encompassing the foot and knee. Two splints should be used, one on each side of the leg. The splints should be padded and held in place by tape, bandages, rope, or similar material. If the area of the fracture is still painful when the victim is moved, the outer splint should be extended above the hip. Some straightening may be necessary before a badly distorted ankle can be splinted, but such manipulation must be held to a minimum and performed only while traction is being applied by pulling the foot downward. A patient with an ankle fracture may be able to move short distances with his uninjured leg and firm support on each side. However, evacuation for distances greater than a few hundred yards usually requires a stretcher.

Leg and Knee

Fractures of the lower leg can be immobilized in a manner similar to that used for fractures of the ankle. Fractures involving the knee require immobilization of the foot, ankle, knee, and hip.

Kneecap

A fracture of the kneecap alone may prevent use of the lower leg because the tendons that pull the leg forward are severed. Patients with such fractures should have a splint placed behind the leg, extending from the level of the ankle to the hip. With the leg and thigh snugly bound to this splint, the victim may be able to walk short distances.

Thigh

For immobilization of a fracture of the long bone in the thigh (femur), traction to overcome the pull of the strong thigh muscles is desirable. These muscles tend to cause the bone ends to override at the point of the fracture, damaging the surrounding tissues. A Thomas splint, or one of its modifications, is probably the best way to apply traction for a broken femur in mountaineering circumstances. However, these splints have been used incorrectly so often that their use is being discontinued and they are rarely available.

The Thomas splint consists of a padded ring attached to a metal frame. The ring fits snugly against the buttock and is held in place by a belt, strap, or similar

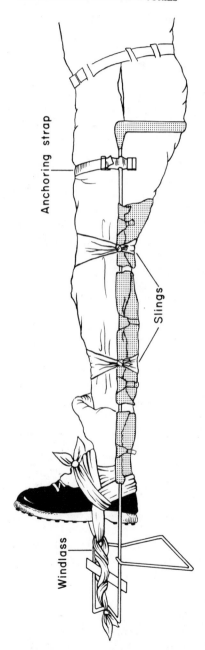

Figure 19. Fractured thigh immobilized by a Thomas splint.

device which passes over the front of the leg at the level of the groin. The frame is composed of two metal rods which extend along both sides of the leg and are joined a few inches beyond the foot by a crosspiece.

When a splint of this type is being applied, the boot should remain in place, and the ankle must be carefully padded to prevent obstruction of the blood supply to the foot. A traction hitch similar to the figure eight bandage used for sprained ankles is placed over the boot and padded ankle. (See Sprains and Strains.) Next, the leg is gently lifted by pulling on the foot and the splint is slipped into place. After the splint is secured at the level of the groin, the hitch should be tied to the crosspiece of the metal frame. A rod or stick is then inserted in the hitch (between the crosspiece and the foot) and twisted to apply traction on the leg. The pull should only be strong enough to prevent the foot and leg from sagging when the splint is lifted, but the hitch may have to be tightened one or two hours after the splint is applied as the thigh muscles relax and lengthen.

Extra bandages should be used as hammocks to support the leg in the splint, and a circular bandage must be added to prevent the leg from swinging from side to side. In addition, the lower end of the splint should be elevated so no pressure is placed on the patient's heel.

Pain in the foot after the splint has been applied indicates the blood supply to the foot has been impaired. The traction hitch must be disassembled at once and the ankle more carefully protected. Permanent damage to the foot, which usually is more crippling than the fractures, frequently results if adequate precautions are not taken to prevent obstruction of the circulation. In view of this danger, Thomas splints probably should not be used by inexperienced persons if evacuation is going to require more than a few hours or if the temperature is below freezing.

A makeshift Thomas splint can be made from two ski poles in an emergency. The wrist straps are hooked together and slipped up against the buttock like the half ring of a Thomas splint. A handkerchief or similar strap is used to tie the hand grips together across the front of the thigh like the belt on the Thomas splint. Bandages tied between the poles support the leg, and the hitch around the ankle is hooked to the baskets or ends of the ski poles.

Ordinary straight splints, as described for fractures of the ankle and lower leg, also can be applied. The outside splint must extend up to the level of the armpit, and the inside splint must extend to the groin. In addition, both legs should be bound together so that the uninjured leg can serve as an additional splint. Padding placed between the thighs reduces discomfort from the inner splint. If both thighs are fractured, the legs should still be bound together to increase the stability of the independent splints.

Hip

Fractures of the hip require no splinting other than binding the legs together. The victim must not be permitted to walk on the injured leg.

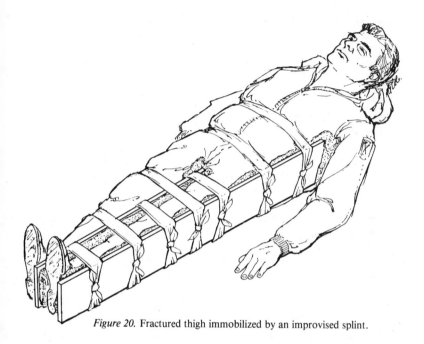

Figure 20. Fractured thigh immobilized by an improvised splint.

SPECIFIC FRACTURES OF THE TRUNK

Pelvis

Fractures of the pelvis should be suspected following violent accidents if side to side or front to back pressure over the pelvis causes pain. Blood loss of major proportions is inevitable with pelvic fractures, but it is rarely evident when the victim is examined. The volume of blood lost into the tissues around the fracture commonly is great enough to produce shock and may prove lethal. Therefore, therapy for shock should be instituted if a pelvic fracture is suspected.

Splinters of bone from pelvic fractures frequently damage the organs within the pelvis, particularly the urinary bladder. This complication should be suspected if the victim fails to void or passes only a few drops of bloody urine after the injury. (Injuries of the bladder are discussed in Chapter Eleven, "Abdominal Injuries.")

No splinting is required for pelvic fractures because the muscles around the pelvis hold the bone fragments in place. The patient should be placed on a stretcher in a supine position and should be evacuated without being permitted to sit up or stand.

No one with a pelvic fracture should be permitted to walk unless absolutely necessary. Furthermore, pain prevents any motion by most victims. However, some individuals may be able to move slowly and carefully with such injuries if circumstances make it essential. Injuries of the back of the pelvis are less dangerous than those in front, if the victim must walk.

Vertebral Column Fractures

Fractures of the vertebral column (spine) in the back and neck are always accompanied by the possibility of injury to the enclosed spinal cord. The higher the level at which the fracture occurs, the greater is the risk of serious nervous system damage, and the more grave are the consequences of the injury.

Pain or tenderness along the spine or anywhere in the neck following a fall should arouse concern about the possibility of a vertebral fracture. Occasionally such fractures present areas of swelling or discoloration similar to fractures elsewhere. Unusual prominence of one of the vertebral spines is sometimes found. However, if pain alone is present, the existence of a fracture should be assumed.

Signs of spinal cord damage include pain that radiates around to the front of the body or down the arms or legs, numbness, tingling, and partial or complete paralysis. However, the absence of spinal cord damage is by no means evidence that a vertebral fracture has not occurred. The vertebral column is commonly fractured without injuring the underlying cord. To risk cord damage by improper treatment is to take a chance of turning an unfortunate accident into a genuine catastrophe. Paralysis resulting from a spinal cord injury is usually permanent.

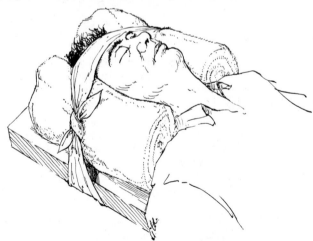

Figure 21. Technique for immobilizing the head for patients with fractured cervical vertebrae.

Approximately fifteen percent of accident victims with a head injury severe enough to produce prolonged unconsciousness have fractures of the vertebrae in the neck. Since they are unconscious and can not complain of pain, these patients routinely must be treated as if cervical fractures were known to be present.

During evacuation of a patient with a confirmed or suspected vertebral fracture, the body must be firmly secured so that it does not roll or twist if it is jostled while going over rough terrain. The patient should be transported on a firm support such as a metal basket or a broad wooden board. A rolled up jacket or a similar object should be placed under the small of the back to support the spine in that area. With injuries of the neck, padding must be placed on both sides of the head and neck to prevent the head from rolling from side to side.

There possibly are mountaineering situations, particularly in extremely exposed and hazardous locations, in which it may be safer to allow an individual with a vertebral fracture but no evidence of spinal cord injury to walk slowly and carefully on his own. His spine may be better protected when splinted by the spasm of the surrounding muscles and a collar of some type, even an improvised collar, than when subjected to the jolting of an improvised stretcher. However, any movement by the victim should be risked only under extreme circumstances and with a full realization of the danger of severe injury from such minor mishaps as stepping on a loose stone.

An accident victim with spinal cord damage and paralysis requires special attention during evacuation, particularly if evacuation takes more than twenty-four hours. The victim should not be moved until a complete examination has been performed and all other injuries have been treated. Good respiratory function must be present and the victim should preferably not be in shock. Finally, adequate personnel and equipment for proper transportation must be on hand.

During prolonged evacuation, special care must be given to the areas that support the body's weight — heels, buttocks, shoulders, and elbows. Pressure on these areas prevents blood from circulating through the tissues. Normally such deprivation of the blood supply results in pain and the person shifts his position. Patients with spinal cord injuries may not be able to feel pain and may not be able to shift position. After a few hours of being deprived of blood, the tissues in these areas die, eventually resulting in extensive ulcers known as "bed sores." To avoid this complication, the pressure points, particularly the heels and buttocks, must be carefully padded. Furthermore, this padding must be rearranged every two hours, day and night. The prevention of bed sores, which heal very poorly and are difficult to cure, requires diligent and devoted nursing care.

Most vertebral fractures that damage the spinal cord paralyze the urinary bladder and large intestine. Bladder care requires repeated catheterizations at least every eight hours or the insertion of an indwelling catheter. The care for bowel paralysis necessitates enemas about every three days and close observation to prevent the development of a fecal impaction. (See Chapter Eighteen, "Gastrointestinal Diseases.")

OTHER FRACTURES

Rib fractures are discussed in Chapter Ten, "Chest Injuries;" skull fractures and fractures of the face and jaw are discussed in Chapter Nine, "Injuries of the Head and Neck."

DISLOCATIONS

A dislocation is an injury in which the normal relationships of a joint are disrupted. Frequently the bone is forced out of its socket, as occurs in dislocations of the shoulder, elbow, or hip. Other joints have no definite socket, and the two joint surfaces are simply displaced. Fractures of the associated bones and injuries of adjacent nerves, blood vessels, and other structures may be present.

The signs of dislocation are similar to those of a fracture: pain that is aggravated by motion, tenderness, swelling, discoloration, limitation of motion, and deformity of the joint. The findings are localized to the area around a joint, but comparison with the opposite, uninjured joint is often necessary to be certain that a definite abnormality is present. Frequently, the dislocated joint appears larger than normal due to overlapping of the bone ends. Pain and muscle spasm usually prevent use of the extremity for climbing.

Correction of a dislocation can be technically difficult; unskilled efforts can easily damage blood vessels and nerves, or even produce fractures. Some injured joints must be splinted or even placed in a cast for three to four weeks or more in order for the injured ligaments around the joint to heal. However, an attempt to correct the deformity is justified in certain circumstances, particularly in remote areas.

Pain, pallor or cyanosis, swelling, numbness, or the absence of pulses beyond the dislocation are indicative of obstruction of the blood supply. Trapping and compression of arteries are particularly likely to occur with dislocations of the elbow or knee. Prompt action may be required to save the limb from gangrene. A steady, firm, but gentle pull in the direction of the limb's long axis, while an associate pulls in the opposite direction from above, may correct the dislocation or, at least, relieve pressure on the blood vessels.

The muscles surrounding a dislocated joint go into spasm rather quickly. The chances for successful correction of the dislocation decrease and the risk of further injury increases with the passage of time after injury. Therefore, attempts at reduction must be made as quickly as possible.

The reduction of any dislocation is facilitated by the administration of medications to relieve pain. Approximately fifteen minutes should be allowed for the drug to take effect. (Finger dislocations usually can be reduced so easily that such drugs are not necessary.)

After any dislocation is reduced, the injured area should be splinted in the same manner as a fracture of that area. The injured extremity may be useless for climbing for at least two to three weeks — usually longer.

Fingers

Dislocations of the fingers, which occur most commonly at the second joint, may be corrected quite easily immediately after the dislocation by pulling on the injured digit. The injured finger can then be splinted effectively by taping it to an adjacent uninjured finger. Dislocations of the thumb are usually accompanied by a fracture of the bone at the base of the thumb. Such injuries are seldom stable when corrected by manipulation alone and are best treated in the field by total immobilization.

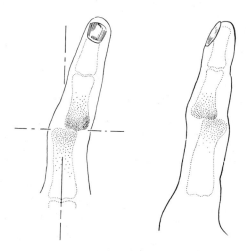

Figure 22. Dislocation of the finger.

Elbow

A dislocated elbow should be reduced as quickly as possible. However, before attempting reduction, the pulse at the wrist should be checked and sensation in the hand, particularly on the palm side of the first three fingers, should be tested. When the dislocation is corrected, the bone sliding back into its normal position may trap and compress the blood vessels and nerves that course very close to the joint. Unless pulse and sensation were known to be present prior to manipulation, the cause of their loss can not be determined.

With one hand above the elbow and one below, a strong enough pull should be applied to separate the bones of the joint. A considerable amount of force is usually needed. As the joint separates, any sideways displacement of the bones should be corrected first. Then the elbow should be gently straightened, possibly even a few degrees beyond 180 degrees. If the joint is not fully restored, gentle bending of the elbow may complete the correction. As soon as normal configuration is obtained, the pulse and sensation must be rechecked. If they are absent, the joint should be separated again with traction and gently rotated to free the entrapped structures.

The arm and hand should be splinted with the elbow at a 90 degree angle. Pulse and sensation should be checked again after the splint is applied. The elbow must not be wrapped circumferentially with tape or bandages because swelling does occur. If confined, it can compress blood vessels and nerves. Fractures of the bones of the elbow commonly occur along with the dislocation. A physician should be consulted as soon as possible, particularly if pain persists.

Shoulder

A shoulder dislocation can usually be diagnosed by the presence of pain and by the absence of the end of the long bone of the upper arm (humerus) in the joint, which is located just lateral to the collar bone and below the shoulder. Loss of the normal rounding or fullness is most apparent when comparing the two shoulders from the front.

The dislocated arm is rotated slightly outward and the elbow is held away from the side of the body. Attempts to bring the elbow to the side, or the forearm across the chest or abdomen, are resisted.

A number of methods can be used to restore the dislocated bone to its normal position. Taping a ten to twenty pound weight to the patient's hand or arm is the safest, but most prolonged method. The patient must be lying face downward on a flat surface with the arm freely dangling straight down. After one-half to two hours the constant pull by the weight usually tires the muscles surrounding the shoulder, causing them to relax and frequently permitting the bone to slip back into its socket. A strong analgesic such as morphine or meperidine often facilitates relaxation and shortens the time needed for reduction. If the dislocation is not corrected within two hours, traction should be discontinued and the victim evacuated.

Other methods for reducing a dislocated shoulder can be tried, but all carry a greater risk of damage to the nerves and blood vessels that pass through the armpit. The patient may sit with the dislocated arm dangling straight down on the opposite side of a vertical support like the back of a chair. A weight is attached to the lower portion or the arm. When the weight has tired the muscles around the shoulder, the arm frequently slips back into its socket. This method requires heavy padding between the support and the armpit to prevent nerve and blood vessel damage.

Reduction of the dislocation can be tried with the patient in a supine position by grasping the lower forearm with both hands and pulling the arm downward alongside the body. If needed, counter traction can be provided by a second person pulling on a well padded sling placed around the upper chest just below the injured shoulder. The direction of counter traction should be toward a spot above the opposite, undislocated shoulder.

Placing the heel of a foot against the chest wall and pulling outward and downward on the arm carries a high risk of injury to structures around the shoulder. If this technique is tried, the foot must push against the chest, not into the armpit.

A dislocated shoulder may be reduced rather easily if the joint has been dislocated on previous occasions. Patients with recurrent dislocations have lax or permanently damaged ligaments which allow dislocation by almost insignificant trauma.

In general, the more vigorous methods of reducing a shoulder dislocation should be tried only in circumstances where days may pass before a physician's help can be obtained. In no instance should force other than traction, particularly force of a levering nature, be used in an attempt to resolve a dislocation.

Following reduction of a dislocation of the shoulder, the arm should be immobilized for at least two weeks, preferably three, with two slings, one supporting the forearm and hand, and the other holding the upper arm against the body. A recurrent dislocation of the shoulder does not require such long immobilization; such injuries are not associated with acute tears of ligamentous structures. Their ultimate treatment is operative correction of the lax ligaments; redislocation may occur with annoying frequency after insignificant trauma until reparative surgery is performed.

Knee

In most instances, major dislocations of the knee pop back into position spontaneously, or quite readily, with traction on the foot or lower leg. Pulses and sensation in the foot must be checked as with dislocations of the elbow. Injury to the large vessels behind the knee occurs frequently and is suggested by painful swelling behind the knee developing immediately or hours after correction of the deformity. Repeated dislocation may occur, so the leg should be securely splinted; recently dislocated knees are usually too unstable for walking over rough terrain.

Jaw

An individual can become so completely relaxed while asleep that his jaw falls downward and slips out of its socket. When the subject awakens he finds that he can not close his mouth. In a remote situation, the resulting inability to swallow could lead to serious difficulties. Usually such complete relaxation follows the use of sleeping pills or overindulgence in alcohol.

Dislocations of the jaw are rather easily and safely reduced. Both thumbs should be inserted over the molars of the victim's lower jaw and pressed directly downward. Considerable force is required to overcome the spasm in the jaw muscles, which are quite strong, but the jaw should slip back into place without too much difficulty. (The thumbs should be heavily padded to prevent serious "bites" as the jaw pops back into its socket.) After reduction, a bandage should be placed over the point of the chin and tied over the top of the head. This bandage should permit the jaw to be opened slightly for eating and talking, but should be tight enough to prevent repeated dislocations. The bandage should be worn continuously for about a week and while sleeping for a month. Persistent pain in the joint, which is located just in front of the ear, may be indicative of a fracture, and a physician should be consulted.

OTHER INJURIES OF BONE AND RELATED STRUCTURES

Contusions of Bone and Subperiosteal Hematomas

A direct blow to a bone that does not produce a fracture or dislocation may still cause sufficient damage to produce swelling in the tissue covering the bone (periosteum) or bleeding between that tissue and the rigid portion of the bone (subperiosteal hematoma). The injured person complains of localized pain, the area is quite tender, and the bone may appear or feel larger than normal.

Treatment consists of the application of cold packs and a pressure bandage for the first twenty-four hours following injury, and splinting to prevent motion. After twenty-four hours, local heat rather than cold should be applied, and activity can be allowed to the limits of pain tolerance. However, if a fracture or dislocation can not be ruled out, immobilization should be continued.

Sprains and Strains

Sprains and strains, which are tearing, avulsing, or severe stretching injuries of ligaments and tendons around a joint, often can not be differentiated from fractures without x-rays. The injury can impair function of an extremity as severely as a broken bone. The signs are similar to a fracture, although grating of broken bone ends and deformity are not present. Swelling is often quite marked and discoloration may also be present. If an injury is obviously severe, the wisest course is to treat it as a fracture.

The application of cold immediately after an injury reduces hemorrhage and swelling. (Cold injuries must be avoided.) Later the reduction of swelling can be speeded by circumferential compression by an elastic bandage. (The circulation must not be impaired.) The blood and damaged tissue are absorbed more rapidly and healing promoted somewhat if the injured area is elevated slightly above the rest of the body. Motion and use speed healing but only when resumed after the initial reaction — primarily swelling and hemorrhage — has subsided and healing has already begun spontaneously.

Sprained ankles are the most common injuries of this type, and circumstances frequently require the subject to walk (or hobble) from the injury site. In most situations the ankle should be supported by a figure eight bandage put on over the boot. The loops of the figure eight should pass around the back of the heel and under the sole of the foot, crossing on top of the foot. The support must be snug but must not obstruct the circulation. The accident victim can no longer rely on the injured ankle to perform normally, and the risk of further, more severe damage is great. He should return to camp and rest until the absence of a fracture is assured.

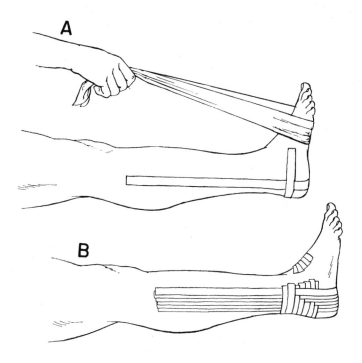

Figure 23. Technique for taping a sprained ankle after healing has begun. (The foot should be held perpendicular to the leg while the tape is being applied. The ankle should be taped for only the first three or four days of use after healing is underway.)

If the ankle is to be taped after the boot has been removed, alternate interlacing layers of tape should be placed under the heel and straight up the leg, and around the back of the heel and straight out over the foot. Tape must not be allowed to completely surround the leg, or subsequent swelling (which could result just from immobilization) would impair the circulation of blood to the foot.

One of the most common downhill skiing injuries is an injury of the tendons and ligaments of the knee. Occasionally the cartilage that covers the joint surface is injured also. A person with this injury should not be permitted to walk on his injured leg. (He rarely can do so.) The knee should be splinted as if it were fractured and the victim evacuated by sled or stretcher. Such injuries frequently require a cast and four to six weeks or more to heal.

Muscle and Tendon Tears

A sudden, strong force with the related bones and joints fixed in position, such as can occur at the end of a fall, may tear a muscle from its insertion or may completely rupture the body of the muscle or tendon. Muscle tears or "pulls" can also result from sprinting at top speed or from sudden movements or changes in direction. A penetrating injury may partially or completely sever a muscle or tendon. A complete separation of the muscle or its tendon and attachments results in a loss of the ability to perform the movements produced by the muscle. An incomplete interruption seldom produces loss of function but does predispose the structures to later complete separation.

Sites at which injuries to the insertions (points of attachment to bone) of muscles or tendons commonly occur are the fingertips behind the nails, the shoulder, the elbow, and the ankle. Ruptured muscles and tendons more commonly occur in the calf of the leg, the front and back of the thigh, and the upper portion of the arm and shoulder. Pain, tenderness, swelling, and loss of motion are the usual findings. Sometimes a defect in the muscle or tendon can be felt.

Treatment consists of the application of cold and immobilization. If possible, the victim should be rapidly evacuated because definitive repair of these injuries is most successful if done within twenty-four hours of the accident.

Muscle Compartmental Syndromes

Some muscles are enclosed in a firm fibrous sheath or "compartment" which forms a tight, only slightly distensible envelope. Bleeding or swelling within the muscle can increase the compartmental pressure to such a level that the circulation of blood to the muscle is impaired or totally blocked. When deprived of its blood supply, the muscle dies and is replaced with nonfunctioning scar tissue, usually resulting in a permanent crippling of that extremity.

Compartmental syndromes are rare but can produce permanent disability, so they should be recognized and promptly treated whenever possible. The anterior tibial muscle, which is located on the outside of the shin bone in the front of the lower leg, is most commonly involved by this type of compartmental compression. Most patients have an obvious injury of the leg, but compartmental syndromes can develop from swelling of the muscle following unaccustomed exercise. Occasionally pressure on the leg during a period of unconsciousness or injuries such as burns or snake bites can produce this disorder, and a few patients have had previous episodes of much milder pain, particularly following vigorous exercise.

The initial symptom is pain in the involved muscles, which typically is much worse than would be expected from the injury or exercise by which it was preceded. Passive movement or stretching of the muscles is also painful. Usually the muscle is obviously swollen and the overlying skin is tense and glossy. However, the most diagnostic feature is severe weakness or paralysis of the involved muscles. With an anterior tibial compartmental syndrome the foot can not be flexed upward and can not resist pressure forcing it down. The foot may be cold and numb, and the pulses may be weak, but such signs are inconsistent and their absence should not be considered an indication that the patient does not have a compartmental syndrome.

In the field two maneuvers may be helpful: any constricting clothing or bandages should be removed, and the extremity should be positioned at or above the level of the heart. However, the only effective treatment is surgically opening the compartment to relieve the pressure. Such therapy is beyond the capability of anyone not familiar with surgical techniques and the anatomy of the involved muscles. Therefore, most victims of this disorder must be evacuated to a hospital.

However, immediate, rapid evacuation is essential. Treatment must be given as promptly as possible to avoid permanent paralysis. In one group of physicians's experience with forty-six compartmental syndromes in forty-four patients, only thirty-one percent of the extremities treated within twelve hours of the onset of symptoms had residual disability, but ninety-one percent of the limbs decompressed more than twelve hours after the onset of pain had permanent functional deficits and twenty percent had to be amputated.[1] The usual functional deficit is an inability to lift or flex the foot upward, which is called a "foot drop" or "drop foot." A person with this disability usually must wear a brace to support the foot when walking on a flat surface. On a wilderness trail his disability would be much greater.

Bursitis, Tendinitis, and Shin Splints

Bursitis, tendinitis, and shin splints are characterized by inflammation of the tendons or the flattened, fluid filled, cystlike spaces (bursae) that cushion and lubricate the movement of the tendons. These disorders are characterized by the gradual onset of pain and stiffness, which is usually related to the unaccustomed use of a muscle or group of muscles for an extended length of time. Frequently the pain is first noticed upon awakening the morning after such activities. The gradual onset and the lack of any relation to a single traumatic incident serve to distinguish these disorders from fractures, dislocations, and sprains, but the associated pain can be quite severe.

Splinting may relieve the immediate discomfort but often prolongs the problem. Moist heat, such as a warm, moist towel, and aspirin every four hours provide some relief. In some instances application of cold may be more effective than heat. The pain, which is rarely disabling, may persist for a long time. Continued use of the joint throughout the full range of motion is necessary to prevent chronic stiffness and pain.

Tenosynovitis

Inflammation and infection of the sheaths that surround tendons and lubricate their movements may result from unaccustomed overuse or a penetrating injury. In the field, such infections may develop several days after the occurrence of a small cut or puncture wound that did not appear serious at the time, particularly on the hands, fingers, or feet. Pain with motion of the involved tendon is the diagnostic finding. When infection as well as inflammation is present, painful swelling, increased warmth, and redness are apparent. Crepitation (a crackling sensation) in the affected tissue may be felt with pressure or movement of the tendon. Whereas sterile inflammatory episodes due to overuse usually subside with rest, an infected tenosynovitis requires the attention of a physician, who quite frequently must surgically drain the tendon sheath. If infection is suspected, broad spectrum antibiotics should be started and the patient evacuated without delay. Failure to obtain surgical treatment can result in permanent loss of mobility of the tendon, extension of the infection to adjacent tendons and body spaces, and loss of function of the involved structures.

Joint Effusion

Swelling, discomfort, and increased warmth and redness may occur in a joint after an injury — sometimes without any preceding trauma. The knee is the most common site for this disorder, but joints such as the elbow or wrist can be involved. The cause may be outside the joint and only appear to involve it, as occurs with "tennis elbow" or a similar condition involving the insertion of the tendons just below and to the side of the kneecap. Within the joint, effusions often result from deterioration of the cartilage following repeated injury. If inflammation is present without infection or pus formation, the discomfort and swelling may respond to rest, wrapping with an elastic bandage, moist heat, and aspirin. An infected joint, manifested by redness, much more severe pain and swelling, and fever that is sometimes high, requires immediate care by a physician, particularly if the patient is febrile.

Ingrown Toenails

Ingrown toenails are best prevented by trimming the toenails straight across without rounding the corners and by wearing well fitted boots and socks. If pain and redness occur in the field, a wedge can be cut from the outer third of the nail on the offending side. The cut should begin towards the middle of the outer edge of the nail, and progress to the side as the cut moves back towards the foot. The offending sharp hook at the corner of the nail must be carefully removed. Warm soaks hasten recovery; elevating the new corner of the nail with a pledget of cotton or foil as it regrows may prevent recurrence.

Corns and Calluses

Prevention by wearing well fitted shoes is best, but if corns or calluses cause discomfort on a hike or longer outing, they can be shaved flat with a razor blade after they have been softened by soaking in warm water.

BACK INJURIES

Strain

Back pain is produced by a wide variety of disorders. Simple strain, which is one of the most common causes, can result from carrying heavy loads, working in an unaccustomed stooped position, or sleeping in an awkward position. However, treatment of a strained back is frequently frustrating. The measures that provide the greatest relief are sleeping on a firm support, such as a mattress with a sheet of plywood underneath, and applying heat to the affected area. When sleeping out of doors a mat that provides insulation but little padding should be used. Warm, moist towels or a hot water bottle applied to the painful area help relieve the muscle spasm. Aspirin can be taken to mask the pain; codeine may also be necessary on some occasions.

Ruptured Disc

The vertebrae of the spinal column are separated by cushions of cartilagenous material which absorb the force from the numerous jolts to which the body is subjected. A ruptured disc is an extrusion of this semisolid material into the spinal canal where it compresses the spinal cord or the nerves coming from the core. The basic defect consists of degeneration and weakening of the ligaments which normally hold this cushion in place. Trauma is only the final incident producing the ruptured disc. Unless this basic defect is present, trauma alone usually fractures the vertebrae instead of causing the disc to rupture.

The nature and location of symptoms in this condition are highly characteristic. Pain begins in the lower back, radiates to one side, and passes through the buttock and down the back of the leg. The pain may also involve the outside of the leg but is rarely present in the front or inner portion of the leg. The discomfort frequently causes the victim to walk with a decided limp. Excruciating back pain when moving to and from a supine position is also characteristic.

Examination of the patient reveals that the vertebral column in the lower back does not bend when he leans as far as possible to either side. This immobilization is produced by spasm in the muscles in the area of injury, resulting from the pain associated with movement. This muscle spasm can usually be palpated by an examiner's fingers. Loss of sensation to pin prick or the light touch of a wisp of cotton may be present over the foot and lower leg on the affected side.

The treatment for a ruptured disc is the same as for strain of the back muscles. However, the two conditions should be differentiated since each has a quite different outlook. Strain, which is rarely disabling, usually clears up in a few days, or perhaps a few weeks, with rest and proper treatment. In contrast, a disc may be incapacitating. Furthermore, the pain of a ruptured disc, although occasionally disappearing in a similar period of time with complete rest, is usually much more prolonged and may be relieved only by surgery. Finally, even though symptoms disappear rather promptly, a recurrence is likely at any time. Under expedition circumstances these prognostic factors must be considered in making plans for future climbing.

Individuals with a previous history of a disc problem should consult an orthopedist or neurosurgeon before undertaking further climbing activities, particularly if evidence of sensory impairment is present.

REFERENCES

1. Leach RE, Hannond G, Stryker WS: Anterior tibial compartment syndrome: Acute and chronic. *J Bone Joint Surg* 1967;49-A:451.

CHAPTER EIGHT

BURNS

Any consideration of burns and their treatment in the wilderness must divide such injuries into minor and major categories. Minor burns are common, particularly burns of the hands or fingers which can result from a hot pot or stove and similar accidents. Such injuries clearly are not life threatening, and their care is relatively simple and straightforward — although they must not be neglected.

Major burns, fortunately, are rare in wilderness settings. Probably the greatest risk of such injury in mountaineering is at high altitudes where snow is the only source of water and must be melted on a stove inside a tent. In these situations fuel spills or even explosions are common, due both to the notoriously poor performance of stoves at high elevations and to the impairment of climbers by hypoxia. Such accidents could be catastrophic because destruction of tents, sleeping bags, and clothing could leave severely burned climbers exposed to a bitterly hostile environment.

Successful treatment and evacuation of a major burn victim from this kind of situation requires an incredible combination of medical knowledge, mountaineering skills, dedication and determination, and sheer luck. Almost never would the intravenous fluids and other supplies needed just to keep the patient alive for the first twenty-four hours be available in such circumstances. However, severe burns can occur in less remote circumstances, and few climbers would not make a concerted effort to provide the best care possible. Therefore, a discussion of the basic principles of medical care for victims of major burns has been provided, even though few opportunities for its successful application can be expected.

EVALUATING BURN SEVERITY

The severity of a burn is determined by three features: its depth, its size, and its location. In the past, burns have been classified according to their depth as first, second, or third degree. First degree burns were superficial, did not kill any of the tissues, and only produced redness of the skin. Second degree burns damaged the upper portion of the skin, resulting in blisters. Third degree burns destroyed the full thickness of the skin and could extend into the underlying tissues. This terminology has been modified, and first and second degree burns are lumped together as "partial thickness" because they are less destructive and generally are treated the same. Third degree burns are labelled "full thickness."

The area covered by the burn is of critical significance. Until recently, few individuals survived full thickness burns that covered more than fifty percent of their body surface, even when treated in specialized burn centers. In contrast, few burns covering less than fifteen to twenty percent of the body are lethal when given proper care.

Location is also important. Burns of the face and neck, hands, or feet are more incapacitating due to the specialized organs and complex anatomy of these areas. Also, burns of the face may be associated with burns of the air passages or lungs, which often are lethal.

BURN SHOCK

The most urgent, life threatening problem associated with major burns is shock — specifically "burn shock." When tissues are burned, the capillaries are damaged and allow the fluid portion of the blood to pour out into the burned tissues. This loss of fluid reduces the blood volume and produces shock just as a major hemorrhage does. The victim of a major burn usually dies in shock within twelve to eighteen hours unless appropriate fluid therapy is instituted. Such fluids almost always must be administered intravenously for three reasons: the burn victim is often unconscious or too stuporous to swallow fluids; victims of such injuries often vomit anything taken by mouth; and even if not vomited, the fluids often stay in the stomach and are not absorbed. Since appropriate fluids are rarely available in wilderness situations, a major burn in a remote area usually requires immediate evacuation by the fastest means available.

EVACUATION

As a general rule, all full thickness burns larger than one inch in diameter eventually require surgical therapy — debridement and skin grafting. Therefore the only decision that must be made for patients with burns of that size or larger is when, or how urgently, they should be evacuated. Help with this decision can be obtained from the following criteria for the classification of burn injuries established by the American Burn Association and the American College of Surgeons:

MAJOR
Blistering partial thickness burns of more than twenty-five percent of the body surface;

Full thickness burns of more than ten percent of the body surface;

Significant burns of the critical areas: face, eyes, ears, hands, feet, or perineum (groin);

Significant associated trauma or coexisting disease.

MODERATE

Blistering partial thickness burns of fifteen to twenty-five percent of the body surface, with less than ten percent full thickness burns, and no involvement of critical areas.

MILD

Blistering partial thickness burns of less than fifteen percent of the body surface, with less than two percent full thickness burns and no involvement of critical areas.

Patients with moderate or major burns require hospitalization and must be evacuated. If therapeutic fluids are not available, emergency evacuation is required.

If any question exists about the severity of the burn, the victim should be evacuated. Experts have difficulty determining whether a burn is partial or full thickness immediately after it occurs, and inexperienced persons almost always underestimate both the depth and the area. Furthermore, the patient is often deceptively alert for several hours until fluid losses reach major proportions.

Many patients with less extensive burns must also be evacuated, particularly patients with burns of the hands or face. (According to the listed criteria such burns are considered severe.) However, speed is not as crucial. Fluid loss occurs with all burns, both partial and full thickness, but in previously healthy young adults does not achieve life threatening proportions in burns that cover less than ten to fifteen percent of the body surface.

Care of a seriously burned patient demands a major commitment of time and personnel. Only a large expedition would have enough members for some to continue climbing while others took care of even one burn victim. Disrupting the expedition to evacuate the patient probably would not significantly reduce the time available for climbing.

TREATMENT OF THE BURN WOUND

The treatment for a minor burn consists almost entirely of care for the burn wound. With a major burn, the wound must be treated and fluids must be administered to prevent or treat shock.

Immediate Care

Immediately after the burn has been incurred, all clothing and jewelry covering the injury should be removed. If the burn is small and not full thickness, immediate application of cold helps reduce the pain. Holding a towel soaked in ice water against the burned area, or immersing it in cold, soapy water usually is effective. However, more extensive partial thickness burns and full thickness burns should not be treated in this manner. Full thickness burns are usually painless because the nerves in the skin have been destroyed.

The burn, like any other open wound, should be cleaned and covered with a dressing. In the field, cleaning can best be done with sterile cotton, liquid soap, and warm, disinfected water. If these materials are not available, the burn should be cleaned in the best way possible. All debris, dirt, and fragments of loose skin must be removed. These measures are surprisingly painless if carried out gently.

The burn should be covered with a thin layer of an antibacterial ointment such as Silvadene (silver sulfadiazene in a petroleum jelly base), over which is layered gauze, a thick bulky dressing, and then a snug bandage that applies a moderate amount of pressure but does not interfere with blood circulation. The dressing or external splints can be used to immobilize a burned extremity and reduce the pain. Burned hands should be splinted in the "position of function," which is the position used to hold a pencil.

Ointments or creams that do not contain appropriate antibacterial agents increase the risk of infection and should not be used.

Subsequent Care

The bandage should be left undisturbed for six to eight days. Changing the dressing in the field increases the risk of introducing dirt and bacteria that would produce an infection. Furthermore, an accurate distinction between partial and full thickness burns can be made only about a week after the injury. If the burn is very superficial (first degree) and no blisters are found when the bandage is removed, no further treatment is required. Subsequent bandaging would be needed only to protect a sensitive area from trauma.

Small unbroken burn blisters generally should be left intact. However, the fluid within blisters is an ideal medium for the growth of bacteria, and blisters larger than eight centimeters (three inches) in diameter should be opened (without contamination) to reduce the potential for infection. Rebandaging with an antibacterial burn ointment and a protective dressing is needed for blistered burns; the bandage can be changed every three or four days until healing is complete.

Full thickness burns six to eight days old are covered by a thick, leathery layer of parched, dead skin which may range in color from white to dark brown or black. This dead skin is usually completely insensitive to touch. If the depth of the burn — whether it is partial or full thickness — is uncertain, gentle testing for anesthesia with a sterile object is a good way of determining whether the burn has extended through the full thickness of the skin.

A full thickness burn should be dressed as described and the patient evacuated. Even under ideal hospital conditions these wounds almost always become heavily infected. They require operative care, including skin grafting, and can not be managed in the field.

FLUID REPLACEMENT

The most urgent aspect of treatment for a major burn is the administration of fluids to prevent or treat shock.

Calculating Fluid Volumes

A convenient formula for determining the volume (in cc) of intravenous fluids to be administered during the first twenty-four hours following a major burn requires the body weight in kilograms (2.2 pounds = 1 kilogram) to be multiplied by the percentage of the body surface covered by the burn and that product to be multiplied by three. The percentage of the body area covered by the burn can be estimated from the accompanying chart.

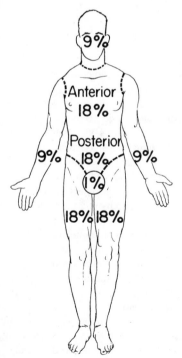

Figure 24. Percentage of total body surface area of various portions of the body.

Weight (kg) X Percent Surface Area X 3 =
Volume of Fluid to be Administered

For example, the fluid requirements for the first twenty-four hours after a burn for an 80 kilogram (176 pound) man with a thirty percent body surface area burn would be:

$$80 \text{ (kg)} \times 30 \text{ (\%)} \times 3 = 7{,}200 \text{ cc}$$

In some burn centers the product of body weight times burn area is multiplied by four instead of three. According to that formula, an eighty kilogram person with a burn covering thirty percent of his body surface — approximately one arm and one leg — would require approximately 10,000 cc of fluid instead of 7,000 cc to prevent shock.

Approximately half of this calculated volume of fluids should be given in the first eight hours of treatment, and the remainder should be given over the next sixteen hours. Although opinions differ about the ideal composition of the fluids, in a wilderness situation saline or Ringer's lactate are almost certain to be the only fluids available.

Patient Monitoring

These calculations illustrate the tremendous volume of fluids required, but the difference in these fluid volumes also demonstrates the imprecision of the formula. The exact volumes derived can not be given indiscriminately because the severity of the vascular injury produced by the burn and the functional capacity of the patient's heart and kidneys vary widely. Careful monitoring of the patient's response to the fluids is just as essential for his care as the calculations. Failure to give enough fluid can lead to shock, but administering too much can overload the vascular system and lead to heart failure, particularly in older individuals who already have some reduction in cardiac reserve. A fine line separates inadequate fluid replacement and overload, and at high elevations the margin of safety is even narrower.

If the patient remains confused or stuporous (in the absence of a head injury), his blood pressure is below normal, his pulse is weak and rapid, and his urinary output is below 50 cc per hour after several hours of treatment, fluids must be administered more rapidly and perhaps in larger quantities. Conversely, excessive fluid administration is indicated by a urinary output greater than 75 cc per hour; subcutaneous fluid accumulation causing swelling in unburned tissues, particularly in the legs or over the sacrum; or pooling of fluid in the lungs producing unusual shortness of breath. If these signs are present, the rate of fluid administration must be slowed, occasionally drastically. An indwelling urinary catheter is very helpful for monitoring urinary output.

Other Considerations

Fluid requirements for patients with burns of more than fifty percent of the body surface should be calculated as if the burn were limited to that area. Larger fluid volumes overload the heart if given within twenty-four hours.

A severely burned patient is usually thirsty, as are most individuals in shock. But thirst should be controlled with intravenous fluids since fluids given orally usually cause vomiting and still greater fluid loss. (Fluids lost by vomiting must also be replaced with Ringer's lactate or saline.)

Subsequent Fluid Therapy

During the first twenty-four hours after a burn, Ringer's lactate or saline solutions should be used to replace the fluid and sodium lost into the burned tissues. Thereafter, five percent glucose should be used for fluid replacement. (Few expeditions would carry such fluids, but in some popular climbing or trekking areas such as the southern approach to Everest — which is not wilderness — fluids are available.)

Once shock has been prevented or corrected, fluid requirements are somewhat greater than normal, but not on the enormous scale of the first day after the burn. Also, the patient may be able to take fluids by mouth with only small (one to two liter) intravenous supplements. As always, urine volume is an excellent indicator of the patient's fluid status.

By the second or third day after the burn, the blood vessels in the burned tissues begin to recover and the fluids lost into those tissues are reabsorbed and excreted by the kidneys. Large volumes of urine may be passed, but in this recovery stage, fluid intake should not be restricted because the urinary output is high. Fruit juices that have a high potassium content may be particularly beneficial at this time.

OTHER CONSIDERATIONS

Control of Pain

Inexperienced persons often are horrified by the appearance of a major burn and mistakenly administer unneeded pain medications, thinking the wound must be painful. However, the pain from a burn is quite variable. Superficial burns hurt at first but are usually relatively painless once they are covered and not exposed to air. Full thickness burns, although more severe injuries, are usually less painful because they destroy the nerves and produce anesthesia in the area of injury. In addition, shock tends to dull the pain. If the patient complains bitterly, pain should be controlled with as little medication as possible. Drugs stronger than codeine are rarely needed. If morphine or meperidine are necessary, smaller doses (one-half to three-fourths the usual dose) should be tried before resorting to a full dose. Morphine and meperidine have a depressive effect on the brain, may aggravate the general effects of the burn, and are almost never needed. Further-more, if the patient is in shock when the drugs are administered, they are poorly absorbed; if they are absorbed later when the shock is corrected, an overdose can result.

Facial Burns

Burns around the face and neck are particularly dangerous because the flames and hot smoke may be inhaled, damaging the lungs. Such patients must be evacuated with extreme urgency. Burns of the face, nose, mouth, and upper respiratory tract cause swelling and obstruction of the airway. Treatment requires intubation with an endotracheal or nasotracheal tube or creation of an alternate airway by tracheostomy or crichothyroidostomy. If the flames and smoke reach the lower portion of the respiratory tract and the lungs are seared, no effective treatment is possible in the field. If the victim survives the initial injury, the burn and smoke cause fluid to collect in the lung in quantities that are often lethal. Subsequently, severe pneumonia is common. Fortunately, such injuries are rare.

Burns of the upper airway should be anticipated after any facial burn, par-ticularly if the skin around the nose and mouth is burned or the nasal hairs are singed. The victim typically becomes hoarse and begins to have difficulty breathing. Wheezes may be heard when listening to his chest. However, the most critical sign of an airway burn is coughing up black, sooty material. This finding should be considered diagnostic of an airway burn. Unfortunately, some of these signs do not become detectable until twenty-four to forty-eight hours after the in-jury, so patients with facial burns must be closely watched.

Oxygen

Oxygen, if available, should probably be administered immediately to all vic-tims of severe burns occurring at high elevations. Burns can reduce respiratory effectiveness, and at high altitude the patient may not be able to breathe rapidly and deeply enough to compensate for the hypoxia of his environment. Fires in enclosed quarters, such as a small tent in which air circulation is reduced by a covering of snow, produce large amounts of carbon monoxide. The victim of a burn in such circumstances has to cope with a reduction in the oxygen carrying capacity of his blood due to carbon monoxide poisoning regardless of the altitude. Oxygen may be lifesaving until he can be evacuated to lower levels, par-ticularly for the first hour or two after the burn while the carbon monoxide is be-ing eliminated.

Additional Measures

To prevent secondary streptococcal infection, penicillin G should be administered to patients with major burns every six hours until the patient is in the care of a physician.

Patients with burns covering more than twenty to twenty-five percent of their body surface usually develop paralysis of the stomach and intestine known as ileus. Since they continue to swallow air and saliva, the paralyzed stomach becomes distended and they vomit. To avoid these problems, a nasogastric tube should be inserted, if one is available, and gastric suction should be instituted. (See Appendix B, "Therapeutic Procedures.") Fluids lost through the nasogastric tube should be replaced with Ringer's lactate or saline.

Dehydration following a burn, caused by the outpouring of fluids into the tissues, greatly increases the risk of thrombophlebitis. This complication should be anticipated and appropriately treated if it occurs. However, prevention by administering the required fluids and avoiding dehydration is far more desirable.

ADDITIONAL READING

Moylan JA: Burn care after thermal injury. *Topics Emer Med* 1980;2:39.
Pruitt BA Jr: In the heat of the emergency. *Emer Med* April 15, 1981;24.

CHAPTER NINE

Injuries of the Head and Neck

BRAIN INJURIES

Brain injuries are probably the most common cause of death in mountaineering accidents. Usually the only care possible for the victims of such injuries outside of a hospital consists of maintaining an open airway. (Injuries to other parts of the body also must be treated.)

Unconsciousness following a blow to the head is a sign that the brain definitely has been injured. The severity of the injury correlates roughly with the duration and depth of coma. A patient who responds in some fashion when called by name, or responds to pinching or similar painful stimuli, usually has not suffered serious brain damage and often regains consciousness in a short period of time. In contrast, a patient who is completely flaccid and has dilated pupils, a slow pulse, and irregular respirations has a much more severe injury. Widely dilated pupils which do not contract when exposed to light usually indicate extensive brain damage which few survive. Bleeding from within the ears is a sign of fracture of the base of the skull, which is very often associated with lethal damage to the brain.

Occasionally a person who has received a blow to the head may regain consciousness only to lapse into coma later as the result of continued bleeding within the skull (see Subdural Hematoma). Considerable perspicacity is required to recognize the subtle changes of this disorder at a time when effective treatment can be instituted.

Treatment

No specific treatment can be given for a brain injury in the field. The patient must be evacuated to the care of a neurosurgeon. An open airway must be maintained during evacuation if the victim is unconscious. The only reason for evacuating an unconscious individual whose airway can not be kept open is for burial!

Evacuating a comatose subject can be so difficult that waiting until the subject has regained consciousness is often highly desirable. In a particularly exposed and hazardous situation, such as on a sheer rock wall, a delay of several hours is fully justified. However, if the victim is not awake at the end of this time or shows signs of deepening coma, he can not be expected to regain consciousness without

142

medical treatment. Even if he does regain consciousness later, his recovery is usually so slow that he can not assist in his rescue, although he may be able to keep his airway open. The absolute necessity for maintaining an airway during evacuation, and the difficulty in doing so during descent from such a position, may require that the victim be left on the wall with one or more of the party to care for him while the rest go for help.

Approximately fifteen percent of all severe head injuries are associated with a broken neck. Therefore, all unconscious patients must have their heads immobilized as if they were known to have that injury.

Injuries to other areas of the body must be found and treated. Diligence is required when the patient is unconscious and not able to point out painful areas. Many serious injuries are neglected for long periods because the victim is lying on his back and no one examines that area. Any lucid interval must be utilized to ensure that no injuries have been missed. Shock rarely results from brain injury alone, and the presence of shock should prompt a search for other injuries, particularly damage to the abdominal organs and fractures of the legs or pelvis.

Oxygen should be administered to all brain injury victims regardless of altitude if it is available. With such injuries, respiratory function is depressed at a time when an adequate supply of oxygen for the brain is essential.

During evacuation the victim should be transported in the supine position with his head slightly elevated to promote drainage of venous blood from the brain and help reduce swelling and congestion. However, if the victim is vomiting, his head must be lower than the rest of his body to prevent aspiration. The presence of severe facial fractures greatly magnifies the difficulty of maintaining an open airway. If a tracheostomy can not be performed, considerable ingenuity may be needed to keep the victim breathing.

A record of pulse, respiration and, if possible, blood pressure should be made at hourly intervals for the first twelve hours after injury and then every four hours until evacuation is completed. Such records are of vital importance for brain injury victims because they often reflect his status more accurately than any other data, even sophisticated electronic monitoring or laboratory results.

If the victim is not hospitalized, either because he regains consciousness promptly and the injury does not appear to be of sufficient severity, or other circumstances prevent hospitalization, he should be closely watched for at least a week after his injury, preferably longer. A blood clot, which produces no signs of symptoms at the time of the accident but can prove lethal a few days or weeks later if not promptly recognized and treated, may be developing within the skull.

SUBDURAL HEMATOMA

Among the brain's unique features is its snugly fitting envelope of bone, the skull. Although the skull is essential for protecting the very soft brain from injury, its presence occasionally is a disadvantage. Bleeding or swelling, which accompany injuries to any tissue, compress the brain within this rigid covering and frequently produce damage and dysfunction far out of proportion to the size and severity of the original injury. A minor hemorrhage, which would be of no significance at another site, is often sufficient to cause death when confined within the skull.

Occasionally a blow to the head, although not severely injuring the brain at the time, tears some of the blood vessels around the brain. Blood from the torn vessels pours out into the narrow space between the brain and the skull and produces a clot which compresses the brain. Death is usually the final outcome in victims who are untreated or treated too late.

The speed with which this clot develops depends on the number and size of the blood vessels that have been damaged. Following severe injuries, bleeding may become apparent within a few hours. In other patients, signs of injury do not appear for two or three weeks, occasionally even longer. (Even though the bleeding stops, the clot can continue to enlarge through the absorption of water due to the osmotic pressure created by the breaking up of red blood cells.) The prognosis for the patient correlates fairly well with the speed with which the hematoma becomes evident. An acute subdural hematoma that develops within twenty-four to forty-eight hours carries a poor prognosis. A chronic subdural that develops two to three weeks after injury is associated with a much more favorable prognosis — if detected and removed promptly.

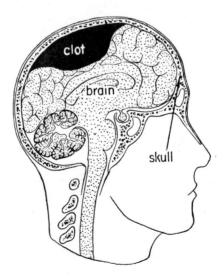

Figure 25. Subdural hematoma.

An epidural hematoma is a similar disorder which usually follows a fracture of the skull. The clot is located between the bone and its covering fibrous membrane, but the effect on the brain is the same. The damaged blood vessels producing an epidural hematoma are usually medium sized arteries rather than the small veins that produce a subdural hematoma. As a result, signs of an epidural usually come on faster and are more severe.

Diagnosis

The typical accident victim who develops a subdural hematoma receives a blow to the head, is unconscious for about thirty to sixty minutes, and then returns to consciousness and apparent normality. Some time later he begins to exhibit signs and symptoms of brain dysfunction. After a variable period of time, he lapses into unconsciousness.

The victim is in critical condition when coma occurs the second time and must be evacuated immediately if he is to have any chance for survival. A much more favorable outcome is usually possible, and evacuation is certainly much easier, if signs of the developing clot can be recognized before unconsciousness ensues.

Few subdural hematomas follow injuries that render the victim unconscious for less than twenty minutes. However, this disorder occasionally does follow less severe injuries and may rarely develop after a blow that does not produce unconsciousness at all. The recipient of any blow on the head must be closely watched. However, the period of twenty minutes is a valuable reference point in evaluating the seriousness of a head injury. Anyone unconscious for a longer time must be considered to have a significant risk of developing a subdural hematoma.

The intellect is the highest function of the brain and is frequently the first to be impaired in central nervous system disorders. Changes in personality, of which irritability is often the first to appear, confusion, and irrational speech or behavior are all signs of cerebral dysfunction. Anyone rendered unconscious by trauma may be mildly confused or irrational for a few hours after regaining consciousness. However, such signs are suggestive of a more serious disorder if they persist for more than twenty-four hours or if they begin to get worse instead of improving.

Headaches may follow almost insignificant injuries. However, headache associated with nausea, with or without vomiting, usually indicates significant, although not necessarily severe, brain injury. Stumbling, loss of coordination, loss of ability to stand with the eyes closed, and weakness are signs of more severe cerebral damage. Inequality of the pupils (which did not previously exist) is a definite and important sign of brain injury which must be sought.

None of these signs in itself is diagnostic of the presence of a subdural hematoma; most can be produced by diseases of other organs. However, deterioration in the victim's condition, an increase in the severity of signs and symptoms of brain injury, or the concurrence of several such signs following a head injury should prompt immediate evacuation. Paralysis, loss of sensation, disturbances of vision or hearing, and loss of consciousness are signs that develop later in the course of the disorder. Evacuation should not be delayed until these late signs have appeared.

Treatment

Treatment for a subdural hematoma consists of its surgical removal, which can not be performed in the field. The only recourse is evacuation of the patient to the care of a neurosurgeon. The more quickly evacuation is accomplished the better are the victim's chances for complete recovery.

A rapidly developing subdural hematoma in a remote area is of such grave significance, and the difficulty evacuating an unconscious subject so great, that the occurrence of a head injury on a weekend outing or similar short trip calls for immediate termination of the outing while the victim is still able to walk to a location where medical care is available. On a more extended expedition, the victim should at least be returned to a point from which he can be evacuated if he becomes incapacitated.

SKULL FRACTURE

Skull fractures are often surprisingly difficult to diagnose. Nonfatal fractures may occur with relatively little brain injury and no detectable deformity. (In contrast, fatal brain injuries occur fairly commonly without fracturing the skull.) A few fractures result in a small portion of the skull being depressed into the brain. Larger depressed fractures and fractures accompanied by other obvious deformities are usually lethal.

With a skull fracture, the typical signs of a fracture in any other bone — pain, tenderness, swelling, and discoloration — are often masked (or mimicked) by contusions or lacerations of the scalp which produce swelling and bleeding in the tissues overlying the skull. Occasionally, signs typical of a fracture are present on the opposite side of the head from the point of impact. In this location, pain, tenderness, swelling, and discoloration are indicative of a fracture. This injury, the so-called *"contre-coup"* fracture, is produced by the coincidence of the forces created by the impact at a point on the opposite side of the skull. Paradoxically, the skull may not be fractured at the point where the blow actually landed.

Fractures of the base of the skull frequently produce bleeding from the ears or nose. (The blood must be coming from within the ears or nose and not from a laceration of the surrounding skin.) Similarly, the clear, straw colored fluid that surrounds the brain, cerebrospinal fluid, may leak from defects in the bones of the ear or nose after a basilar skull fracture. However, so much force is required to produce a fracture of the base of the skull that the associated brain injury proves fatal immediately or within two or three days for all but a few victims.

Fractures of the skull may also involve the bony orbit of the eye. When this type of fracture is present, the eye on the injured side typically drops back into its socket and appears sunken when compared with the opposite eye.

The safest course is to assume that any head injury that has resulted in unconsciousness has also fractured the skull. X-ray examination should be obtained to determine whether a fracture is present. Under expedition circumstances, the persistence of headache for more than two or three days, the appearance of other signs of fracture or brain injury, or the presence of blood or cerebrospinal fluid leaking from the nose or ears should prompt immediate evacuation to an area where x-ray studies can be made and definitive treatment instituted.

No specific treatment for skull fractures can be given in the field. The victim should be evacuated promptly with special precautions to prevent further injuries to the head. Injuries to other parts of the body must receive attention. If blood or cerebrospinal fluid is leaking from the nose or ears, penicillin should be given every six hours to reduce the possibility of infection spreading from these areas to the brain.

SCALP INJURIES

Scalp injuries differ from other soft tissue injuries in two respects. First, the scalp contains a large number of blood vessels that produce profuse bleeding from small injuries. Secondly, infected scalp wounds are potentially more dangerous due to the proximity of the brain and the danger of spread of infection to that organ. Fortunately, the scalp is more resistant to infection than most other soft tissues.

The treatment of scalp injuries is similar to the care for soft tissue injuries located anywhere else on the body. Bleeding can be controlled by pressing down firmly with the finger tips or with a gauze pad on both sides of the injury. Special care must be taken to flush all loose foreign material out of the wound.

A foreign body embedded in the skull or brain must not be disturbed. The wound should be bandaged with the object in place. Thick dressings must be applied to prevent dislocation of the object during transport, and the victim must be evacuated immediately. If evacuation requires more than a day, the patient should be given penicillin or a penicillinase resistant penicillin, intravenously if possible, in twice the usual dose every six hours.

During the cleansing of a scalp wound, the underlying bone should be examined, but not probed, for evidence of a fracture if the bone is visible. If a fracture is found or suspected, similar antibiotic therapy should be given and the patient evacuated.

FACIAL INJURIES

Soft Tissue Injuries

The tissues of the face have a greater blood supply than most other areas, tend to heal faster, and have greater resistance to infection. Tags of skin around facial wounds should not be trimmed away unless they are so badly damaged that survival is obviously impossible. Many such skin fragments can be saved and may reduce the need for skin grafting at a later date. Scarring may also be reduced by preserving these fragments.

Fractures

Facial fractures are uncomfortable but do not require splinting and seldom interfere with locomotion. Delayed treatment is often the preferred method of caring for hospitalized patients with such injuries. Therefore, specific treatment for facial fractures is rarely an urgent problem. However, such fractures can make the maintenance of an open airway quite difficult, particularly in unconscious patients. A fractured jaw may permit the tongue to drop back into the throat, completely obstructing the passage of air. Extensive fractures of the nose and adjacent bones can allow the nasal air passages to collapse, blocking the flow of air. Blood from fractures about the nose runs back into the throat where it is often aspirated, causing obstruction of the smaller air passages in the lung.

Brain injuries, skull fractures, and fractures of the neck frequently accompany facial fractures and must receive care.

Fractures should be suspected after any forceful blow to the face. Pain, tenderness, swelling, and discoloration tend to confirm such suspicions. Facial fractures rarely cause any obvious deformity, except for some fractures of the nose or jaw. Some discontinuity of the bones can occasionally be felt. A broken nose frequently produces rather profuse nose bleeds. Double vision is a sign of fractures of the bones about the eye.

Except for fractures of the lower jaw, facial fractures do not require splinting. A broken jaw can be splinted with a bandage which passes under the chin and over the top of the head, binding the lower jaw to the upper. However, individuals splinted in this manner usually have difficulty breathing, particularly if they are stuporous or comatose. Fractures of the jaw should not be splinted if the victim needs to breathe through his mouth.

The maintenance of an open airway in a patient with facial fractures may require diligence and perseverance. A finger must be swept through the mouth of an unconscious patient with a broken upper or lower jaw to remove tooth or bone fragments and prevent them from entering the airway. If a tracheostomy can not be performed and an oral airway is not available or not tolerated by the victim, he may have to be transported in a face down position, particularly if severe bleeding or swelling is present. Obviously, his face must be kept free of pillows, sleeping bags, and the stretcher while he is in this position. A hole can be cut in a fabric stretcher for the victim's nose and mouth — one of the few occasions such stretchers offer a significant advantage over basket stretchers.

Nose Bleeds

Nose bleeds are very common following minor injuries to the nose; fractures of the nasal bones are usually accompanied by rather severe bleeding. Nose bleeds without any antecedent trauma are even more common and may be severe. Anyone with repeated or severe nose bleeds should consult a physician since such incidents may be signs of a serious disorder.

The patient should be placed in an upright position, seated or standing, with his head and body leaning forward. He should not lean backwards or lie down, as this permits the blood to drain back into the throat where it is swallowed, usually producing nausea and vomiting.

Many different maneuvers for stopping nose bleeds have been devised. Almost all are equally ineffective. However, most nose bleeds stop spontaneously and no specific treatment is needed. Pinching the nostrils together along their full length is probably as effective as any other maneuver.

If bleeding persists, a cotton pledget can be moistened with neosynephrine nose drops or spray and formed into an elongated roll. After both nostrils have been blown clear of clots or mucus, the cotton roll should be inserted in the side that is bleeding. The nose should be held closed with gentle pressure for three to five minutes. After the pressure has been released, another two or three minutes should be allowed to pass, and then the cotton roll can be gently removed. If bleeding persists, this procedure can be repeated as often as necessary until the bleeding is controlled. This technique is usually effective eventually, even with nasal fractures.

EYE INJURIES

Eye injuries must always receive immediate and careful attention. Apparently trivial injuries can cause total loss of vision if neglected. Eyelid injuries can be almost as devastating as injuries of the globe.

Injuries to the Globe

Eye injuries are usually obvious, particularly for the victim, but may be overlooked in an unconscious patient. Such injuries must always be suspected in the presence of head or facial injuries, or injuries of the opposite eye.

Penetrating or lacerating injuries of the eye produce visible damage. Contusions can produce hemorrhage within the eye and loss of vision with no externally visible sign of injury. Injuries of the nerves and muscles of the eye, or of the surrounding bone, can produce double vision or, occasionally, loss of vision. Because the eye is located within a socket of bone which protects it from most injuries, those that do occur are often associated with damage to the adjacent bone and soft tissues.

The treatment in the field for all visible or suspected eye injuries (including sudden, unexplained loss of vision) consists of bandaging the eye and evacuating the victim to an ophthalmologist. Attempts to remove foreign bodies or any other manipulations almost inevitably produce greater damage. Extensive experience has demonstrated that delays of ten to fourteen days in treating such injuries usually make no difference in the final results.

All dirt and debris should be washed away as gently as possible with lukewarm, disinfected water or saline. No attempts should be made to remove blood clots attached to the eye, because distinguishing between blood clots and retina that has been extruded through a wound is usually impossible. Eyelid injuries must also receive careful attention.

During evacuation the eye must be covered. The uninjured eye also should be covered by an opaque shield containing a small hole in the center. This type of shield permits the wearer to see only straight ahead and minimizes eye movements, thereby tending to splint the injured eye.

Penicillin should be given orally every six hours to patients with penetrating injuries if evacuation requires more than one day. Aspirin and codeine or morphine may be given every four hours for pain; medications for sleep or tranquilizers may be required, because such injuries often arouse much anxiety. The patient should be kept quiet during evacuation. He must not be permitted to touch his injured eye or finger its bandage.

Eyelid Injuries

Vision can be destroyed by injuries of the eyelids as well as by injuries to the eye itself. If the eye is not continuously moistened by the tears that the lid spreads over its surface, it rapidly dries. Drying kills the superficial cell layers of the cornea and can lead to scarring and blindness.

The torn or lacerated eyelid, after being washed free of all dirt and foreign material, should be returned as closely as possible to its original position. The eye must be completely covered. A snugly fitting bandage should be applied to hold the fragments in place. The opposite eye should also be snugly bandaged to prevent blinking or other movements that would disturb the alignment of the injured lid.

Rarely, the entire lid may be ripped away. If the lower lid is lost, the upper lid can be pulled down with adhesive tape to cover the entire eye. If the upper lid or both eyelids are lost, the exposed eye should be covered with a thick layer of ophthalmic ointment. A sterile dressing of soft material should be placed over the eye and held in place with a snug bandage.

Patients with such severe eyelid injuries should be evacuated as fast as possible. Antibiotics are not necessary and should not be given unless the injury is unusually contaminated. The tears contain a substance (lysozyme) that is antibacterial and is quite capable of eliminating most bacteria.

Minor lacerations, scratches, or abrasions that do not perforate the eyelid are not serious injuries and should be treated in the same manner as similar skin injuries anyplace else.

Foreign Bodies

Foreign bodies in the eye are very common, are usually easily removed, and are rarely followed by significant complications. Such objects are most commonly adherent to the inner surface of an eyelid and can be removed by pulling the eyelid over the lashes of the other. If necessary, the eyelid can be folded outward over a match stem or similar object, and the foreign material can be brushed away with the edge of a clean handkerchief or a wisp of sterile cotton. Occasionally the foreign material produces a mild conjunctivitis which should be treated as described in Chapter Twenty-two, "Disorders of the Eye, Ear, Nose, and Throat."

A foreign body may become embedded in the superficial layer of the eye itself. An ophthalmologist preferably should remove the offending object, but in circumstances where a physician is not available, attempts can be made to brush the object away with a sterile cotton swab or the corner of a folded handkerchief. If the object can not be brushed away, it can occasionally be removed with the tip of a needle. Obviously great care must be exercised. If these measures are not successful, the eye should be bandaged and medical assistance obtained. The patient should be treated for conjunctivitis even though evidence of infection is not present.

Foreign objects that appear to actually penetrate the eye should never be removed or manipulated by anyone other than an opthalmologist.

EAR INJURIES

Ear injuries are uncommon. Most are simple skin injuries which should be treated like similar injuries located anyplace else. More severe injuries are often associated with severe head or brain injuries.

One important cause of ear injuries is the use of keys, toothpicks, hair pins, or almost anything to clean the external canal. The ear should not be cleaned in this manner. The old adage "never put anything in your ear smaller than your elbow" is a wise one, particularly in a remote area. If an accumulation of wax, a foreign body, or even a small insect causes problems, the object should be removed by irrigating the ear with lukewarm water, preferably with a soft rubber bulb designed specifically for this purpose.

Occasionally a traumatic injury causes a blood clot beneath the skin of the external portion of the ear. If the clot is large enough to cover one-third or more of the ear, it can cause a permanent "cauliflower ear" if allowed to persist. Such clots should be drained to avoid this type of scarring. First the skin should be cleaned and coated with an antiseptic. Then one or more one-eighth inch (3 mm) incisions should be made and the blood expressed with gentle pressure. Removal of all of the blood is not necessary and would probably aggravate the underlying injury.

BAROTRAUMA

The middle ear and the paranasal sinuses are lined by thin mucous membranes and filled with air. These chambers have narrow openings to the nose or throat through which air can move to equalize the pressure within the chamber with the atmospheric pressure. From the middle ear, the opening is the eustachian tube, which is much longer than the openings into the sinuses. As a result, barotrauma is more common in the ear.

As atmospheric pressure decreases during an ascent to higher altitudes, air leaves these chambers without difficulty. However, increasing atmospheric pressure during a descent to lower elevations tends to close the chamber openings. Active measures such as swallowing or yawning may be required to open the eustachian tube. A light "pop" is often heard as the pressure is suddenly equalized. However, at a pressure differential of 90 mm Hg (which represents a change in altitude of about 3,750 feet (1,150 m) near sea level) the eustachian tube can no longer be opened by swallowing.

If the pressure within the chambers is not equalized with the atmosphere, a sense of fullness or pain develops. Hearing is diminished if the middle ear is involved. A cold or nasal allergy may cause swelling of the mucosa around the eustachian tube or the ducts into the nasal sinuses, partially obstructing the openings and hindering pressure equalization. As the pressure differential increases, the ears and sinuses become more and more painful. Involvement of the middle ear also can cause sensations of noise, lightheadedness, and hearing loss. However, such large pressure differentials can only develop when descent is rapid, as occurs in unpressurized aircraft or sometimes in automobiles on steep mountain roads.

As soon as an individual becomes aware of symptoms in his nose or ears, he should begin trying to equalize the pressure. Scuba divers, for whom barotrauma is a constant threat, commonly hold their nose and try to exhale against the obstruction to open their eustachian tubes. Subjects with colds or hay fever should be aware of their increased risk from barotrauma and should be prepared with decongestants to help reduce the mucosal swelling. A neosynephrine spray or similar preparation is usually adequate. Care must be taken to apply the spray a second time after an interval of several minutes so the spray can enter the deeper recesses of the nose. A systemic decongestant can also be taken in advance of the descent. However, such drugs are often combined with antihistamines. Such combinations should not be taken if drowsiness is likely to create problems.

If precautions are not successful or are neglected, or the individual is unconscious, an aerotitis media or aerosinusitis may develop. Hemorrhage from the mucosa may occur. These disorders are usually quite painful. However, they rarely cause any other problems, and the pain usually disappears within twenty-four hours or less. The patient should be given a systemic decongestant to promote drainage of the ears or sinuses. Aspirin with codeine may also be given to help relieve the pain.

NECK INJURIES

Injuries to the neck can damage vital structures. Massive hemorrhage usually follows injury of the large blood vessels. Hoarseness, coughing up blood, or diffuse, severe swelling that feels spongy or is crepitant indicates injury to the air passages. Patients with such injuries must be evacuated without delay. Swelling associated with the injury may lead to airway obstruction, so the patient must be closely watched and preparations made for a tracheostomy. The bandage over the wound must not encircle the neck. Soft tissue swelling after the bandage has been applied could result in strangulation.

CHAPTER TEN

Chest Injuries

Chest injuries are of particular importance because they interfere with the vital function of respiration. At high altitudes, where oxygen content of the air is low, even minor injuries to the chest may be life threatening. In contrast to abdominal injuries, however, definite help can be given to victims of chest injuries in mountaineering circumstances.

THE MECHANICS OF RESPIRATION

During inspiration the chest is expanded by the muscles in the chest wall that pull the ribs upward. Simultaneously the diaphragm, a large, flat muscle, contracts and pulls itself downward. Air is drawn into the lungs by the negative pressure created through this bellows action of the chest and diaphragm. Expiration is essentially a passive action involving no muscular contractions. Elastic tissue in the lung is stretched by the expansion of the chest during inspiration. When the muscles relax at the end of inspiration, the chest wall and diaphragm are pulled back into their original positions by this elasticity.

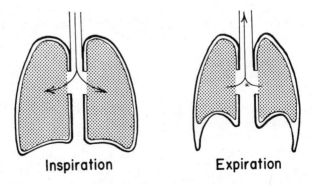

Inspiration   Expiration

Figure 26. Normal pulmonary function. (Figures 26, 27, 29, 30, 32, and 59 are adapted from *Surgery of the Chest,* 3rd ed., by Julian Johnson and Charles K. Kirby. Copyright 1964, Year Book Medical Publishers, Inc. Used by permission. Drawings by Edna Hill.)

Each lung is enveloped by a thin membrane called the visceral pleura. A continuation of this membrane, the parietal pleura, lines the inner surface of the rib cage. The space between these two layers of pleura is called the pleural cavity. Normally the lungs fill the entire thorax so that the two layers of pleura are in intimate contact with each other and essentially no space is present in the pleural "cavity." When the chest wall is perforated or the lung is punctured, air enters the pleural space. The elasticity of the lung causes it to collapse, extruding or pulling more air into the pleural space, depending on the site of the opening. Subsequent expansion of the chest cavity serves only to pull air in through a hole in the chest (or to pull air out through a hole in the lungs) into the pleural cavity and does not expand the lung itself. This condition is known as pneumothorax. At high altitude, where the cardiopulmonary system is already working near capacity, the resulting loss of pulmonary function could prove fatal.

CLOSED CHEST INJURIES

Broken Rib

A forceful blow to the chest may break one or more ribs, but the ribs are so enmeshed by muscles that they do not need to be splinted or realigned as do other broken bones. Other than producing discomfort, most rib fractures are not serious injuries. However, pain from the fracture can interfere with movement of the underlying lung. Fluid and secretions then collect in the immobile segment of lung, producing congestion or even pneumonia.

Very rarely a broken rib is displaced by the force producing the fracture. The displaced bone end can puncture the lung or, if low in the chest, injure a kidney, the liver, or the spleen.

A broken rib should be suspected when a blow to the chest is followed by unexpected pain and tenderness at the point of impact, particularly if the pain is aggravated by deep breathing. Usually a defect can not be palpated at the point of fracture since the ends of the rib are held in position by their surrounding muscles.

The victim should rest for a day or two, as dictated by the pain. Adhesive strapping over the rib is not advisable at altitudes over 10,000 feet (3,000 m) because such immobilization of the chest wall produces even more interference with movement of the lung on that side. Impaired function in the segment of lung underlying the fracture could have serious effects under such conditions. At lower elevations, if the pain can not be controlled with moderate doses of codeine, four or five strips of one or two inch adhesive tape can be applied to the chest to minimize movement of the injured area. The strips of tape should lie over and parallel with the fractured rib and should run from the midline in front past the vertebral column in back. Taping usually gives some relief from pain but must be removed in two to three days. Similar immobilization can also be provided by wrapping the chest with an elastic bandage, but since both sides of the chest are restrained, this technique must not be used at high altitudes.

Flail Chest

Fractures of a number of adjacent ribs in two or more places can produce a mobile, almost free floating plate of chest wall which moves back and forth during respiration — a flail chest. When the chest is expanded, the negative pressure pulls the loosened segment of chest wall inward instead of pulling air into the lung; during expiration the loosened plate is forced outward. If the area of flail chest is large, the movement of air into and out of the lungs may be so impaired that death ensues. Even if the damaged area is smaller, severe respiratory insufficiency results. Such injuries require immediate treatment.

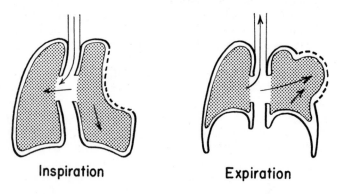

Inspiration   **Expiration**

Figure 27. Pulmonary function with a flail chest. (Adapted from
Surgery of the Chest, 3rd ed.)

The victim typically has a history of having received a severe blow to the chest followed immediately by pain and difficulty with breathing. He is usually fighting for air and breathing very rapidly; his lips, skin, and nails may be cyanotic due to poor oxygenation. Careful examination of the chest discloses a mobile segment of chest wall which moves "paradoxically" with each respiration. When the rest of the chest expands on inspiration, the loosened segment of chest wall is pulled inward; when the chest contracts during expiration, the flail segment is pushed outward.

Flail chest must be differentiated from a simple broken rib, which produces pain with breathing but does not interfere with the movement of air. Traumatic pneumothorax, which is discussed below, must also be anticipated.

The treatment of flail chest centers upon immobilization of the loosened segment of chest wall, thus reestablishing normal respiratory function. In an emergency, the victim can simply lie on the injured side with a rolled up piece of clothing beneath the loose segment of rib cage. The pressure effectively immobilizes the loosened portion of the chest wall and allows more adequate respiration. Such a simple measure may often prove life saving.

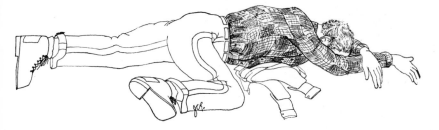

Figure 28. Patient lying on a rolled up garment to support a flail chest.

More permanent fixation of the rib cage can be achieved with adhesive tape immobilization of the loose fragment of chest wall or through external pressure on the broken rib segments by a sand bag or even a smooth rock properly padded. The loosened segment of chest wall must not be allowed to move; any reasonable means of providing such immobilization benefits the patient's respiratory function.

The lung underlying a flail chest is usually bruised and is poorly aerated. Fluid and secretions often accumulate in the damaged lung because drainage is impaired. To avoid pneumonia the patient must be encouraged, or even forced, to clear his lungs frequently by coughing.

The need for oxygen therapy can be determined by the degree of respiratory distress and the general condition of the patient. If the patient has a severe flail and can not be moved to a physician's care immediately, penicillin should be given every six hours to reduce the danger of bacterial pneumonia. At altitudes over 10,000 feet (3,000 m), both antibiotic and oxygen therapy should be administered, even for relatively minor chest injuries that would not require such vigorous therapy at lower altitudes.

The advisability of emergency evacuation depends on the situation and the condition of the patient. Even with an extensive injury, the chest wall becomes relatively stable within about one week. However, during this period pneumonia and progressive hypoxia of life threatening proportions can develop. If such complications develop with fractured ribs, flail chest, or pneumothorax, oxygen should be administered and the patient evacuated. He must be hospitalized where he can be placed on a mechanical ventilator if required.

Following any chest injury in which breathing is difficult and oxygenation marginal, propping the patient in a sitting position provides some help. While lying down, the heavy abdominal organs press on the diaphragm and squeeze the lungs into the upper part of the chest. Such encroachment is more likely to occur in fat people. In a sitting position these organs pull down on the diaphragm, giving the lungs more room for expansion, and improving ventilation. Even rolling a fat person on his side helps, for the weight of his belly and abdominal organs rests on the ground, not against his lungs.

Pneumothorax

A broken rib may be displaced and puncture the underlying lung, allowing air to enter the pleural space through the injury and causing the lung on that side to collapse. The tear in the pleura may act as a one way valve, allowing air to enter the pleural space during inspiration, but closing and not allowing air to leave the space during expiration. Considerable pressure can be built up in the pleural space, a condition known as tension pneumothorax. As a result, the lung is further collapsed and respiration is severely impaired.

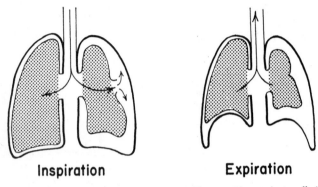

Inspiration   **Expiration**

Figure 29. Pulmonary function with a punctured lung and intact chest wall. (Adapted from *Surgery of the Chest,* 3rd ed.)

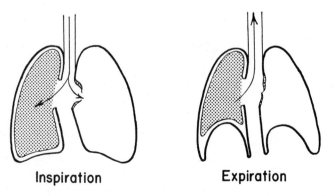

Inspiration   **Expiration**

Figure 30. Pulmonary function with a tension pneumothorax. (Adapted from *Surgery of the Chest,* 3rd ed.)

The patient usually has received a forceful, nonpenetrating blow to the chest, followed by respiratory distress. (Pneumothorax occasionally occurs spontaneously, the onset marked by the sudden appearance of chest pain and respiratory difficulty.) Pain and tenderness are present over the fractures, as with an uncomplicated rib fracture, but chest wall instability or flail is usually absent. When listening to the chest, preferably with a stethoscope, the breath sounds are greatly diminished or absent over the entire chest on the side of the injury, a highly significant diagnostic finding. The pressure within the pleural space may push the heart to the opposite side, causing the point at which the heart beat is felt to shift away from the injured side. Also, the trachea in the lower part of the neck may be pushed to the side opposite the pneumothorax.

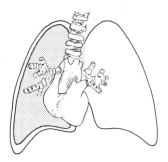

Figure 31. Collapse of the left lung and shift of heart and trachea to the right with left pneumothorax.

Although oxygen partially alleviates symptoms of pneumothorax, the only definitive treatment is to remove the air trapped in the pleural cavity and allow the lung to expand. This procedure should be performed under sterile conditions in a hospital where the chance of infection is minimal. If, however, the patient appears to be in critical condition, tube thoracostomy may have to be performed in more primitive circumstances. Only a person who has witnessed a thoracostomy, or preferably practiced it under the tutelage of a physician, should attempt tube drainage of the chest. The possible dangers — infection, puncture of the heart or a major blood vessel, missing the chest and puncturing the liver or spleen, and others — outweigh the potential benefits in totally untrained hands. (See Technique for Tube Thoracostomy in Appendix B, "Procedures.")

A chest tube is available fitted with a one way flutter valve (Heimlich valve) which permits air and blood to leave the chest but stops air from entering. This apparatus does not require underwater bottle drainage and therefore is well adapted for use in the mountains on the rare occasions when tube thoracostomy is necessary. The Heimlich valve can be used for a patient who is being evacuated, a great advantage over older techniques.

Decompression of a pneumothorax produces immediate relief of respiratory distress. However, considerable hazard for the patient still exists. The presence of a tube in the chest wall creates an opening through which bacteria can enter the pleural space. To reduce the risk of infection the area around the tube must be kept clean and covered with a sterile bandage. Penicillin may be administered every six hours if the probability of infection appears great.

Usually the hole in the lung seals within one to four days, at which time air no longer bubbles from the end of the chest tube when it is placed under water. When no bubbles have been seen for six hours or more, the tube should be clamped. The patient must be watched closely for several hours in case respiratory distress returns. If he remains in satisfactory condition, the tube should be left clamped for twenty-four hours. If no air bubbles from the tube when the clamp is released at the end of this time, the tubing may be withdrawn. If bubbles are seen, the entire procedure should be repeated twenty-four hours later. The patient must be closely attended during the time the tube is clamped so that the clamp can be released if respiratory difficulty develops.

Tube thoracostomy is not to be undertaken lightly and should be attempted only if the victim appears to be dying and the proper equipment is on hand. **The person performing the procedure must have had prior experience with the technique under the guidance of a surgeon.** However, since the technique may prove life saving, particularly in cases of traumatic pneumothorax at high altitude, it should be utilized if adequately trained personnel and proper equipment are available.

Hemothorax

An injury to the chest may damage blood vessels in the chest wall or in the lung, resulting in bleeding into the pleural space, particularly if a rib is fractured and displaced. The hazards of a hemothorax, as an accumulation of blood in the chest is called, are: (1) the consequent collapse of the lung as the blood fills the chest; (2) the occasional instances in which the blood loss is sufficiently large to produce shock; (3) the tendency of the clot to become infected; and (4) constriction of the lung as the clot retracts weeks or months after the injury.

Blood accumulating in the chest after an injury should be removed; however, removal can wait until the patient is evacuated. The desperate respiratory disturbance that occurs with a tension pneumothorax rarely occurs with hemothorax and there is little danger that the patient will die from bleeding into his chest.

Hemothorax usually follows a severe, nonpenetrating injury to the chest and may produce signs and symptoms that simulate pneumothorax. However, tapping on the bare chest produces a dull, solid sound over the accumulating blood instead of the resonant sound heard over air filled lungs. If the patient can be placed in a sitting position, breath sounds may be absent over the lower part of the chest and yet present over the upper portion. (The breath sounds may be difficult to hear without a stethoscope.)

Bleeding into the chest cavity usually stops spontaneously within a few hours. If shock does appear, it should be treated. Nothing can be done to stop the bleeding without surgical intervention, and even that is impossible in hospitals that are not equipped to handle chest surgery. Evacuation should be carried out as soon as the patient's blood pressure, pulse rate, respiratory rate, and his general condition look as though he can tolerate being moved.

If a patient is in such a remote area that he can not be evacuated for several days or weeks and bleeding is so severe that the lung can not expand properly, tube thoracostomy may be necessary to remove the blood from the chest.

PERFORATING CHEST INJURIES

A fall onto a pointed object such as an ice ax (particularly during an ice ax arrest) may actually punch a hole in the chest wall, producing one of the few medical emergencies in which minutes can determine success or failure. A hole in the thoracic wall allows air to be sucked through the wound into the pleural cavity, causing the lung to collapse. Subsequent respiratory efforts move air back and forth through the hole in the chest wall rather than through the trachea. Air does not reach the portion of the lungs in which oxygen and carbon dioxide are exchanged and the patient rapidly suffocates.

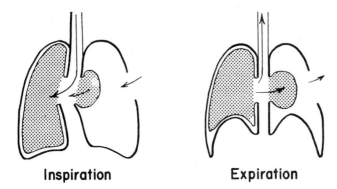

Inspiration   **Expiration**

Figure 32. Pulmonary function with a punctured chest wall. (Adapted from *Surgery of the Chest,* 3rd ed.)

The victim almost always has an obvious penetrating injury of the chest wall, producing a "sucking wound" — so called because air is sucked in through the wound during inspiration. Due to the impairment in respiration, the patient begins fighting for air almost immediately and soon becomes cyanotic, loses consciousness, and goes into shock if untreated.

The hole in the chest must be tightly closed at the earliest possible moment in order to restore respiratory function. The best method of closing such a wound is with sterile, fine mesh, vaseline impregnated gauze and an outer, thick, sterile dressing. However, the cleanest available substitute must be utilized immediately. A clean handkerchief, or even a parka can be stuffed over the opening. **The hole must be closed immediately or without exception the patient will die.** A more ideal dressing may be applied later, but air must not be permitted to enter the chest while the coverings are being switched.

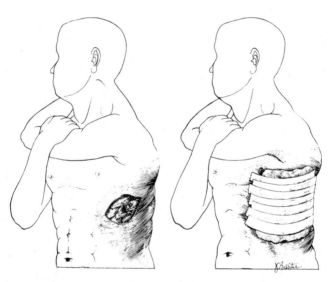

Figure 33. Open chest wound before and after bandaging.

Oxygen therapy should be instituted at the earliest opportunity and discontinued only when the patient's condition has definitely stabilized. Decompression of the chest as described for pneumothorax may be necessary. Shock almost invariably accompanies a large penetrating wound of the chest, and should be anticipated and treated. A penicillinase resistant penicillin or a cephalosporin should be given every six hours until evacuation is completed if the patient is not allergic to penicillin.

All patients with penetrating injuries of the chest must be evacuated at the earliest possible moment so that the hole in the chest wall can be permanently closed by surgery.

CHAPTER ELEVEN

Abdominal Injuries

The definitive treatment for a severe abdominal injury consists of surgery, which is out of the question in mountaineering surroundings. Therefore, management of severe abdominal trauma in such situations consists of recognizing the severity (or triviality) of an injury and deciding whether immediate evacuation is required. As with all injuries, a conservative approach should be adopted; if there is any question about the diagnosis, the worst should be assumed.

Under no circumstances should pseudoheroic attempts at surgical intervention be made. The results would be uniformly fatal without proper anesthesia, sterile operating conditions, or the proper instruments. Operative intervention under primitive conditions by untrained hands would be more deadly than most injuries. Even the most severe trauma can occasionally be successfully managed without surgery.

DIAGNOSIS

Before any decision can be made concerning the care for an accident victim, an accurate diagnosis must be made. The first step is obtaining an account of the accident. Exact details of the mishap, including the site and direction of a blow to the abdomen, are helpful in diagnosing the abdominal injury. A blow to the left upper quadrant of the abdomen or lower part of the chest may rupture the spleen; on the right side, a blow to the corresponding area would injure the liver. Trauma to either flank or the back may damage a kidney.

The abdomen must be carefully examined as described in Chapter Nineteen, "Acute Abdominal Pain." Close attention should also be given to blood pressure, pulse rate, respiratory rate, color of the skin and fingernails, and other signs of shock. The vital signs should be measured at least hourly for the first twelve hours and must be recorded. The urine should be examined for blood.

Attention must not be focused on the abdomen to the extent that other injuries are overlooked or neglected. At some time in the patient's care, preferably early, a complete examination must be performed.

If the patient is to be evacuated to a physician, a written account of the accident and all diagnostic findings, along with a detailed record of subsequent events,

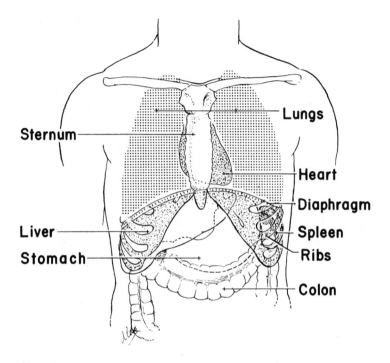

Figure 34. Location of the liver and spleen in relation to the lower ribs anteriorly.

should accompany him. The exact time of the accident, all medications and the time they are administered, hourly measurements of pulse and respiratory rates, and observations about the victim's general condition must be written down.

TREATMENT

Most abdominal injuries occur out of camp. Since the victim may require immediate evacuation to a surgical facility, he should be carried with all reasonable haste to base camp. The sooner such patients are brought to a camp or evacuation point, the better they withstand the subsequent rigors of bleeding or peritonitis that result from the accident. Patients with severe abdominal injuries usually require litter evacuation of some kind.

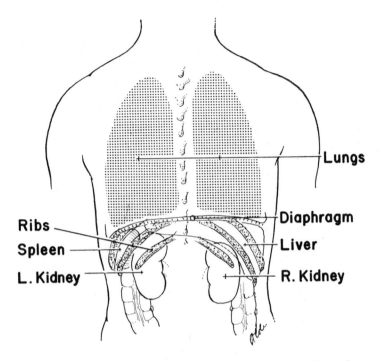

Figure 35. Location of the liver, spleen, and kidneys in relation to the lower ribs posteriorly.

Abdominal trauma frequently produces rather severe pain, but the pain may not be proportional to the severity of the injury. Even minor abdominal trauma may be quite painful at first, although the discomfort usually subsides in the hours that follow. In general, the patient should be kept comfortable by the administration of codeine or morphine. However, if injected intramuscularly, these drugs may not be properly absorbed if shock is present, and an overdose may occur after the circulation is restored. Intravenous administration may be necessary. The patient should be made comfortable but not "snowed under." If the patient is to be evacuated promptly to a surgeon, morphine or other analgesics should not be given, since such medications tend to mask some vital diagnostic signs. If evacuation is not necessary or must be delayed, more liberal use can be made of morphine.

Severe abdominal trauma may produce bleeding into the peritoneal cavity, rupture of abdominal organs, or both. Peritonitis inevitably results, although the inflammation following hemorrhage is due to irritation by the blood rather than infection. Gastric distension, absence of bowel sounds, nausea and vomiting, and other signs of peritonitis are usually present. (The diagnosis and treatment of peritonitis are described in greater detail in Chapter Nineteen, "Acute Abdominal Pain.")

Shock usually follows abdominal trauma, particularly trauma that causes intra-abdominal hemorrhage, and should be anticipated and treated.

NONPENETRATING INJURIES

Blunt or nonpenetrating injuries to the abdomen may produce:

1. Contusion of the abdominal wall;
2. Internal bleeding due to a ruptured spleen, liver, or kidney;
3. Rupture of other internal organs such as the urinary bladder or, rarely, the intestines;
4. Any combination of the above.

Contusion of the Abdominal Wall

Any blow to the abdomen causes a bruise which may be very painful. However, although the area of impact may be quite tender, the abdomen around it is not so sensitive. If the internal organs have been injured, tenderness is usually diffuse. In the first hour after injury deciding whether a severe blow has produced merely a bruise or serious intra-abdominal damage may be quite difficult. Therefore, a delay of several hours may be necessary before a diagnosis can be made with certainty. A large black and blue area may blossom forth twenty-four to thirty-six hours after the injury as blood lost at the time of the accident works its way out under the skin. This discoloration is of no significance, does not require treatment, and subsides spontaneously in time regardless of its extent.

After a tumbling fall, as may occur on a steep ice slope, bruises often appear in areas that the victim had not realized were injured. Frequently the subject feels far more sore and stiff a day or two after a fall than he did immediately after the injury. If there is no associated injury, the victim usually recovers after a few days of rest and mild analgesia with aspirin and codeine every four to six hours.

Internal Bleeding

A blow to the abdomen may rupture the liver, spleen, kidney, or a combination of the three. Rupture is more likely if the blow falls immediately over the organ.

The liver lies in the right upper quadrant; the spleen in the left upper quadrant. Both are tucked under the rib cage but can be injured by blows to the upper abdomen or to the lower part of the chest. The kidneys, which lie on either side of the backbone, may be damaged by a blow from the back. These organs are solid and may shatter when hit directly. Blood from an injured liver or spleen flows unimpeded into the abdominal cavity. The hemorrhage usually does not stop without surgical intervention. In contrast, the kidney is enveloped in a tough, fibrous sheath which contains the bleeding. However, blood from a ruptured kidney does appear in the urine.

Ruptured Kidney

A ruptured kidney is usually manifested by:

1. A history of a blow in the flank;
2. Pain, tenderness, and discoloration at the point of injury;
3. Blood in the urine.

Most kidney injuries cease bleeding spontaneously; only rarely must the kidney be removed to stop the hemorrhage. The presence of large amounts of blood in the urine for more than six hours, a drop in blood pressure, or a consistently elevated pulse rate are indications that bleeding has assumed dangerous proportions. The patient should be treated for shock and evacuated as rapidly as possible. If the bleeding does stop, the victim must still wait ten to fourteen days before resuming vigorous activity.

Ruptured Liver or Spleen

The patient characteristically has a history of a blow to the upper abdomen or lower chest. Pain, tenderness, and evidence of contusion are usually found in the area of impact, and one or more ribs may be broken. Shortly after the injury intra-abdominal pain appears, first in the region of the injury and later more diffusely throughout the abdomen. The pain is usually aggravated by breathing deeply and may be associated with pain in the shoulder.

A patient with either of these injuries typically appears in reasonably good condition at first. As hours go by his condition deteriorates. The pulse becomes weak and rapid, and pallor, restlessness, and other signs of shock appear. With the spread of pain, the abdomen becomes tender, and rebound tenderness, distension, absence of bowel sounds, and other signs of peritonitis develop.

A patient with an injury of the spleen may recover from the initial accident only to bleed massively when a clot breaks loose from the splenic surface several days or even a week later. The signs of intra-abdominal hemorrhage appear rapidly following this development.

Patients with such injuries must be evacuated to the care of a surgeon as rapidly as possible. The hemorrhage very rarely stops spontaneously; most victims bleed to death if they do not receive surgical treatment. The sooner an operation can be performed, the better are the chances of survival.

During evacuation shock must be anticipated — if it is not already present — and treatment should be started. Pulse, respiratory rate, and blood pressure should be recorded every hour to assist the surgeon who is to assume care of the patient.

Ruptured Abdominal Organ

Severe blunt abdominal trauma may rupture one of the hollow intra-abdominal organs such as the intestines or the urinary bladder. The contents of the damaged organ are spilled into the abdominal cavity, producing peritonitis. Rupture of the urinary bladder usually occurs only if the patient has a full bladder when he is injured. It is usually associated with a fractured pelvis.

Following injury, the pain gradually becomes worse and spreads over the entire abdomen as peritonitis becomes generalized. Diffuse tenderness, abdominal distension, vomiting, and fever soon appear. If the bladder is ruptured, no more urine is voided except for a few drops, which are mostly blood.

Treatment is the same as for peritonitis of any cause described in Chapter Nineteen, "Acute Abdominal Pain."

PENETRATING ABDOMINAL INJURIES

Perforating injuries of the abdomen, which are rare in mountaineering, are occasionally caused by a skewering ski pole, an aberrant ice ax, or even a gunshot wound. These injuries are extremely serious and require operative treatment. Not only are the abdominal organs injured, but the abdominal cavity is contaminated from external sources, causing severe peritonitis.

The diagnosis is usually quite obvious. However, a perforating abdominal wound may be overlooked following a shotgun injury. Attention must not be limited to the area of most obvious injury. The patient should be stripped of all clothes and the entire abdomen and back carefully checked for pellet holes.

Evacuation should be carried out as quickly and rapidly as possible. During evacuation the patient should be treated for peritonitis. Shock should be anticipated and treated.

A sterile dressing should be placed over the wound. In contrast to the usual care given soft tissue injuries, the wound should not be washed or cleaned up, because such efforts only introduce more infection. Any loops of bowel protruding through the wound should be pushed back into the abdomen with the cleanest technique possible. The dressing over the wound should be sufficiently snug to prevent the bowel from popping back out again. This dressing should not be changed once it is in place because further contamination of the wound would result and no benefit can be expected.

SECTION THREE
ENVIRONMENTAL INJURIES

CHAPTER TWELVE

Medical Problems of High Altitude

Medical problems associated with high altitude include a number of uncomfortable symptoms and some life threatening conditions. All are primarily the result of a decreased oxygen concentration in the blood caused by the lower atmospheric pressure at high altitude.

Oxygen diffuses from the alveoli (air sacs) of the lung into the blood because the amount of oxygen (pressure or partial pressure) in the alveoli is greater than that in the blood. At high altitudes, the composition of the atmosphere is the same as at sea level, about twenty percent oxygen, but the pressure of oxygen (and the quantity or number of molecules present in a specific volume of air) is reduced in parallel with the reduction in atmospheric pressure. At 18,000 feet (5,500 m) the atmospheric pressure and the pressure of oxygen in the air is only half that at sea level.

The human body operates most efficiently when the pressure of oxygen in arterial blood is 80 to 90 mm Hg, which provides the red blood cells with almost all the oxygen they can carry. (Ninety-five percent of the hemoglobin is saturated with oxygen.) At high altitudes the lower pressure of oxygen results in a lower oxygen pressure in the blood. Without compensatory changes, at 18,000 feet (5,500 m) the pressure of oxygen in the blood would be only 40 to 45 mm and the hemoglobin saturation only about seventy percent. An increase in the rate and depth of breathing at high altitude increases the blood oxygen pressure, but not to sea level values, and all the tissues of the body must function at a lower oxygen pressure. Oxygen consumption by the body at high altitude, however, remains essentially the same as at sea level for the same amount of physical work.

ALTITUDE LEVELS

The altitudes encountered in mountaineering can conveniently be divided into the following three levels that have physiologic significance:

High Altitude — 8,000 to 14,000 Feet (2,400 to 4,300 Meters)
This altitude range is encountered by tourists and climbers in the continental United States. However, very few cities frequented by tourists anywhere in the

world are located at elevations higher than 14,000 feet (4,300 m). Because a large number of individuals visit locations within this range of altitudes, most cases of altitude illness occur at these elevations. Eight thousand feet (2,400 m) is a rough threshold above which altitude illness occurs. While acute mountain sickness may occur in some unusually susceptible individuals below 8,000 feet (2,400 m), high altitude pulmonary edema is very rare below this altitude.

Very High Altitude — 14,000 to 18,000 Feet (4,300 to 5,500 Meters)

In this range of elevations are located most high altitude base camps. Except for some Himalayan trekkers, such elevations are usually encountered only by experienced, well conditioned climbers. Rapid ascent to such altitudes without prior acclimatization is dangerous and can cause all types of altitude illness.

Table Two. Gas Pressures at Various Altitudes (mm Hg)*

Meters	Feet	BarP	PiO2	PaO2	PaCO2	SaO2(%)
0	0	760	149	94	41	97
1,500	5,000	630	122	66	39	92
2,400	8,000	564	108	60	37	89
3,000	10,000	523	100	53	36	85
3,700	12,000	483	91	52	35	83
4,600	15,000	412	76	44	32	75
5,500	18,000	379	69	40	29	71
6,100	20,000	349	63	38	21	65
7,300	24,000	280	52	34	16	50
8,500	28,000	250	42	28**	7**	30**
9,100	30,000	226	37	--	--	--

ABBREVIATIONS: BarP = Barometric Pressure; PiO2 = Pressure of Inspired Oxygen; PaO2 = Arterial Oxygen Pressure; PaCO2 = Arterial Carbon Dioxide Pressure; SaO2(%) = percentage arterial hemoglobin oxygen saturation; mm Hg = millimeters of mercury.

* Hecht HH: A sea level view of altitude problems. *Amer J Med* 1971;50:703-708.

**Estimated

(Gas pressures have not been measured in humans at altitudes exceeding 24,000 feet [7,300 m]. However, the 1981 American Medical Research Expedition to Everest measured the pressure on the summit [29,028 feet or 8,850 meters] as 253 mm Hg. The discrepancy from these calculated values was attributed to the increased thickness of the atmosphere near the equator.)

Extreme Altitude — 18,000 to 29,000 Feet (5,500 to 8,800 Meters)

At this range of altitudes most climbers are acclimatized, those who are susceptible to altitude illness usually have been weeded out, and altitude problems consist largely of altitude deterioration. A prolonged stay above 18,000 feet (5,500 m) usually results in loss of physical conditioning rather than increasing fitness and acclimatization.

DECREASED PHYSICAL PERFORMANCE AT HIGH ALTITUDES

At high altitude the maximal amount of work or exercise that can be performed is lower than at sea level, even for well conditioned and acclimatized athletes or climbers. The decreased performance is directly related to altitude and is illustrated by reduced climbing rates. Physical performance is lowest upon arrival at high altitude but can be progressively improved. Several changes are responsible for the diminished capacity for physical work at high elevations.

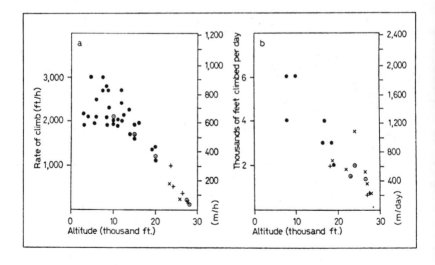

Figure 36. Rate of ascent and daily altitude gain at various altitudes.

Decrease in Cardiac Output

After several days at high altitude, the volume of blood pumped per minute by the heart (cardiac output) at any level of exercise is lower than during comparable exercise at sea level. In addition, the maximum heart rate that can be attained during heavy exercise is lower at high altitude.

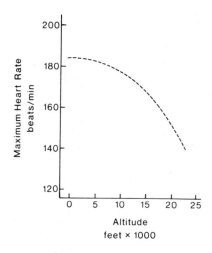

Figure 37. Decline of maximum heart rate with altitude.

Decreased Oxygen Saturation

During maximal exercise at sea level the arterial oxygen saturation remains normal, and exercise is not limited by the capacity of the lungs to transfer oxygen from air to blood. During exercise at high altitude, the lower oxygen pressure in the atmosphere and in the lungs results in incomplete loading of red blood cells with oxygen. For this reason, blood (or hemoglobin) oxygen saturation decreases during exercise at high altitude. This decrease is proportional to the exercise level and the altitude. This phenomenon may account for the frequent rest stops climbers make at extreme altitudes. Exercise decreases oxygen saturation and resting allows the saturation to rise again.

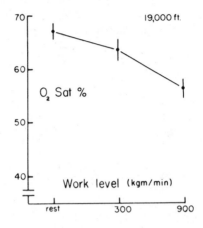

Figure 38. Blood oxygen content (saturation) under varying working conditions at 19,000 foot altitude.

Work of Breathing

During heavy exercise at sea level the work of moving air in and out of the lungs by the muscles of the chest wall and diaphragm consumes only a small part (about five percent) of the oxygen used by the body. During heavy exercise when the body is consuming 3,000 ml of oxygen per minute, only about 150 ml per minute is needed for the work of breathing. At high altitude, the volume of air moved in and out of the lungs during exercise is increased, which increases the work of breathing. (The lower air density at high altitude reduces the work of breathing somewhat, but the net effect during heavy effort is a moderate increase.) Maximum oxygen consumption by the body is reduced at very high altitudes; on the summit of Everest the oxygen cost of breathing requires so much of the total oxygen intake that little is left for vital organ function and climbing. Habler and Messner described this problem vividly in their account of their ascent of the last 480 meters to the summit of Everest. "We can no longer keep on our feet to rest. . . every 10-15 steps we collapse into the snow to rest, then crawl on again."

Very high breathing rates at high altitude may result in fatigue of the respiratory muscles, a lower respiratory effort, a decrease in ventilation, and a decrease in arterial oxygen saturation.

Decrease in Blood Volume

Rapid ascent to high altitude is accompanied by a prompt decrease in blood (or plasma) volume because fluid moves out of the blood vessels into the tissues and cells. The decrease in blood volume may persist for several weeks. The magnitude of the decrease is five to ten percent of the sea level volume or the equivalent of about one to two pints of blood. Inadequate fluid intake at high altitude may further decrease blood volume. Maximal work capacity is significantly impaired by a blood volume reduction of this magnitude.

Sleep Hypoxia

A decrease in arterial oxygen during sleep is now recognized as an important cause of high altitude discomfort and illness. During sleep at sea level a slight drop in arterial hemoglobin oxygen saturation occurs due to a decrease in the rate and depth of breathing. During sleep at high altitude, this decrease in ventilation of the lungs is more marked and fluctuates widely, and arterial oxygen saturation may reach very low levels.

Sleep hypoxia may account, in part, for the inability of many individuals to sleep well at high altitude. It may also explain why headache and other symptoms of acute mountain sickness are more severe in the morning hours, and why high altitude pulmonary edema often becomes more severe during the night. Part of the beneficial effect of acetazolamide for acute mountain sickness probably results from amelioration of sleep hypoxia.

At sea level the arterial hemoglobin is ninety-four to ninety-six percent saturated with oxygen, and the saturation falls only slightly during sleep. At 14,000 feet (4,300 m) the hemoglobin oxygen saturation is about eighty-six percent, but during sleep it may fall to seventy-five percent with occasional drops to sixty percent. Acetazolamide may not change the waking saturation but limits the decline during sleep to about eighty-two percent and eliminates the severe drops. Barbiturates, sedatives, tranquilizers, and other drugs that promote sleep intensify sleep hypoxia and should be avoided at high altitudes.

Sleep hypoxia probably decreases physical working capacity during the day, which provides a physiologic explanation for the wisdom behind the mountaineer's dictum "sleep low and climb high." Climbers also have noted better physical performance when low flow oxygen has been used during sleep.

For these reasons, lower work and climbing rates should be expected at high altitude. Studies of the ability of Sherpas to carry varying loads at different speeds at 12,000 feet (3,700 m) suggest that only thirty to forty percent of maximal sea level work capacity should be undertaken routinely at that altitude (55 to 75 lb loads at about 2 mph or 25 to 35 kg loads at 3.0 to 3.5 km/hr). At higher work rates, the subjects became exhausted after short work periods. Even these low rates must be further reduced at higher altitudes.

PHYSIOLOGY OF ACCLIMATIZATION

Man's survival and effective function at 18,000 feet (5,500 m) and toleration of 29,000 feet (8,800 m) without supplemental oxygen vividly demonstrates his ability to adapt or acclimatize to high altitudes. The most significant processes in acclimatization are an increase in respiratory volume, an increase in pulmonary artery pressure, an increase in cardiac output, an increase in the number of red blood cells, an increase in the oxygen delivering capability of red blood cells, and changes in body tissues to promote normal function at low oxygen pressures.

Increase in Respiratory Volume (Ventilation)

An increase in the depth and to a lesser extent the rate of respiration usually begins at about 3,000 feet (900 m) and may not reach a constant value for several days after arrival at a high altitude. As a result of this change, more oxygen is delivered to the alveoli of the lung to be absorbed into the blood. The increase in ventilation is most obvious during exercise. The new arrival at high altitude may experience unusual shortness of breath during only moderate exertion.

Increase in Pulmonary Artery Pressure

In response to a reduced concentration of oxygen in the alveoli from any cause, including the hypoxia of high altitude, pressure in the pulmonary arteries is elevated. The capillaries in all portions of the lung, many of which are closed during quiet respiration at sea level, are "forced" open and are perfused with blood, "maximizing" the capacity of the pulmonary circulation to absorb oxygen.

Increased Cardiac Output

During the first few days at high altitude the volume of blood pumped by the heart at rest or at any exercise level is higher than at sea level, which increases the amount of oxygen delivered to the tissues. However, after seven to ten days the cardiac output for any level of exercise is less than at sea level, and more time is required for any specific amount of work, whether running a mile or carrying a specified load a designated distance.

Increased Number of Red Blood Cells

Shortly after arrival at high altitude a slight increase in the concentration of red cells in the blood results from loss of water from the blood into the tissues. Later, red blood cell production by the bone marrow increases and the blood actually contains more red cells than at sea level.

The increased number of red cells should permit the blood to carry more oxygen, but whether this change is really beneficial has been questioned. Dilution of the blood of four acclimatized climbers at the Everest base camp (17,700 ft or 5,400 m) in 1981 with an albumin solution, which reduced the concentration of red blood cells from 58.3 percent to 50.5 percent of the blood volume, resulted in no changes in exercise tolerance or maximal oxygen uptake.

Changes in Oxygen Delivery Capacity

Red blood cells contain the enzyme 2,3 diphosphoglycerate (DPG) which facilitates the release of oxygen from hemoglobin to the tissues. The concentration of DPG in the blood increases during ascent to high altitudes. This increase may allow oxygen to be released to the tissues more easily, at least at altitudes below 20,000 feet (6,100 m).

Changes in Body Tissues

Prolonged residence at high altitude is accompanied by changes that permit normal function by the oxygen consuming tissues, particularly muscle, at very low oxygen pressures. These changes include an increase in the number of capillaries within the muscle, an increase in the intramuscular oxygen carrying protein myoglobin, an increase in the concentration of intracellular oxidative enzymes, and an increase in the number of mitochondria, the intracellular structures within which oxidative enzymes are located.

Other Considerations

The time required for the different adaptive processes varies. The respiratory and biochemical changes are complete in six to eight days. In contrast, the increase in the number of red blood cells requires six weeks to reach ninety percent of maximum. In general, about eighty percent of adaptation is complete by ten days, and ninety-five percent is complete at six weeks. Climbing at high altitude probably increases the strength and size of muscles used in respiration over a six week period. Longer periods of acclimatization result in only minor increases in altitude tolerance but may improve muscular strength and endurance.

ACHIEVING ACCLIMATIZATION

Individuals vary widely in their ability to acclimatize, not only in the degree of acclimatization they can achieve, but in the time required. Three examples of the way acclimatization could be achieved are:

INTERMEDIATE STAGING

Prior to climbing and sleeping at altitudes of 10,000 to 14,000 feet (3,000 to 4,300 m), gradually increasing exercise such as walking and climbing can be carried out at an intermediate altitude of 6,000 to 8,000 feet (1,800 to 2,400 m) for three to four days. Such staging provides sufficient acclimatization to prevent most altitude problems at higher elevations. Prior to going to 15,000 to 18,000 feet (4,600 to 5,500 m) a second stage of two to three days at 12,000 to 13,000 feet (3,700 to 4,000 m) is helpful. For example, when climbing the volcanoes in Mexico (17,600 to 18,700 ft or 5,365 to 5,700 m) two to four days should be spent in Mexico City (7,300 ft or 2,225 m) followed by two to three days at the well equipped Tlamacas Lodge on Popocatepetl (13,000 ft or 4,000 m) before ascending to the summit (17,887 ft or 5,452 m).

ONE STAGE ASCENT

Ascending to 10,000 to 12,000 feet (3,000 to 3,700 m) without stopping requires rest with minimal activity at that elevation for three to four days before heavy work such as climbing is begun. The risk of altitude illness after such an ascent is high. This method is the least satisfactory way to acclimatize and is no faster than spending the three or four days at 6,000 to 8,000 feet (1,800 to 2,400 m).

GRADED ASCENT

In areas such as the Himalayas, long approach marches are often required to reach high elevations (although commercial airline flights to landing strips at relatively high elevations are now available to trekkers). During such gradual ascents, acclimatization and some physical conditioning are achieved. At altitudes above 14,000 feet (4,300 m) ascents should be limited to 500 to 1,000 feet (150 to 300 m) per day, and every third day should be a rest day. To ascend to altitudes greater than 14,000 feet (4,300 m) and begin climbing immediately is foolhardy and dangerous.

Individuals who have difficulty sleeping or experience other altitude related discomforts during the first few days at high elevations may try taking acetazolamide. This drug should be taken twice daily beginning on the day before ascent and continuing for three to five days after arrival at high altitude. If no discomfort is expected at altitude, acetazolamide should not be used.

Other Considerations

The altitude at which individuals sleep strongly influences the occurrence of altitude illness. Skiers and climbers who sleep below 8,000 feet (2,400 m) can ascend to 14,000 feet (4,300 m) with only minor altitude discomfort. Sleeping above 8,000 feet (2,400 m) increases the risk of altitude illness, particularly acute mountain sickness and high altitude pulmonary edema.

Acclimatization is lost at about the same rate it is gained. Therefore, acclimatization to significant altitudes requires continuous exposure. The amount of acclimatization achieved by weekend sojourns above 10,000 feet (3,000 m) is minimal. An acclimatized individual can spend a few days at sea level and return to high altitude without much loss of tolerance. However, if the sea level stay is longer than one or two weeks, altitude problems occur just as frequently as during the initial ascent.

Prolonged high altitude exposure at yearly intervals has been observed to provide some benefits in succeeding years, although the benefit may consist largely of greater knowledge of methods for coping with altitude. Individuals over twenty-five years old are less likely to develop acute mountain sickness or high altitude pulmonary edema than younger persons. Physical fitness does not confer any protection against acute mountain sickness and does not facilitate acclimatization, although physical training before ascent to high altitudes does permit more effective climbing.

No artificial aids to acclimatization are known. Breathing a low oxygen mixture several times daily is of no value. No drugs promote or speed up acclimatization. Neither vitamins nor supplemental iron is beneficial.

Altitude Tolerance

Climbers who have reached the summit of Everest without oxygen have enjoyed certain physiologic advantages that can not be entirely predicted by sea level studies or performance. Some of these are:

1. Unusual ability to perform sustained physical work for long periods of time;
2. Highly developed mountaineering skills that permit efficient, fast climbing with minimal energy expenditure;
3. A high pulmonary diffusing capacity;
4. A normal or increased ventilatory response to hypoxia;
5. Effective muscular function during severe hypoxia, possibly due to unique peripheral tissue characteristics;
6. Effective brain function during severe hypoxia.

Summit of Mt. Everest

The barometric pressure on the summit of Everest, as measured for the first time in 1981 by Chris Pizzo, was 253 mm Hg or about one-third sea level atmospheric pressure. The pressure was 17 mm higher than had been predicted, apparently due to the greater thickness of the atmosphere around the equator. The pressure may vary by the equivalent of 100 to 300 feet (30 to 90 m) due to weather related changes in atmospheric pressure. At the summit of Everest the oxygen pressure in the blood is about 28 to 32 mm Hg or approximately one-third that of sea level.

ACUTE MOUNTAIN SICKNESS

Acute mountain sickness is a term applied to a group of unpleasant symptoms related to high altitude. Their primary cause is probably the direct effect of low oxygen on the brain. However, changes in the circulation of blood to the brain may also be important. Blood vessels in the brain dilate when blood oxygen saturation is decreased, which occurs at high elevations. These blood vessels constrict when the blood carbon dioxide concentration is decreased, which occurs as the result of increased pulmonary ventilation at high altitude. Either dilatation or constriction of blood vessels in the brain may cause headache. The hydration or water content of the body does not seem related to the symptoms of acute mountain sickness.

The occurrence of acute mountain sickness depends upon the elevation attained, the rate of ascent, and individual susceptibility. Symptoms usually start twelve to twenty-four hours after arrival and begin to decrease in severity on about the third day. The most common symptoms are headache, dizziness, fatigue, shortness of breath, loss of appetite, nausea and vomiting (particularly in children), disturbed sleep, and a general feeling of being unwell (malaise) which has been compared to "flu" or a hangover. Drowsiness and frequent yawning are common. Anxiety attacks and hyperventilation may occur. Cheyne-Stokes breathing may be present during the day and is common at night, when it may interfere with sleep. (Cheyne-Stokes breathing is described in Chapter Sixteen, "Diseases of the Respiratory System.")

A cerebral form of mountain sickness due to oxygen lack and possibly edema (the presence of abnormal quantities of fluid) of the brain may be manifested by headache, dizziness, and impaired mental function evidenced by loss of memory, forgetfulness, or the inability to solve simple problems such as reading a clock from a mirror. In severe cases disturbances in gait, psychotic behavior, or hallucinations may occur. The cerebral form of acute mountain sickness is more commonly observed at altitudes above 14,000 feet (4,300 m). Prompt treatment is essential.

Acute mountain sickness occurs with increasing frequency during unbroken ascents to higher altitudes and can be prevented by gradual acclimatization at intermediate altitudes. After rapid ascents from near sea level to between 8,000 and 10,000 feet (2,400 to 3,000 m) occasional individuals have symptoms. After rapid ascents from near sea level to 14,000 feet (4,300 m) almost everyone has symptoms. In 1975, sixty-nine percent of trekkers who flew from Katmandu to 9,275 feet (2825 m) and started hiking to the Mt. Everest base camp at 17,500 feet (5,350 m) experienced acute mountain sickness. (Two years later, an educational prevention campaign by the Himalayan Rescue Association had reduced the incidence to forty-three percent.) Children are very susceptible to acute mountain sickness. They frequently become very sleepy and develop striking cyanosis of the lips and tongue at high altitude.

Individuals with acute mountain sickness should avoid heavy exertion, although light outdoor activity is preferable to complete rest. Sleep is definitely not helpful because respirations are slower during sleep, which may make symptoms worse. At night, sedatives should be avoided since they also decrease respirations. Victims should drink extra fluids and eat a light, high carbohydrate diet. Aspirin can be taken for headache. Tobacco and alcohol should be avoided.

Individuals may be forced to rest if acute mountain sickness is severe and may require oxygen (two liters per minute through a mask that covers nose and mouth). To obtain full benefit from oxygen it should be used continuously for at least fifteen minutes. Oxygen is of no value if it is inhaled for only a few minutes a few times a day. If the supply is adequate, oxygen can be used for twelve to forty-eight hours. If severe symptoms persist despite oxygen (or oxygen is not available), descent to a lower altitude usually results in prompt relief, even if the descent is only 2,000 to 3,000 feet (600 to 900 m).

Occasionally, an individual who has recently arrived at high altitude becomes unusually drowsy or very weak. He may rest in a semisleeping condition, becoming increasingly cyanotic and beginning to hallucinate or behave in an irrational manner. Improvement can be quickly achieved by awakening the individual, helping him walk around in the open air, and encouraging him to to breathe deeply. Because his respirations are decreased during sleep, the oxygen concentration in the blood can fall to low levels, but the oxygen content increases rapidly when the individual is awake, active, and breathing deeply.

Some temporary relief from the symptoms of acute mountain sickness can be achieved by voluntarily taking ten to twelve deep breaths every four to six minutes. However, if overdone, this maneuver can cause dizziness and tingling of the lips and hands due to "blowing off" too much carbon dioxide.

Acetazolamide (Diamox) has been found to reduce the severity of acute mountain sickness in several well controlled studies. A physician should provide the prescription because this drug is contraindicated in the presence of certain kidney, eye, or liver diseases. The usual dose is 250 mg twice daily beginning one day before ascent and continuing for three to five days after arrival. Side effects, especially if acetazolamide is taken for more than five days, include tingling of the lips and finger tips, blurring of vision, and alteration of taste, but these symptoms subside when the drug is stopped.

No physiologic tests can determine in advance whether an individual is susceptible to acute mountain sickness, nor can any specific measurements diagnose the presence or severity of the disorder. Psychologic factors, including suggestibility, may affect the symptoms significantly.

HIGH ALTITUDE PULMONARY EDEMA

High altitude pulmonary edema is the most dangerous of the common types of altitude illness. This disorder results from filling the alveoli of the lungs with fluid that has oozed through the walls of the pulmonary capillaries. As more alveoli fill with fluid, oxygen transfer from air to the pulmonary capillaries is blocked. A drop in the concentration of oxygen in the blood results, eventually causing cyanosis, impaired cerebral function, and finally death by suffocation.

High altitude pulmonary edema is not the result of heart failure or pneumonia, although prior to the recognition of this disorder in 1960, most episodes in climbers were incorrectly diagnosed as pneumonia. The cause lies in the pulmonary circulation. High altitude, sleep hypoxia, hypoxia from any other cause, and heavy exercise are all associated with a rise in pulmonary artery pressure. Normally, constriction of the smallest pulmonary arteries (called arterioles) protects the capillaries from excessive pressure and high flow rates. In individuals susceptible to high altitude pulmonary edema, arteriolar constriction may not be uniform throughout the lungs. Arterioles in some areas constrict, but arterioles in other areas do not. In the areas where no constriction occurs, high pressure and flow are transmitted directly to the capillaries. When the capillary pressure exceeds 20 mm Hg, fluid is forced out of the capillaries into the alveoli of the lung.

Some individuals are unusually susceptible to high altitude pulmonary edema and have had repeated episodes of this disorder. Such subjects may have an abnormal rise in pulmonary artery pressure at high altitudes, particularly during exercise. This abnormal rise in pressure appears to be the first event leading to high altitude pulmonary edema.

When severe enough to cause physical incapacity, high altitude pulmonary edema has usually followed rapid ascents by unacclimatized individuals who engaged in heavy physical exertion after arrival at high altitudes. Very rapid ascents may result in high altitude pulmonary edema even in acclimatized individuals. However, this disorder rarely occurs below 8,000 feet (2,400 m).

The chances of developing symptomatic high altitude pulmonary edema after a rapid ascent to 12,000 feet (3,700 m) are about one in two hundred (0.5 percent) in individuals more than twenty-one years old but may be six to twelve times higher in individuals ten to eighteen years old. (Episodes of high altitude pulmonary edema producing only mild or no symptoms and spontaneously subsiding without specific treatment may also occur, but their incidence and related features are unknown.) Probably no one is completely immune; high altitude pulmonary edema does occur in experienced mountaineers. Acclimatized individuals who live at high altitude may develop high altitude pulmonary edema if they descend to a lower elevation for seven to fourteen days (or more) and rapidly ascend again.

Symptoms of high altitude pulmonary edema usually begin one to four days after arrival at a high elevation and consist of undue shortness of breath with moderate exertion, a sense of "tightness in the chest" or a feeling of impending suffocation at night, weakness, and marked fatigue. The individual with pulmonary edema is typically much more tired than other members of the climbing party. Headache, loss of appetite, nausea, and vomiting are frequently present, particularly in children. Coughing is an important early sign, although it is probably more frequently caused by drying of the throat than pulmonary edema. The cough is usually dry and intermittent at first, but with pulmonary edema the cough becomes persistent, and white, watery or frothy material is coughed up. Later the sputum may be streaked with blood. In rare instances high altitude pulmonary edema may be manifested first by disturbances of consciousness or coma with little or no shortness of breath.

The pulse rate is usually rapid (110 to 160 per minute), even after several hours of rest, and is associated with rapid respirations (20 to 40 per minute). The lips and nail beds are cyanotic, and the skin may be pale and cold. Bubbling or crackling sounds (rales) may be heard when listening to the lungs with the unaided ear or with a stethoscope. The symptoms and signs often become worse during the night.

An important indication of the severity of high altitude pulmonary edema is the level of mental acuity. Confusion, delirium, and irrational behavior are signs of a pronounced reduction in the oxygen supply to the brain and are indicative of severe pulmonary edema. If the patient becomes unconscious, death may follow within six to twelve hours unless prompt descent or oxygen therapy are initiated.

Grading the severity of high altitude pulmonary edema may be useful. Patients with a disorder of only grade one severity usually have only mild symptoms such as fatigue or exertional dyspnea. Listening to the chest usually discloses fine rales. If an x-ray of the chest is taken, small infiltrates may be present, particularly in the right midlung field. Patients with grade one pulmonary edema usually recover after descending to a lower altitude for two to three days. Patients with more severe grades of high altitude pulmonary edema should be considered medical emergencies and require more vigorous treatment.

Trip leaders and physicians must actively look for the early signs of high altitude pulmonary edema, particularly during the first week of climbing above 8,000 feet (2,400 m). Young, ambitious, physically fit climbers may conceal symptoms. A useful method of detecting early high altitude pulmonary edema is to evaluate each party member at the end of each day's climbing after the individual has rested quietly for fifteen to twenty minutes. His climbing performance should be evaluated; symptoms of undue fatigue, weakness, or shortness of breath should be sought. The heart rate and respiratory rate should be determined, and the chest should be examined by the ear or stethoscope for crackling or bubbling sounds during inspiration. Unusual fatigue, a resting heart rate greater than 110, a resting respiratory rate of greater than sixteen per minute, or rales or bubbling sounds in the chest may indicate the presence of high altitude pulmonary edema. If these signs and symptoms persist through the night, the patient should descend to lower altitude, preferably while he is in good enough condition to walk under his own power. High altitude pulmonary edema may progress very rapidly, particularly during the night, and frequent examination of patients with mild signs is necessary. Any worsening of the condition is an indication for prompt descent.

Table Three. Severity Classification of High Altitude Pulmonary Edema

Grade	Clinical Signs and Symptoms	Pulse	Resp.	Chest X-Ray
I Mild	Minor symptoms. Dyspnea on moderate or heavy exertion. May have rales.	<110/min	<20/min	Minor infiltrates, <25% of one lung field.
II Moderate	Dyspnea, weakness, fatigue on ordinary effort. Headache, dry cough, rales present.	110-120	20-30	Infiltrates in 50% of one lung, usually RML.
III Serious	Dyspnea, weakness, headache at rest. Anorexia. Persistent productive cough.	120-130	30-40	Infiltrates in half of both lung fields.
IV Severe	Stupor or coma. Hallucinations. Can not stand. Severe cyanosis. Rales prominent. Copious sputum, often bloody.	>130/min	>40/min	Infiltrates in >50% of both lung fields.

The most important method of treatment is descent to a lower altitude. If the patient can not walk, litter evacuation may be necessary. A descent of as little as 2,000 to 3,000 feet (600 to 900 m) often results in prompt improvement. After arriving at a lower altitude, the patient should rest for two to three days. Physical activity increases the severity of high altitude pulmonary edema, and several days are required for the fluid to be absorbed from the lungs.

If oxygen is available, it should be administered without delay. Rescue parties, particularly helicopter evacuation units, should bring oxygen to the victim and begin using it at once. Deaths have occurred during evacuation when oxygen has not been carried. However, descent to a lower altitude is essential even if oxygen is available.

The oxygen should be given at a flow rate of four to six liters per minute for the first fifteen minutes, after which the flow rate can be reduced to two liters per minute to conserve oxygen. A snugly fitting face mask is essential for administration. (Light weight oxygen cylinders and attachments are available from Nageldinger, 1 Mahan Street, West Babylon, New York 11704.)

Improvement is usually rapid after oxygen is begun in mild cases. However, administration should be continued for at least six to twelve hours if possible. Oxygen should be continued after arrival at a lower elevation. Twenty-four to

Table Four. Analysis of Thirty-Three Cases of
High Altitude Pulmonary Edema in Climbers

	Average	*Range*
Age	30 years	20-43
Altitude of Occurrence	13,670 feet (4,166 m)	8,600-24,000 feet (2,630-7,315 m)
Duration of Ascent	3.9 days	1-11
Interval Before Onset of Symptoms	3 days	1-11
Most Common Features	Cough (24) Shortness of Breath (20) Fatigue (16) Confusion, Mental Changes (16) Gurgling in Chest (14)	
Pulse Rate	115/min	96-170
Duration of Edema	5.2 days	2-10
Prior Episodes of High Altitude Pulmonary Edema	4 (12%)	
Deaths	9 (27%)	

forty-eight hours of low flow oxygen therapy (two liters per minute) may be required for prompt and complete recovery. Oxygen should not be given for less than fifteen minutes; continuous low flow oxygen for six to twelve hours is more beneficial than intermittent short periods at high flow rates. An oxygen mask is preferable to nasal prongs.

As soon as the victim reaches a medical facility, a chest x-ray should be obtained, since diagnostic pulmonary densities may persist for several days after apparent recovery. Residual weakness and fatigue may persist for one to two weeks.

Many drugs have been employed in the treatment of high altitude pulmonary edema, including steroids, digitalis, antibiotics, and diuretics such as furosemide (Lasix). Controlled studies have provided no evidence that such drugs are of any benefit. Furosemide has been used with the concept that it would help remove fluid from the lungs, but the only type of pulmonary edema in which fluid can be removed from the lungs by a diuretic is that due to heart failure. (In heart failure, the drug lowers the pressure in the left ventricle and thereby lowers the pulmonary capillary pressure. The lower capillary pressure stops the movement of fluid into the alveoli and permits absorption of the edema fluid.) Since high altitude pulmonary edema is not due to heart failure, a diuretic would not be expected to be helpful. In some patients a diuretic can cause a large urine output, resulting in a drop in blood volume and collapse. A walking patient, able to descend with minimal assistance, can be converted into a litter case. The role of acetazolamide in the treatment of early or mild cases of high altitude pulmonary edema is unknown and needs to be studied. Morphine may be helpful, particularly for patients who are very apprehensive and have marked shortness of breath, but should only be given by a physician.

Measures for preventing high altitude pulmonary edema are identical to those for preventing acute mountain sickness: gradual ascent and acclimatization. Heavy physical exertion should be avoided for the first few days after a rapid ascent to high altitude. A low salt intake is recommended.

Individuals with a prior history of this disorder must be particularly careful, and preventive measures can not be stressed too strongly. Such persons may be helped by acetazolamide, which should be started on the day before ascent and continued for three to five days after arriving at high elevations. Patients who have the rare congenital abnormality of the lung in which a pulmonary artery is absent are very susceptible to high altitude pulmonary edema and may develop this disorder at altitudes below 8,000 feet (2,400 m).

In the central Peruvian Andes, over 300,000 people live at altitudes exceeding 12,000 feet (3,700 m) and travel to the seacoast and jungle frequently. In the 1960s twenty to forty cases of high altitude pulmonary edema were seen annually at one Andean hospital located at 12,400 feet (3780 m). As people became aware of the problem, preventive measures were instituted. For susceptible subjects treatment with acetazolamide was started prior to ascent and oxygen was administered for six to twelve hours after arrival. Exercise was forbidden for the first two days after arrival. If signs or symptoms of high altitude pulmonary edema were present, the patient was put to bed and given low flow oxygen at home. As a result of these measures, high altitude pulmonary edema has become a rare occurrence in this hospital.

Case Study One

A thirty-eight year old healthy, experienced mountaineer was climbing in the Cordillera Blanca of Peru. In three days he climbed with a heavy pack from 9,000 to 14,000 feet (2,700 to 4,300 m) over a series of ridges, one of which was 16,000 feet (4,900 m) high. On the evening of the third day he was more tired than other members of the party and had Cheyne-Stokes respirations. The following day he engaged in little activity but on the fifth day climbed steeply with a heavy pack to a higher camp. He was far more short of breath than other members of the party. Upon arrival at the 16,000 foot (4,900 m) camp he was tired and listless and could not eat. He began to cough and one of his companions stated that he "obviously had fluid in his lungs." He was comfortable only in a seated position. Because he was thought to have pneumonia, he was given penicillin. His breathing rapidly became more labored and his cough more severe and frequent. His companion, who was not a physician, wrote in his diary, "the next few hours his breathing became progressively more congested and labored. He sounded as though he were literally drowning in his own fluid with an almost continuous loud bubbling sound as if breathing through liquid." During the night the victim's breathing became far worse and he lost consciousness. He died at dawn on the second day of his illness. His companion's diary stated, "a couple of hours after his death, when we got up to carry on the day's activities, I noticed that a white froth resembling cotton candy had appeared to well up out of his mouth." An autopsy disclosed severe pulmonary edema.

At the time of this incident high altitude pulmonary edema had not been recognized. Prompt evacuation to a lower altitude would have been life saving.

Case Study Two

A thirty year old salesman from the San Francisco Bay area was an avid skier, skiing nearly every weekend from late November to the middle of April in the Lake Tahoe area. A late snowfall in May enticed him to ski over the Memorial Day weekend. He drove to Mammoth Lakes (8,000 ft or 2,400 m) where he spent the next three nights. He skied the next two days on Mammoth Mountain between 8,000 and 11,000 feet (2,400 and 3,400 m). On the afternoon of the second day at Mammoth he noted increasing shortness of breath, fatigue, and weakness. He continued to ski even though he barely could climb up the loading ramp to the chairlift. That night he developed a cough and more intense shortness of breath, and he noted gurgling sounds in his chest. Early the next morning he was coughing up bloody sputum and a physician was called. He was given an injection of penicillin and advised to drive home. The following day, eighteen hours after arrival at sea level, he still felt weak and short of breath and saw his family physician. He had a respiratory rate of twenty-four per minute and a heart rate of ninety-two. Persistent crackling sounds were present in the lower portion of the right lung. A chest x-ray disclosed fluid in the lower portions of both lungs. The patient was hospitalized and treated with oxygen. He improved rapidly and was discharged four days later after complete clearing of the pulmonary fluid.

This study illustrates several important aspects of high altitude pulmonary edema:

1. Two days of skiing between 8,000 and 11,000 feet (2,400 and 3,400 m) and three nights of sleeping at 8,000 feet (2,400 m) were sufficient to produce pulmonary edema in this physically fit man. Shorter periods of skiing, or sleeping at a lower elevation, might have prevented the episode.
2. He continued his physical exertions on the second day of skiing in spite of his symptoms, a common occurrence in patients who develop severe high altitude pulmonary edema.
3. His symptoms became worse at night, a frequent event probably caused by lower blood oxygen concentrations during sleep.

HIGH ALTITUDE CEREBRAL EDEMA

Signs and symptoms of brain dysfunction occasionally appear in some individuals exposed to altitudes exceeding 12,000 feet (3,700 m). Although this condition has been referred to as high altitude cerebral edema, the cause of the signs and symptoms may be damage to the brain tissue by hypoxia, and the swelling or edema of the brain may be entirely secondary to such injury. The cerebral hypoxia results from decreased quantities of oxygen in the blood and is related to altitude. Clearly, more than just hypoxia is necessary. Local circulatory factors, such as excessive vasoconstriction in portions of the brain, may be required.

For an unacclimatized person, exposure to an altitude greater than 20,000 feet (6,100 m), as might occur in a pressure chamber, results in loss of higher mental functions, unsteady gait and posture, collapse, and finally coma within a few minutes. The cause is lack of oxygen in specific areas of the brain. Return to sea level pressures or the administration of oxygen quickly relieves the symptoms.

High altitude cerebral edema has an insidious, often unexpected onset and may occur in a fit, well functioning climber who has gradually ascended to a very high altitude over many days. While edema of the brain due to hypoxia occurs in many cases, it is not always present. Obviously, certain brain functions may be impaired more than others, and this impairment may last for many months after return to sea level.

Most episodes occur after several days at altitudes greater than 12,000 feet (3,700 m). The most common symptoms are headache, abnormal mental function, and ataxia (unsteadiness or muscular incoordination). Headache is usually present, although in some patients it is curiously absent. The usual headache is severe and constant, and the patient may require codeine or morphine for relief. Mental dysfunction can range from confusion, loss of memory, and inability to exercise proper judgment to hallucinations, psychotic behavior, and coma, the most severe sign. The patient can not be aroused and does not respond to names, commands, or even painful stimuli.

Ataxia is typical of high altitude cerebral edema. The most common form of ataxia is truncal ataxia, with which the patient is unable to maintain a balanced body position. In severe cases he can not walk or stand without falling. A sensitive test for truncal ataxia is to determine whether the patient can walk a straight line. In severe cases of ataxia of the upper extremities, the subject may be unable to tie his shoes, hold a cup or plate, or feed himself.

High altitude cerebral edema can cause death or (rarely) permanent brain damage. As in high altitude pulmonary edema, early diagnosis and treatment are important. Trip leaders should carefully check the condition of their party members in the evening and in the morning, when signs and symptoms may be more severe. Any confusion or ataxia combined with a severe persistent headache should raise the possibility of cerebral edema. Individuals with such signs should be given oxygen if available and be forced to descend. Assistance must be provided during descent because ataxia may progress rapidly and the patient may fall and be injured. Once hypoxic brain injury occurs, even if recovery is rapid at a lower altitude, further climbing is not advisable. Some individuals appear to be unusually susceptible to this disorder and have had more than one episode.

Patients who are unconscious must be hospitalized as soon as possible. Standard methods of treating cerebral edema at sea level should probably not be employed for two reasons: cerebral edema may not always be present, and intravenous mannitol and diuretics may reduce the circulation to the brain and impede recovery. Steroids such as dexamethazone may be beneficial and have the advantage of not decreasing blood flow to the brain.

High altitude cerebral edema may occur in the absence of acute mountain sickness or high altitude pulmonary edema. However, many patients with severe high altitude pulmonary edema may be unconscious and may exhibit all the signs and symptoms of cerebral edema. For this reason, the heart rate and respiratory rate should be determined, and the chest should be examined carefully in all patients with central nervous system abnormalities at high altitude. A chest x-ray should be obtained as soon as a medical facility has been reached to determine whether pulmonary edema is present. In rare instances, high altitude pulmonary edema may appear as coma or unconsciousness without cough or shortness of breath and may simulate cerebral edema.

Case Study Three

A twenty-two year old experienced climber was a member of an expedition to Makalu. Three years earlier he had developed mild confusion and stumbling at 17,500 feet (5,350 m), but these symptoms disappeared after descending to 14,500 feet (4,450 m). On Makalu he had spent twelve days climbing to 16,400 feet (5,000 m), where he stayed two days. On successive days he carried loads to 17,500, 18,500, and 20,000 feet (5,350, 5,650, and 6,100 m). At 20,000 feet (6,100 m) he noticed that he was dizzy and had poor balance on delicate pitches. He slept at 20,000 feet (6,100 m) and then carried a load to 21,000 feet (6,400 m). That evening he felt very sleepy and dozed off between the courses of his evening meal. He was not short of breath and had no headache. During the night, he was observed to be snoring loudly and could not be awakened. The following morning he was unconscious. His eyes were open and staring, and he frequently made involuntary, convulsive movements. Over the next several days he was carried down to 14,750 feet (4,500 m), where he became conscious but was confused and hallucinating. He crawled aimlessly around his tent and could not recognize his own sleeping bag. He still made convulsive movements and frequent facial grimaces. Eighteen days after his collapse he became mentally clear for the first time. A month afterward retinal hemorrhages persisted. He could not perform delicate hand and foot movements and was unable to maintain his balance. Abnormal reflexes were present, indicating persistent nervous system injury.

This young man had a serious episode of high altitude cerebral edema with residual nervous system abnormalities, but he did survive. Others have not been that fortunate. Apparently the longer a high altitude cerebral edema victim remains at high altitude, the more severe and prolonged are the symptoms, and the greater is the risk of permanent nervous system damage or death.

HIGH ALTITUDE RETINAL HEMORRHAGE

Hemorrhage (or bleeding) into the retina, the layer of sensitive light receptors in the eye, occurs commonly at altitudes above 14,000 feet (4,300 m) and has been found in thirty to one hundred percent of climbers at an elevation of 17,600 feet (5,365 m). Such bleeding is rare below 14,000 feet (4,300 m). In most instances the hemorrhages cause no visual difficulty, are painless, and can be found only by examining the retina with special instruments. Occasionally the hemorrhages are larger, involve the central part of the retina, and cause clouding of vision or the inability to see in certain directions with one eye. Individuals with such large hemorrhages should descend to a lower elevation since further exposure to high altitude can worsen the condition. The hemorrhages usually clear up completely four to six weeks after descent. Only rarely have minor visual defects been permanent.

The hemorrhages are probably related to dilatation and increased blood flow in the blood vessels of the retina due to reduced blood oxygen concentrations. The high pressure may produce small openings in these thin walled vessels, resulting in bleeding.

Whether to descend after the discovery of small retinal hemorrhages that cause no visual difficulty is a decision that must be made for himself by each individual climber.

HIGH ALTITUDE SYSTEMIC EDEMA

Swelling of the feet and hands may occur after ascent to high altitude, particularly in women. Swelling of the face and eyelids may be troublesome in the mornings. Urine output is usually low despite an adequate fluid intake. A weight gain of eight to twelve pounds may occur within a few days. High altitude systemic edema may not be associated with symptoms of acute mountain sickness. Recurrent episodes are common. Although this condition sometimes is a nuisance, it is harmless and clears up within a few days after returning to sea level. A copious urine output and rapid loss of the extra weight usually signal its disappearance after descent.

The edema results from retention of salt and water by the kidneys, but the cause is not understood. Prolonged exercise at sea level may also result in water retention, but the edema is less severe.

Salty foods, salt tablets, or sodium containing antacid tablets should be avoided because an increased sodium intake aggravates the condition. A diuretic such as furosemide taken once or twice daily for three to six days usually eliminates the excess fluid. Acetazolamide may be given if symptoms of acute mountain sickness are severe and persistent. However, diuretics must be used with caution at high altitude because an excessive urine output can cause a decrease in blood volume, resulting in weakness and dizziness.

PERSISTENT MOUNTAIN SICKNESS

Subacute Mountain Sickness

Although acute mountain sickness disappears within two to six days after acclimatization has been achieved, a few individuals continue to have symptoms for days to months, sometimes at the relatively moderate elevations between 10,000 and 14,000 feet (3,000 and 4,300 m). The inability to obtain sound, restful sleep is common and ranges in severity from mild insomnia to an almost total inability to sleep which forces the victim to return to lower altitude. Cheyne-Stokes respiration is responsible for sleeplessness in a few individuals. Nocturnal restlessness, awakening after short intervals of sleep, and disturbing dreams are more frequent.

A particularly difficult problem for individuals with subacute mountain sickness is their decreased capacity for sustained physical work. Fatigue persists throughout the day and recovery does not occur with sleep. Weakness and lethargy are common; undue shortness of breath during exertion may be troublesome.

Loss of appetite and insomnia are largely responsible for the weight loss of ten to twenty pounds experienced by nearly everyone spending a significant amount of time at high altitude. Distaste for tobacco may accompany the loss of appetite.

Some subjects exhibit predominantly neurologic symptoms and signs. Headaches, usually in the back of the head, can be intense and are occasionally associated with neck pain. Ringing in the ears, numbness and tingling sensations, particularly in the extremities, or severe pain in the arms and legs, joints, or low back may appear. Paralysis of the extremities and paralysis of one side of the body have occurred. Depression, inability to carry out sustained mental work, forgetfulness, and a decreased ability for conceptual thinking are common. Irritability and personality changes are occasionally noticed.

Measures that ameliorate the symptoms of subacute mountain sickness are prior acclimatization, periodic visits to lower altitudes for recuperation, oxygen administration, proper diet with an adequate fluid intake, and the judicious use of drugs, including acetazolamide, to promote restful sleep. No therapy can completely eradicate or prevent subacute mountain sickness. If disability persists, a return to lower altitude is necessary.

High Altitude Deterioration

Acclimatized man can live a normal life span at elevations up to approximately 17,000 feet (5,200 m). Above this altitude even acclimatized individuals experience a slow, progressive deterioration in physical fitness and persistent symptoms of acute mountain sickness. The causes are not clear, but chronic hypoxia is the probable culprit.

Dehydration is common because fluid losses are increased and the sense of thirst is diminished. Loss of appetite and progressive weight loss may occur. The concentration of red cells in the blood may increase to almost double the usual sea level values, which greatly increases the viscosity of blood. This concentrated, viscous blood flows slowly, almost like syrup, and can cause poor perfusion of vital organs such as the brain. Such viscous blood also has a greater tendency to clot within blood vessels, which can result in serious disorders such as a stroke or a pulmonary embolus.

High altitude deterioration can be minimized by spending as little time as possible at extreme altitudes and periodically descending to lower altitudes for several days for recovery. An adequate fluid intake is essential. The urine volume must be greater than 500 cc every day, preferably two to three times greater, and urine color should be clear and light yellow, not deep yellow or orange. Efforts must be made to eat an adequate amount of food in spite of a poor appetite. An adequate caloric intake is needed more than specific nutrients. Nutritional deficiencies do not develop in healthy individuals during the short periods expeditions are at high altitudes. Oxygen during sleep at a flow rate of two liters per minute through a face mask is beneficial. The value of acetazolamide or respiratory stimulants such as progesterone is unknown.

German physicians have recommended diluting the blood by removing one to three pints and replacing it with a fluid that resembles plasma but contains no red cells, thereby reducing blood viscosity. The results of the few attempts to utilize this technique have been equivocal. Climbers have not been impaired but have not clearly benefited either. The procedure could be dangerous as it could cause allergic reactions or even high altitude pulmonary edema.

Chronic Mountain Sickness

Chronic mountain sickness is entirely different from acute and subacute mountain sickness. It is characterized by marked cyanosis of the lips and nails and by episodes of pronounced sleepiness and mental depression. Coma may occur. The feet and abdomen may be swollen due to heart failure. Chronic mountain sickness is suggestive of serious disease of the lungs or heart, but complete recovery usually occurs within six weeks or less of returning to sea level.

The basic disturbance in chronic mountain sickness is a failure by the body's chemical receptors to react to lower blood oxygen concentrations and stimulate faster, deeper respirations. As a result, aeration (or ventilation) of the lungs is inadequate for blood oxygenation. An individual with chronic mountain sickness usually can never return to high altitude. However, chronic mountain sickness has been observed only in persons who have lived at a high altitude for many years. It apparently never occurs in climbers, even after weeks at high elevations.

Thrombosis, Strokes, and Pulmonary Embolism

At high altitude blood has an increased tendency to clot (thrombose) in veins and arteries. Factors (in addition to altitude and hypoxia) contributing to this tendency include dehydration, long periods of immobility in tents during bad weather, an increased number of red cells in the blood, and possibly an increase in the factors that promote clotting.

Blood clots in the leg veins may be detached and carried to the lungs, where they obstruct the pulmonary arteries (pulmonary embolism). Warning signs of thrombosis of the leg veins are swollen, painful, tender legs and feet, particularly after long periods of immobility. (See Chapter Sixteen, "Diseases of the Respiratory System.") Blood may clot in arteries in the brain and cause a stroke. Temporary or permanent paralysis, commonly limited to one side of the body, is the usual result. (See Chapter Twenty-One, "Diseases of the Nervous System.") Any of these disorders is a serious problem which may cause death or serious disability, and is an indication for prompt descent, oxygen therapy, and hospitalization. Recurrent episodes are likely upon return to high altitude.

Pre-Existing Medical Problems at High Altitudes

Medical conditions which are aggravated or complicated by high altitude include:

1. Chronic lung disease with low arterial oxygen saturation;
2. Pulmonary hypertension;
3. Congenital absence of a pulmonary artery;
4. Cyanotic congenital heart disease;
5. Previous stroke or pulmonary embolus;
6. Pregnancy;
7. Heart failure;
8. Severe angina;
9. Anemia;
10. Sickle cell disease.

Anyone with these conditions should consult his physician before going to higher elevations. Moderate altitudes — 6,000 to 8,000 feet (1,800 to 2,400 m) — may be well tolerated if precautions are taken. After arrival such persons should rest for two to three days. Oxygen should be used if altitude related symptoms cause discomfort or sleep is disturbed. After three to four days, the severity of symptoms usually diminishes and customary activities can be resumed.

NUTRITION AT ALTITUDE

The maintenance of an adequate food and water intake is particularly difficult at high altitudes. Appetites are poor and high altitude climbers usually eat and drink much less than they need. Much of the fatigue and weakness experienced at high altitudes is due to inadequate nutrition, dehydration, and possibly potassium loss accompanying very high energy expenditure. British Himalayan parties have reported that the average caloric intake during approach marches was 4,200 calories per day, but intake fell to 3,200 calories between 19,000 and 22,000 feet (5,800 and 6,700 m) and to 1,500 calories above 24,000 feet (7,300 m). The American party that ascended the west ridge of Everest attributes a large part of its success to continuous conscious efforts to consume adequate amounts of food in spite of a lack of appetite.

Impairment of food absorption in the gastrointestinal tract has been suggested as a cause for the weight loss, which reportedly can not be prevented by forced feeding. The tastelessness of the freeze dried foods carried by most expeditions may be more significant. The 1983 German-American Everest Expedition purchased all of their food supplies from community grocery stores and had no problems with weight loss. One member even gained weight!

Climbers often go hungry at high altitude rather than eat food that they do not crave. Menus should consist largely of foods known to be enjoyed by all the party members, but foods to satisfy individual tastes must also be carried. Diets should contain large amounts of sweets, which are usually consumed in large quantities at high altitudes. Fatty foods or highly condensed rations may not be tolerated.

On prolonged expeditions where fresh vegetables and fruits are not available, possible vitamin C deficiency can be prevented with ascorbic acid. However, most packaged drinks such as lemonade or orange juice contain vitamin C. Furthermore, about six months are required for signs of vitamin deficiency to appear in individuals who previously were in good nutritional condition. If vitamin intake appears inadequate, one or two multivitamin tablets per day can be taken. A high vitamin intake or special vitamins such as E or B complex vitamins are of no benefit at high altitudes (or anywhere else). Vitamin requirements are only minimally increased by the rigors of an expedition, and a standard diet contains much more vitamins than are required. Any excess is simply excreted in the urine. Excess vitamin A and D — possibly others — are definitely harmful.

FLUID BALANCE AT ALTITUDE

Almost everyone is dehydrated at high altitudes as the result of inadequate fluid intake and increased fluid losses. This problem is discussed under Fluid Balance in Chapter Three, "Special Problems."

ACKNOWLEDGMENT
Charles S. Houston, M.D. provided valuable advice and suggestions in the preparation of this chapter.

ADDITIONAL READING

MONOGRAPHS

1. Hackett P: *Mountain Sickness: Prevention, Recognition and Treatment.* New York, American Alpine Club, 1980.
2. Heath D: *Man At High Altitude.* Edinburgh, Churchill Livingston, 1977.
3. Houston C: *Going Higher: The Story of Man and Altitude.* New York, C.S. Houston and American Alpine Club, 1983.
4. Mosso A: *Life of Man on the High Alps,* Kiesow E, trans. London, T. Fisher Unwin, 1908.
5. Ward M: *Mountain Medicine.* London, Crosby, Lockwood, Staples, 1975.
6. West JB, Lahiri S: *High Altitude and Man.* Baltimore, The Williams & Wilkins Co., 1984.

PAPERS

1. Evans WO, Robinson SM, Horstman DH, et al: Amelioration of the symptoms of acute mountain sickness by staging and acetazolamide. *Aviat Space Environ Med* 1976;47:512.
2. Houston CS: Altitude illness — recent advances in knowledge. *Amer Alpine J* 1979;22:153.
3. Houston CS, Dickinson J: Cerebral form of high altitude illness. *Lancet* 1975;2:758.
4. Hultgren HN: High altitude medical problems. *West J Med* 1979;131:8.
5. Hultgren HN: Sickness in high places. *Emergency Med* 1980;12:24.
6. Hultgren HN: Treatment and prevention of high altitude pulmonary edema. *Amer Alpine J* 1965;14:363.
7. Nag P, Sen R, Ray U: Optimal rate of work for mountaineers. *J Appl Physiol* 1978;44:1952.

8. Sutton J, Gray G, et al: Retinal haemorrhage at high altitude. *Amer Alpine J* 1980;22:513.
9. Sutton J, Houston CS, et al: Effect of acetazolamide on hypoxemia during sleep at high altitude. *New Eng J Med* 1979;201:1329.
10. West JB: Human physiology at extreme altitudes on Mount Everest. *Science* 1984;223:784.
11. West JB, Lahiri S, Gill M, et al: Arterial oxygen saturation during exercise at high altitude. *J. Appl Physiol* 1962;17:617.

CHAPTER THIRTEEN

Cold Injuries

The most common major injuries produced by cold are hypothermia and frostbite. Hypothermia is a decrease in the core temperature of the entire body which becomes significant when muscular and cerebral functions are impaired. Frostbite is an injury, usually localized, characterized by freezing of the tissues. Immersion foot (or "trench foot") produces similar damage, but the tissues are not frozen.

HYPOTHERMIA

The body temperature falls when the amount of heat being lost to the environment exceeds that being produced within the body by metabolism, particularly that associated with muscular activity. Understanding why and how hypothermia occurs requires an understanding of the way heat is produced and lost by the body.

HEAT PRODUCTION

Man is a "warm blooded" (or homothermic) mammal who has a relatively constant normal body temperature. He is also considered "endothermic" because most of the heat that maintains his constant temperature originates within his body from the metabolism of food. Most heat producing metabolism takes place within muscles contracting to perform work and within the liver where an incredible array of biochemical processes are continually occurring.

When needed, heat production by the body can be increased to a significant but limited extent. Shivering is an involuntary, seemingly purposeless muscle activity which generates heat by increasing the metabolism within the muscles. The amount of heat produced by shivering is equivalent to that produced by walking fast. Much more heat can be generated by heavier muscle activity, particularly that which exercises the large muscles in the leg. Furthermore, such exercise can serve a useful purpose if it helps a hypothermia victim escape from his predicament. However, heat producing exercise can not be continued indefinitely, nor can enough heat be produced to compensate for severe heat loss such as that occurring with cold water immersion or in a cold terrestrial situation in which the individual is inadequately protected.

HEAT LOSS

Heat is lost to the environment by four routes: Radiation, evaporation, convection, and conduction.

Radiation

Radiation is by far the largest source of heat loss in temperate climates. Radiation or emission of energy, much of which is in the form of infrared radiation, transfers heat directly to the environment. Radiant loss is greater in a cold environment because the amount of heat lost is determined by the difference in temperature between the heat source — the body — and the heat receptacle — the atmosphere or surrounding objects such as rocks, snow, or trees. In a hot environment radiant heat is absorbed by the body. The inability to lose heat by radiation in a hot environment can contribute to heat illness.

Heat loss by radiation is not stopped by clothing. The heat radiates from the body to the clothing and from there to the atmosphere. Efforts to construct clothing of material that would reflect the heat back to the body have met with little success.

However, radiant heat loss becomes a major problem only in extremely cold situations (below -20° to -30° F or -29° to -35° C). Clothing that reduces heat loss by other routes, particularly convection, can largely compensate for the increased radiant heat loss encountered in most climbing circumstances.

Evaporation

Perspiration is continuously being produced in small amounts, even in cold climates. This "insensible" perspiration evaporates from the skin, causing the loss of about 580 calories of heat per cc evaporated. Additional heat is lost from the respiratory passages and lungs as inspired air is warmed to body temperature and moistened to 100 percent relative humidity. In temperate conditions twenty to thirty percent of total heat loss occurs through evaporation, about two-thirds of which takes place on the skin.

Heat and water loss from the lungs becomes much larger at high elevations where breathing is deeper and more rapid to compensate for the lower quantity of oxygen in the atmosphere. As much as four liters of water and 2,000 kilocalories of heat can be lost through the lungs each day at high altitudes. (1,000 calories = 1 kilocalorie).

When clothing becomes saturated with water through immersion or even excessive sweating, evaporative heat loss is increased, but wet clothing is a greater hazard because it no longer provides insulation and permits much greater heat loss by convection.

Heat loss from the respiratory tract can not be reduced in any practical manner. Mouth breathing does increase fluid and heat loss somewhat, but the amount of heat is insignificant compared with the quantity lost through other sources. Climbers must be aware that this heat and water loss is occurring and must eat enough food to regenerate the heat through metabolism and drink enough liquids to replace the water.

Heat loss from insensible perspiration also can not be limited, but excessive sweating can and should be avoided. (The inability to lose heat by perspiring in a humid, hot climate is a major contributor to the development of heat illness.)

Convection

Air in contact with skin extracts enough heat to be warmed to the skin's temperature. When the warmed air is displaced by movement of the body or the surrounding air (wind), it is replaced by cool air, which extracts more heat. Such convective heat loss is an almost continuous process, but the amount of heat required to warm the air (the specific heat of air) is so small that little heat is lost by this route in temperate climates. In a cold atmosphere convective heat loss is greater because more heat is required to warm the colder air.

The greatest convective heat losses occur when the air is moving. Even a mild breeze greatly increases heat loss because the layer of warm air next to the skin is constantly being replaced with cooler air. The amount of heat extracted by moving air increases as the square of the velocity, not in direct proportion to its speed. A wind of eight miles an hour removes four times as much heat, not twice as much, as a wind of four miles an hour. A strong wind can remove tremendous amounts of heat.

The increased heat loss that occurs with moving air has been referred to as "wind chill." The accompanying chart illustrates the additional cooling produced by wind in a cold environment. For instance, a temperature that poses little threat in still air, such as 15 °F (-9.5 °C), can be life threatening in a wind of twenty to twenty-five miles per hour (32 to 40 kilometers per hour).

Because convective heat loss can increase so enormously, it is the major cause of hypothermia in wilderness circumstances. Fortunately, clothing can greatly reduce this type of heat loss. Insulating clothing such as down or wool forms myriads of small pockets in which air is trapped — the essence of thermal insulation. Windproof outer garments help prevent displacement of the air within and between layers of clothing.

Convection is a major source of heat loss for individuals immersed in cold water. The water next to the skin extracts heat and becomes warm, but efforts to swim or other movements displace the warmed water and it is replaced by more cold water. Because the specific heat of water is so high, tremendous amounts of heat can be lost through convection, much more than can be generated by physical activity, even by strong, excellently conditioned swimmers. Individuals accidentally immersed in cold water can stay warmer by holding still to reduce

Table Five. Wind Chill Chart

Temperature (Fahrenheit / Centigrade)

Wind	35 / 2	30 / -1	25 / -4	20 / -7	15 / -9	10 / -12	5 / -15	0 / -18	-5 / -21	-10 / -23	-15 / -26	-20 / -29	-25 / -32	-30 / -34
CALM / CALM														

Equivalent Temperature (Fahrenheit / Centigrade)

Wind														
5 MPH / 8 KPH	33 / 1	27 / -3	21 / -6	16 / -9	12 / -11	7 / -14	1 / -17	-6 / -21	-11 / -24	-15 / -26	-20 / -29	-26 / -32	-31 / -35	-35 / -37
10 MPH / 16 KPH	21 / -6	16 / -9	9 / -13	2 / -17	-2 / -19	-9 / -23	-15 / -26	-22 / -30	-27 / -33	-31 / -35	-38 / -39	-45 / -43	-52 / -47	-58 / -50
15 MPH / 23 KPH	16 / -9	11 / -12	1 / -17	-6 / -21	-11 / -24	-18 / -28	-25 / -32	-33 / -36	-40 / -40	-45 / -43	-51 / -46	-60 / -51	-65 / -54	-70 / -57
20 MPH / 32 KPH	12 / -11	3 / -16	-4 / -20	-9 / -23	-17 / -27	-24 / -31	-32 / -36	-40 / -40	-46 / -43	-52 / -47	-60 / -51	-68 / -56	-76 / -60	-81 / -63
25 MPH / 40 KPH	7 / -14	0 / -18	-7 / -22	-15 / -26	-22 / -30	-29 / -34	-37 / -38	-45 / -43	-52 / -47	-58 / -50	-67 / -55	-75 / -59	-83 / -64	-89 / -67
30 MPH / 48 KPH	5 / -15	-2 / -19	-11 / -24	-18 / -28	-26 / -32	-33 / -36	-41 / -41	-49 / -45	-56 / -51	-63 / -53	-70 / -57	-78 / -61	-87 / -66	-94 / -70
35 MPH / 56 KPH	3 / -16	-4 / -20	-13 / -25	-20 / -31	-27 / -33	-35 / -37	-43 / -42	-52 / -47	-60 / -51	-67 / -55	-72 / -58	-83 / -64	-90 / -68	-98 / -72
40 MPH / 64 KPH	1 / -17	-4 / -20	-15 / -26	-22 / -30	-29 / -34	-36 / -38	-45 / -43	-54 / -48	-62 / -52	-69 / -56	-76 / -60	-87 / -66	-94 / -70	-101 / -74

water movement and limit heat loss than they can by swimming to generate heat. (Unless the shore or a boat is a very short distance away, active swimming should be avoided.) Positions that limit the area of the body surface exposed to the water also help reduce heat loss. Two or more persons should huddle together to limit their contact with the water.

Conduction

Heat is conducted or drained away from the body when it is in contact with water, snow, rocks, or any cold object that is a good conductor. Air is not a good conductor. Water is an excellent conductor, and conductive heat loss is a major contributor to hypothermia during immersion in cold water.

Conductive heat losses can become significant in mountaineering circumstances when a climber must remain seated on ice, snow, or a cold rock while belaying a climbing partner. A more common source of conductive heat loss may be sleeping on the ground without adequate insulation. Simple insulating devices such as foam pads can eliminate most conductive heat loss from these sources. (Air mattresses, which allow air to circulate freely, provide much less insulation than foam pads.) Although conductive heat loss alone is rarely a major cause of hypothermia, additional heat loss by this route can aggravate the effects of large convective heat losses and should be avoided.

Conductive heat losses can become large when clothing is wet. The small pockets usually filled with air, a poor heat conductor, are filled with water, an excellent conductor. Not only does the clothing lose its insulating properties but it becomes a major source of heat loss. Immersion victims may be warmer with no clothes on, particularly if they can be protected from the wind, than clad in wet garments. In any case, wet clothing should at least be temporarily removed and as much water wrung out as possible.

PHYSIOLOGIC LIMITATION OF HEAT LOSS

The body's involuntary physiologic mechanisms for increasing heat dissipation are much better developed than those for reducing loss. (Conversely, intellectually developed methods for reducing heat loss are far superior to those for increasing loss.) Physiologic mechanisms for limiting heat loss are largely limited to the constriction of blood vessels in the skin, which reduces blood flow and allows the tissues to cool. Since the skin temperature is lower, less heat is lost by convection, and the cool tissues form a protective shell which limits heat transfer from the body core to the environment.

The arms and legs, as the result of their long narrow shape, have a greater relative surface area than the body and tend to lose heat more readily. Narrowing of blood vessels in the extremities reduces blood flow and heat loss and also tends to keep the heart and brain supplied with warm blood so they can function after the rest of the body has become significantly chilled.

INTELLECTUALLY DEVISED PROTECTION FROM COLD

A human's greatest protection against the cold is his intellect. At ambient temperatures below about 82° F (28° C), an unclothed human body loses more heat to the environment than its heat generating processes can continuously produce and its heat preserving mechanisms can retain. Almost everywhere they live, humans are dependent upon intellectually devised clothing and shelter to insulate them from the environment and reduce heat loss to levels for which metabolism and physiologic mechanisms can compensate.

Informed, intelligent behavior is even more essential in the severe cold of high altitudes and high latitudes. Threatening situations must be recognized in time for effective countermeasures; preparations may be even more essential. Clothing adequate for such climates can rarely be improvised. Even when available, such clothing must be worn properly. Shelter often can be improvised, but a climber equipped with a snow shovel is far more capable of improvising a truly satisfactory shelter than a climber without one.

PREVENTING HYPOTHERMIA

Preventing hypothermia requires water, food, and clothing.

Water

Water is needed to replace losses through the kidneys, skin, and lungs. Failure to replace that water results in dehydration, which decreases the blood volume and, in a cold environment, handicaps efforts to produce heat by exercise. In addition, dehydration can be accompanied by weakness, fatigue, dizziness, and even a tendency to faint when standing. A person impaired by such symptoms is less able to deal rationally with a threatening environment.

Dehydration contributes to other problems. Constriction of the peripheral blood vessels (so the remaining blood goes to more vital organs) increases the probability of frostbite. Severe shock may develop following even minor injuries. Clots tend to form in the legs and can result in pulmonary embolism. (See Chapter Sixteen, "Diseases of the Respiratory System.")

Thirst is not experienced or is greatly diminished in the presence of dehydration, and a conscious effort to consume adequate fluids is needed. Water intake with mild exertion should be at least two quarts per day; with heavier exertion or at high altitudes, three or four quarts are required. In a world of snow and ice, fuel is required to melt snow for drinking water. Eating snow or ice rarely provides an adequate volume of water, and additional body heat is required to warm water from these sources to body temperature.

An adequate fluid intake is indicated by urine that has a light yellow color and a volume of at least one liter every twenty-four hours. Few climbers would measure or can accurately estimate urine volume, but they should be able to appreciate a reduced frequency for voiding, particularly if they do not need to void when first awakening after a night's sleep. All should be capable of recognizing the deep yellow or orange color of concentrated urine indicative of dehydration, particularly when voiding into a snow bank. Orange "snow flowers" are an ominous sign.

Food

Food is needed to replenish body energy stores essential for physical activity and heat production. Eating small amounts of food at frequent intervals rather than two or three large meals helps prevent depletion of energy stores during the day. Experienced climbers often seem to be munching almost continuously and have developed various mixtures of nuts, dried fruits, candies, and other high calorie ingredients that go under the collective name of "gorp."

In a survival situation, experience has demonstrated that food is one of the most important ingredients of success. Any source of food, even wild animals such as birds or rodents, which may have to be eaten uncooked, is preferable to the ketosis and acidosis — and the accompanying fatigue and depression — that result from not eating and can contribute significantly to hypothermia.

Clothing

In cold climates, outdoorsmen must have clothing that not only protects them from the cold but also can be modified to compensate for changes in temperature and heat production. The best clothing systems for coping with these changes are composed of multiple layers. The outer layers can be opened or removed when the environmental temperature or heat production increases; additional layers can be added as the temperature falls or the person becomes inactive.

For a multilayered clothing system to provide the greatest protection from cold requires attention to two details. First, each succeeding layer must be larger than the one beneath. If the layers are the same size, the outer layers compress the deeper layers and reduce their insulation value. Each layer must be large enough to allow an air space about one-quarter of an inch thick between it and the layer beneath. The outer layer should be windproof. Second, sweating must be avoided as completely as possible. Sweat moistens the clothing, greatly reducing its insulation value. Furthermore, more heat is lost as the perspiration evaporates. The outer layers must be opened or taken off as soon as activity begins, not after the individual has become hot and begun to perspire. The outer layers must be put back on or closed as soon as activity ceases, not after the individual has become cold and requires more heat to warm him again.

Clothing Material

Wool is the oldest and still one of the best insulating materials for cold weather clothing. It is one of the few materials that maintains its insulating properties when wet. Its only disadvantage is its somewhat greater weight.

Down (or more specifically goose down) is the best available insulating material for its weight — when it is dry. When wet, down mats together and loses most of its insulating properties. However, for climates where precipitation is largely in the form of dry snow, which is typical of high altitudes, down provides at least equal insulation and is lighter than the artificial fibers.

Polyester fibers of various types provide insulation similar to down and retain their insulating properties when wet. Their disadvantages are their greater weight (about fifty percent heavier) and their lack of compressability.

Recently, polypropylene has been introduced in a variety of garments, particularly underwear. This material provides a greater sensation of warmth because it "wicks" moisture from the skin to the surface of the fabric where it evaporates without cooling the skin. This material also retains most of its insulating properties when wet.

Hand and Footgear

When the body is cooled, the blood vessels in the hands and feet are constricted, reducing heat loss through those tissues, but also reducing their temperature and commonly causing severe discomfort. The only effective way to prevent cold extremities is to keep the body warm, a lesson many outdoorsmen seem to have great difficulty learning.

For the hands, mittens are much warmer than gloves. Heat is lost from the surface of protective garments; the larger the surface area, the more heat that is lost. Because the fingers are such narrow cylinders, increasing the thickness of gloves to more than one-quarter inch increases the surface area to such an extent that the increased heat loss eliminates any benefit from the increased insulation. Because mittens do not have such a relatively large surface area, their thickness can be increased to a much greater extent without a concomitant increase in heat loss.

One of the warmest types of footgear yet devised is the U.S. Army double vapor barrier boot known as the white Korean boot. However, this type of footwear is too soft for kicking steps in hard snow and is difficult to fit with crampons. Additionally, the rubberized material does not "breathe" and perspiration from the feet can not evaporate. The excessive moisture can lead to maceration of the skin without precautions such as frequently changing to dry socks and using antiperspirants.

Plastic boots do not expand. When constructed with felt liners, which do expand when wet by perspiration, they are hazardous. The combination of an expanding liner and a nonexpanding boot increases the pressure on the foot and lower leg, interferes with the blood flow, and greatly increases the risk of frostbite.

For the severely cold climates typical of high altitudes, double or triple boots are usually worn. The outer boot is usually constructed of a hard, protective material, and the inner boots are made of a softer insulating material. Some double boots have plastic outer boots. Recent studies of climbers on Mount McKinley found that wearers of plastic double boots had a higher incidence of frostbite, which also may reflect the inability of plastic to expand.

Leather, which does breathe and can expand enough to avoid compressing feet and ankles swollen as an effect of altitude (or even just an upright position), still appears to be the most suitable footgear material for climbers in severely cold climates.

Headgear

The large volume of blood that flows to the head makes this part of the body a potential source of major heat loss. Effective headgear, such as wool caps, is essential. Balaclavas, which cover the neck and part of the face, are desirable for severe conditions. Hooded parkas do not fit closely enough to be as effective but do provide additional protection when worn over caps, particularly if the hood is insulated.

RECOGNITION OF HYPOTHERMIA

Awareness of its causes and the rapidity with which it can develop is essential if hypothermia is to be diagnosed at a time when it can be corrected promptly and effectively.

Hypothermia can arbitrarily but conveniently be divided into two forms: mild and severe. A person with mild hypothermia has a low body temperature but is not so incapacitated that he can not stand or walk with assistance. Usually his temperature is above 90 ° F (32 ° C). The victim of severe hypothermia is either unconscious or so disabled that he can not walk and must be evacuated. His body temperature is usually below 90 ° F (32 ° C), although the temperature at which such severe impairment appears may vary several degrees.

Table Six. Stages of Hypothermia

MILD HYPOTHERMIA

98° - 95° F   Sensation of chilliness, skin numbness; minor impairment in muscular per-
37° - 35° C   formance, particularly in fine movements with the hands; shivering begins.

95° - 93° F   More obvious muscle incoordination and weakness; slow stumbling pace;
35° - 34° C   mild confusion and apathy.

93° - 90° F   Gross muscular incoordination with frequent stumbling and falling and in-
34° - 32° C   ability to use hands; mental sluggishness with slow thought and speech;
retrograde amnesia.

SEVERE HYPOTHERMIA

90° - 86° F   Cessation of shivering; severe muscular incoordination with stiffness and
32° - 30° C   inability to walk or stand; incoherence, confusion, irrationality.

86° - 82° F   Severe muscular rigidity; semiconciousness; dilation of pupils; inapparent
30° - 28° C   heart beat or respirations.

Below 82° F   Unconciousness; death due to cessation of heart action.
Below 28° C

Mild Hypothermia

Every member of a climbing party is responsible for recognizing mild hypothermia in other members. The two keys to early recognition are awareness of the possibility for hypothermia and the speed with which it can develop, and close observation of each other by members of the group. A feeling of chilliness is the most typical early symptom. A hiker or climber who feels chilled when he is physically active and generating heat must become colder when that activity ceases unless he is protected from the environment. He can not produce enough heat to warm himself and must have more clothing, shelter, or an external heat source. However, at this stage, a sweater, head covering, or windproof jacket may be all that is needed to prevent more severe hypothermia.

If his body temperature continues to fall, the individual begins to lose muscular coordination. Typically he is unable to perform fine movements with his hands, but if he is hiking and not using his hands, such loss may not be detectable. The first sign of incoordination may be slowing of his pace or stumbling, particularly when crossing rough ground or loose rocks. As hypothermia becomes more severe, stumbling becomes worse and the individual may fall. Characteristically he lags behind, which should provide an unmistakable warning for the rest of his group. If he is left unattended, subsequent deterioration in his condition may go unobserved. Shivering, which usually appears when body temperature has dropped two to four degrees, may further impair his ability to walk over rough terrain.

The intellect is also impaired as hypothermia develops. A common early sign is refusal to admit that anything is wrong. Subsequently the victim becomes apathetic and often is unconcerned about his deteriorating condition. Mental sluggishness may be manifested by slow thought and speech. Confusion and retrograde amnesia subsequently appear and indicate a greater decline in body temperature.

At this point the presence of hypothermia should be obvious, unless the other members of the group are hypothermic also. Failure to take corrective measures could be expected to result in progression to severe hypothermia.

Severe Hypothermia

Severe hypothermia should be defined by the victim's condition, not by a specific body temperature. However, the signs typical of severe hypothermia usually appear when the temperature has fallen to about 90° F (32° C).

As the body temperature approaches this level, shivering gradually disappears, an arbitrary but easily recognizable indicator of severe hypothermia. Muscular incoordination is severe, and the victim usually can not walk without assistance. As his temperature drops further, he becomes unable to even stand without support.

Intellectual impairment is also greater. A common and important sign of severe hypothermia is neglect or carelessness about protection from the cold. Coats (and pants) are left unzipped; hoods are not pulled up; caps or mittens are not worn. Sleeping bags or blankets are not snugged up around the head; fires are neglected. However, mental impairment may be quite subtle. Individuals who seemed to be acting quite sensibly have made gross errors in judgment which have caused problems for the entire group. A pattern typical of hypothermia is the individual who appears to be capable of cooperating with other members of the group but does not do so.

Eventually confusion and irrationality progress to incoherence and semiconsciousness. Finally the victim loses consciousness entirely and, as his temperature continues to drop, becomes totally comatose and does not respond to any stimulus.

As the victim begins to lose consciousness, he may develop a sensation of extreme warmth and, if unattended, may actually remove his clothing or climb out of a sleeping bag. Such bizarre behavior, labeled paradoxical undressing, is relatively common, and individuals unfamiliar with this phenomenon have suspected that the person has been assaulted, particularly when the victim has been female. The real nature of paradoxical undressing should be recognized as a characteristic effect of hypothermia so the victim can be treated.

As the severely hypothermic individual's mental function deteriorates, his other body functions also slow down drastically. Breathing may be so slow and shallow that it appears absent. The heart rate also slows dramatically and can become so weak that it can not be detected.

Unquestionably, a number of individuals in severe hypothermia have been considered dead and have been denied medical assistance when they were actually still alive. No hypothermic individual should be pronounced dead while his body is cold. Only after he has been warmed can death be certain.

No one should be considered cold and dead until he has been warm and dead!!!

TREATMENT OF HYPOTHERMIA

Mild Hypothermia

The treatment of mild hypothermia is relatively simple and easy. Recognizing its presence is usually the most critical aspect. Once an individual has been determined to be hypothermic, a variety of effective corrective measures are usually available. These measures fall into two categories: decreasing heat loss and increasing heat production.

Decreasing heat loss by convection or conduction can be achieved by putting on more clothing: sweaters, caps, mittens, jackets, parkas, windpants, or whatever is available. Replacing wet clothing with dry clothing restores insulation and reduces evaporative heat loss. Protection from the wind by jackets or windpants, rocks or trees, natural shelters such as caves or even crevasses, or manmade shelters such as cabins or snow caves reduces convective heat loss or "wind chill." The warmer environment provided by a fire — or just body heat within a windproof shelter — reduces radiant heat loss.

Heat production is increased by exercise. Vigorous activity that employs large muscles such as those in the legs is most effective. If these muscles can not be used to escape the threatening environment, then movement in place, such as repeatedly stepping up onto stones or a log, can be used to generate heat. A metabolic energy source — food — is also needed if increased heat production is to be maintained effectively for more than a few minutes.

Once hypothermia has been corrected, measures to prevent its recurrence are essential. It should be obvious that thrusting the affected individual back into the same environment with no additional protection would have the same result. Hypothermia would probably recur even faster since his energy stores would have been depleted.

Severe Hypothermia

Severe hypothermia is a much more complex problem for which the simple measures used for mild hypothermia are largely ineffective. The major difficulty is the inability of a victim of severe hypothermia to generate enough heat to rewarm himself. Such individuals are so incapacitated they require assistance just to stand upright. They are not capable of the vigorous exercise required for internal rewarming.

However, rapidly rewarming a severely hypothermic individual with external heat is hazardous. When the body is cooled the blood vessels in the extremities constrict and the circulation of blood falls to very slow rates so that heat can be conserved for the central organs. The stagnant blood in the cold extremities becomes even colder, and its oxygen content falls to very low levels. Metabolism, although greatly reduced, does continue in the hypoxic tissues of the extremities, but in such conditions large quantities of lactic acid and similar products accumulate.

If heat is applied to the extremities, the blood vessels dilate, blood circulation accelerates, and the cold, acidotic blood is returned to the central part of the body. If the central organs, particularly the heart, have not been previously rewarmed, the effects can be disastrous. The cold blood from the extremities further reduces the temperature of the heart while subjecting it to an acid bath. In such circumstances, ventricular fibrillation, an abnormality of heart rhythm during which effective pumping action ceases, is quite common. In a severely hypothermic individual this event is almost always fatal because the chilled heart does not respond to resuscitation. Although the heart is not very sensitive to acidosis at normal temperatures, its sensitivity is greatly increased by hypothermia.

To prevent such accidents, the central organs of the body must be rewarmed first. In hospitals, central rewarming can be accomplished by peritoneal dialysis or "heart-lung machines," but such facilities are not available in a wilderness environment.

Attempts to develop techniques for central rewarming in the field have as yet met with limited success. The most widely publicized method employs inhaled heated air saturated with water vapor to rewarm the blood in the lungs. Actually, the quantity of heat carried by the air is quite small, a reflection of the small amount of heat required to raise the temperature of air (specific heat).

The amount of heat that could be transferred by heated air, according to the most optimistic calculations, is about 200 Calories per hour. However, those calculations are open to question. If the air is not saturated with water, the evaporation of water from the respiratory tract would extract as much or more heat from the body than the heated air could supply. Most of the transfer of heat to the body occurs as the result of condensation of the water vapor when it contacts the cold lung tissues. However, the lung tissues lack bulk and are probably warmed quite promptly, greatly reducing water condensation and heat transfer. Furthermore, the depth and rate of respirations are greatly reduced with severe hypothermia, and the volume of air that would be inhaled may be significantly less than assumed for the calculations.

The value of a system providing only 200 Calories per hour is also questionable. In many — perhaps most — wilderness situations producing severe hypothermia more heat would be lost to the environment. Delaying evacuation to attempt rewarming by this technique would usually result in a further decline in the victim's temperature.

A second problem with severe hypothermia is created by the heart's tendency when cold to develop irregularities of its rhythm, the most significant of which is ventricular fibrillation. The tendency for acidosis to trigger this disorder has been described, but in the presence of severe hypothermia ventricular fibrillation also can be initiated by almost insignificant bumps and jolts. A well documented example was an individual who began fibrillating when he was rolled from his side onto his back on the deck of a boat after being rescued from cold water. A jarring, bouncing stretcher evacuation over rough terrain could be expected to initiate fibrillation more often than not.

The victim of severe hypothermia in a wilderness area may very well be in a hopeless situation. He can not be evacuated smoothly enough to avoid fibrillation, and he can not be rewarmed where he is because facilities for central rewarming are not available and the risk of fibrillation with peripheral rewarming is too great. However, two or three possible solutions are available in most circumstances. The most likely to be successful is evacuation by helicopter. Rewarming should not be attempted before or during transport, although a further decline in body temperature should be prevented.

If a helicopter is not available but evacuation can be accomplished in a few hours, it probably should be attempted, even though travel over rough terrain is required. The hypothermic individual is in a "metabolic icebox" and can often survive several hours of absent or ineffective heart action (fibrillation) without permanent effects, even though an individual with normal temperature suffers irreversible brain damage after five to ten minutes without circulation.

If evacuation requires so much time that the victim's survival is unlikely (more than four to six hours), the only recourse is to try to gradually rewarm the victim where he is. He should be placed in the warmest environment possible, preferably some type of heated shelter, to reduce heat loss. (An environment actually warmer than his body temperature would be almost impossible to achieve.) He also should be insulated as thoroughly as possible, not only to reduce heat loss, but also to promote central rewarming from the limited metabolism taking place in his body. External heat sources, such as hot water bottles or padded, heated stones, should be placed against the sides of his neck, chest, and abdomen. (Body to body contact is not a particularly good source of heat and tends to warm the entire body.) His arms and legs should be insulated but not warmed; they must not be rubbed to promote the flow of blood. If he becomes conscious enough to do so safely, he should be encouraged to drink fluids, particularly warm fluids.

In spite of informed, conscientious efforts, most severe hypothermia victims can not be effectively cared for in the wilderness. Many do not survive even when hospitalized. Hypothermia is to be avoided, not treated!

FROSTBITE

Frostbite is a cold injury produced by freezing of the tissues. The hands and feet, which are farthest from the heart and have a more tenuous blood supply, and the face and ears, which are usually exposed, are most commonly affected.

Constriction of blood vessels in the extremities to conserve heat for the central portions of the body can be so severe that circulation to those areas almost ceases. Cold also damages the capillaries in the affected areas, causing plasma to leak through their walls. The fluid within the tissues interferes with the exchange of oxygen and nutrients, and its loss causes the blood to sludge inside the vessels, further impairing circulation.

As the circulation becomes severely impaired, the skin and superficial tissues exposed to severe cold begin to freeze. With continued cooling, the frozen area enlarges and extends to deeper levels. Ice crystals form within and between the cells and grow by extracting water from the cells. The cells are injured physically by the ice crystals, as well as by dehydration and the resulting disruption of osmotic and chemical balance.

Prevention

Frostbite can occur in any environment in which the temperature is below freezing but is usually associated with hypothermia and impaired circulation. The hypothermia associated with frostbite is no different from hypothermia occurring alone, and its causes, prevention, and treatment are the same. Impairment of the circulation is most often caused by boots that are too tight. Encircling, tight fitting garments also compromise circulation, but boots are the most common offenders, particularly plastic boots which can not expand as the wearer's feet swell or as the lining absorbs perspiration and expands.

Frostbite is best prevented by avoiding the conditions by which it is produced. Prevention of hypothermia has already been described. However, clothing that keeps the trunk warm also keeps the extremities warm by eliminating the need for blood vessel constriction to preserve heat. "If your feet are cold, put on a sweater," is excellent advice. Also essential is footgear that does not constrict the circulation.

Cigarette smoking constricts the blood vessels in the skin and may aggravate local cold injuries such as frostbite.

Diagnosis and Prognosis

The typical early signs of frostbite are sensations of cold or pain and pallor of the affected skin. However, some victims may suffer little pain, and pain typically disappears as the tissues begin to freeze. As freezing progresses, the tissues usually become even whiter in appearance and all sensation is lost. With deep frostbite the tissues become quite hard. An entire hand or foot and lower leg may be involved, and with such extensive frostbite the tissues often have a dull purple color instead of being pale.

Frostbite of the face, tip of the nose, or ears can be recognized by pain and the pallor of the affected tissues.

The extent and severity of frostbite are notoriously difficult to judge accurately during the early stages, particularly while the tissues are still frozen. After thawing some prognostic signs appear. With minor frostbite, which only involves the tips of the fingers or toes, or a small area of the ears, nose, or face, the tissues may only be red for a few days after thawing. With more severe injuries, blisters commonly develop after rewarming and may cover entire fingers or toes. If the blisters contain clear fluid, the underlying tissues are usually still alive and can be expected to recover almost completely. When the blisters are filled with bloody fluid, portions of the underlying tissues are usually dead and can not recover. The most severe frostbite injuries are not followed by blisters, probably because the circulation to the tissues is too poor. Such tissues commonly retain a deep purple color.

After a week or longer the dead frostbitten tissues develop a thick black covering called an "eschar." With time, usually weeks or months, the dead tissue, including entire fingers or toes, usually separates spontaneously. Surgery is usually required only for reconstruction of hands or feet, or occasionally to complete separation of these larger structures.

Treatment

The preferred treatment for frostbite is rapid rewarming in a relatively large water bath. Treatment should be administered in a hospital where facilities for optimal rewarming and sterile supplies for later care are available. Treatment in a wilderness environment should be attempted only when the following conditions can be met:

1. The victim can be kept warm during rewarming and afterwards for as long as recovery requires.
2. Adequate facilities for prompt rewarming, including abundant supplies of warm water and accurate methods for maintaining the temperature of the rewarming bath, are available.
3. The victim does not need to use the frostbitten extremity until healing is complete. More specifically, the victim does not need to walk on a foot that has been frostbitten and thawed.

If the patient's body is cold, the blood vessels in his extremities are constricted. Rewarming frostbitten extremities in such circumstances can leave badly injured tissues without an adequate blood supply at the time it is most needed. However, the greatest tissue damage occurs when frostbitten tissues are thawed and then refrozen. Far less damage is produced by walking on a frostbitten foot.

A particularly difficult situation may be encountered when a climber with frostbite descends from the ice and snow of the high Himalayas or Andes to the tropical climate at the base of many of these peaks. In such circumstances, prevention of slow thawing of frozen tissues may be impossible. Probably the least tissue damage would result from rapid rewarming, even if optimal facilities are not available. The climber would subsequently have to be carried to a site where motorized transportation was available.

During rewarming, the water temperature should be maintained between 100° and 108° F (38° and 42° C). Higher temperatures further damage the tissues; the water must not be hot enough to feel uncomfortable to an uninjured person's hand. A large water bath permits more accurate control of the temperature and also warms the frozen extremity more rapidly, often resulting in less tissue loss, particularly when freezing has been deep and extensive.

During rewarming, hot water must be added to the bath periodically to keep the temperature at the desired level. (A frozen hand or foot is essentially a block of ice and does tend to cool the water.) The injured extremity should be removed from the bath and not returned until the water has been thoroughly mixed and the temperature measured. An open flame must not be used to keep the water bath warm. The frostbitten extremity may come in contact with the heated area and be seriously burned because sensation in the tissues has been lost.

For rewarming, the extremity should be stripped of all clothing and any constricting bands, straps, or other objects that might impair the circulation. The injured member should be suspended in the center of the water bath and not permitted to rest against the side or bottom. Warming usually requires thirty to sixty minutes and should be continued until the tissues are soft and pliable. During rewarming, the frostbitten tissues usually become quite painful. Aspirin and codeine, or morphine or meperidine if needed, may be given during rewarming or afterward for pain.

Following rewarming, the patient must be kept warm and the injured tissues must be elevated and protected from any kind of trauma or irritation. Sleeping bags or bedclothes should be supported by a framework to avoid pressure or rubbing on the injured area. Every effort should be made to avoid rupturing blisters, which invites infection.

The victim should be evacuated immediately. Healing requires weeks to months, depending upon the extent of the injury. Subsequent care in the field should be directed primarily toward preventing infection. Cleanliness of the frostbitten area is extremely important. Soaking the extremity each day in disinfected, lukewarm water to which a germicidal soap has been added may be helpful. A small amount of dry, sterile cotton may be placed between fingers or toes to avoid maceration. Antibiotics should not be given routinely, but if infection appears to be present, ampicillin or cloxicillin should be administered every six hours until a physician's care is obtained.

Smoking should be strictly prohibited because it reduces the already deficient blood supply to the damaged area. Movement of the extremities should be encouraged but should be limited to movements that can be carried out without assistance from others or manipulation by the patient. Most frostbite victims need continuing reassurance and emotional support.

Individuals who have suffered frostbite usually have increased sensitivity to cold and are more susceptible to cold injury because the blood vessels in the injured tissues have been permanently damaged.

IMMERSION FOOT

Immersion foot (or "trenchfoot") is a form of cold injury that is more of a problem for military personnel than for climbers or hikers. However, its effects can be just as devastating as frostbite. In the Falkland Islands fighting fourteen percent (70 of 516) of the hospitalized British battle casualties had immersion injuries. Furthermore, only soldiers with the most severe injuries were hospitalized; the number with lesser injuries was so far greater that a precise count could not be made.

Immersion foot results from exposure to cold water for prolonged periods of time. The cold induces intense vasoconstriction, which deprives the feet of an adequate blood supply. After a period of days or weeks permanent damage results, particularly to the nerves, and can be so painful that amputation is required. Sensitivity to cold is usually life long.

Prevention of this injury requires avoidance of prolonged immersion in cold water, which may not be possible in some battlefield situations. However, actual immersion in water is not required. Cold, wet socks and boots can produce this injury, and socks can usually be changed daily, even on a battlefield. Opportunities to dry boots and socks can usually be provided, but officers and their subordinates must be aware of the need for such precautions to avoid real casualties.

Climbers and hikers also must be aware of the potential for developing cold injuries in wet, nonfreezing weather. They must carry dry socks and must take time to change their socks and to dry their feet and boots when circumstances demand. Certainly their activities do not place the restraints upon such precautions that warfare does.

CHAPTER FOURTEEN

Heat and Solar Injuries

INJURY BY SOLAR RADIATION

Sunlight is beneficial to health and plays a major role in Vitamin D synthesis, but many harmful effects can be produced by excessive exposure. Sunburn is well recognized; less well known are the long term effects of repeated overexposure that produces degenerative changes in the skin that can eventually lead to cancer. Every year in the United States 300,000 new cases of skin cancer are diagnosed and that number is increasing.

In the spectrum of solar radiation much of the energy is of shorter wavelength (ultraviolet) or longer wavelength (infrared) than visible light. Most biologic damage is caused by ultraviolet radiation of wavelengths less than 400 nanometers (nm). (1 centimeter $= 10^7$ nanometers $= 10^8$ Ångstroms.)

Ultraviolet exposure in mountaineering may be much greater than at sea level. At high altitudes the atmosphere is thinner and filters out less sunlight, particularly in the harmful wavelengths. In addition, snowfields and glaciers reflect about seventy-five percent of the incident ultraviolet radiation, and climbers or skiers are exposed to reflected as well as direct rays of the sun. Under certain conditions, such as in a cirque or bowl, reflection can increase the radiation even more. Wind may also increase the harmful effects of ultraviolet radiation.

Even when a climber is shielded from the direct rays of the sun, much ultraviolet radiation can still reach him due to atmospheric scattering. This "sky radiation" may contribute half of the total ultraviolet radiation and tends to be greater when high, thin cirrus clouds are present. Indeed, total ultraviolet radiation may even be greater on an overcast day than on a cloudless day. Such radiation can be particularly dangerous since it is so inapparent.

Sailors, like mountaineers, are exposed to large amounts of direct radiation and large quantities (up to 100 percent) of reflected radiation. The recent popularity of high altitude board sailing on lakes near ski resorts has resulted in even greater ultraviolet exposures.

Two-thirds of the day's ultraviolet radiation is received during the four hours in the middle of the day; protection from solar injury is most essential during this interval.

SUNBURN

Individuals vary considerably in their sensitivity to sunlight. Redheads particularly and blue eyed blondes are more susceptible to sunburn than brunettes. Individuals of northern European ancestry are more sensitive than Mediterranean, Indian, black, or other peoples whose skin contains more of the dark protective pigment melanin. Children are more susceptible than adults.

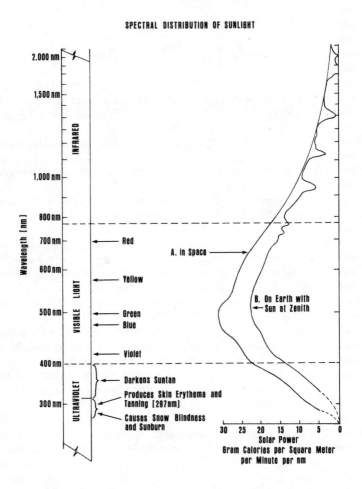

Figure 39. Quantity of light of different wavelengths in sunlight.

Sensitivity to sunlight may be increased by many drugs including sulfonamides and their derivatives such as trimethoprim-sulfamethoxazole (Bactrim and Septra); oral antidiabetic agents; the phenothiazine tranquilizers (Thorazine, Compazine, Phenergan, and Sparine); thiazide diuretics (Diuril); most tetracyclines, particularly doxycycline (Vibramycin) which has been recommended for preventing traveller's diarrhea; and the barbiturates. The many other substances increasing sensitivity to sunlight include biothionol, which is used in soaps, many first aid creams, and cosmetics; green soap; many plants and grasses such as fig leaf, certain meadow grasses, wild parsnip, celery, and others; certain dyes used in lipstick; and coal tar or coal tar derivatives.

Excessive exposure to ultraviolet radiation of 290 to 320 nm, the "B" band, damages the superficial skin layers. Mildly excessive exposure produces redness and slight swelling; more prolonged exposure tends to cause pain and blistering. Severe burns may be associated with chills, fever, or headache. Sunburn of the lips is often followed by painful *Herpes simplex* infections ("fever blisters" or "cold sores"), which may cover most of the surface of the lips.

Longer ultraviolet wavelengths in the range of 320 to 420 nm, the "E" band, increase pigmentation and also increase the thickness of the outer layer (corneum) of the skin. The resulting suntan has a protective value because the increased pigment and the thickened skin markedly reduce the penetration of harmful ultraviolet radiation.

Prevention

The best way to prevent sunburn is through gradually increasing exposure to sunlight, which permits natural tanning and thickening of the skin. For many redheads and some other light skinned individuals adequate tanning is impossible. Such persons may benefit from the use of trioxsalen (Trisoralen), but this is a potent drug which must be taken only under the close supervision of a physician, preferably a dermatologist.

Protective creams or lotions are the most convenient methods for protecting exposed skin from sunlight. They should be applied liberally and frequently, particularly when sweating or wiping the neck and face tends to remove the preparation. The nose, cheeks, neck, and ears are most frequently sunburned; the lower surfaces of the nose and chin are commonly burned by reflected radiation, particularly on snow, and should not be neglected.

Products currently marketed in the United States for use with sun exposure fall into three different groups. The preparations that contain no sunscreens and provide no protection at all from ultraviolet radiation appear to have been generally recognized to have only cosmetic value and to have fallen in popularity. Baby oil, mineral oil, olive oil, lanolin, and coconut oil are among the products in this category.

The largest group of preparations are those containing effective sunscreens that filter out ultraviolet radiation of the skin damaging wavelengths (290 to 320 nm) but allow radiation of longer wavelengths to pass through and produce tanning. The most effective of these sunscreens is para-aminobenzoic acid (PABA). A solution of five percent PABA in fifty to seventy percent ethanol provides excellent protection from sunburn. PABA sunscreens stay on longer than other products when exposed to moisture from sweating or swimming. However, on clothing these products may leave a yellow stain that is not removed by washing. Esters of PABA also provide good protection from sunburn and do not stain clothing. These products also resist moisture fairly well, although they are more easily removed than nonesterified PABA sunscreens.

Rarely PABA products cause contact dermatitis (see Chapter Twenty-Four, "Allergies"); individuals allergic to thiazides or sulfa drugs may also be allergic to PABA or PABA esters.

A sun protection factor (SPF) system used in Europe for many years has recently been adopted in the United States. The SPF scale runs from two (minimal sun protection) to fifteen (almost complete sun screening) and provides an approximate indication of the effectiveness of different products. The SPF number indicates how much longer an individual can tolerate direct sunlight when protected by that product than he could with no protection at all.

Individual tolerance to sunlight has been crudely calibrated in terms of the amount of sun exposure required to just redden the skin — the minimal erythemal dose, or MED. About four times the MED causes painful sunburn; about eight times the MED produces blistering. A product with an SPF of four permits a person with a MED of twenty minutes to tolerate exposure for eighty minutes before turning red.

A comparable system has also been used to classify skin types. These skin categories and characteristics, along with recommended sun protection, are listed in Table Seven.

The third group of protective agents are those that block out all ultraviolet radiation. The best known contain opaque pigments such as titanium dioxide (A-Fil) or zinc oxide (Zincofax Cream). Red Veterinary Petrolatum (R.V.P., Paul B. Elder Co.) is also a very effective sunscreen. Such agents are used on the nose, lips, ears, or similar areas which tend to become easily sunburned and are not covered by clothing. (Products containing benzophenones, such as Uval and Solbar, also screen out all ultraviolet radiation but are easily removed by sweating. Such agents were developed primarily for individuals with skin diseases that require such complete protection.)

Treatment

If prevention has been neglected or has been inadequate, application of cold, wet dressings soaked in a boric acid solution (one teaspoonful per quart of water) or a one to fifty solution of aluminum acetate may relieve discomfort. Soothing

Table Seven. Skin Types and Recommended Sun Protection

Skin Type	Sunburning and Tanning Qualities	Other Characteristics	Recommended Protection (SPF)
I	Burns Easily, Never Tans	Red or Blonde Hair, Blue Eyes, Freckles	8-15
II	Burns Easily, Tans Minimally	Red or Blonde Hair, Blue Eyes, Freckles	6-12
III	Burns Moderately, Tans Slowly to Light Brown	Red or Blonde Hair, Blue Eyes, Freckles	4-8
IV	Burns Minimally, Tans to Moderate Brown	Darker Coloration	2-6
V	Rarely Burns, Tans to Dark Brown	Darker Coloration	2-4
VI	Never Burns	Deeply Pigmented	None

creams may be helpful if swelling is not severe. Anesthetic sprays or ointments (Solarcaine) are effective but carry a significant risk of allergic reactions. Steroid preparations, such as one-quarter percent hydrocortisone ointment or an aerosol spray containing prednisolone such as Meti-Derm, are helpful in reducing inflammation if applied early. However, steroid preparations must be used sparingly. Reducing the inflammation may reduce pain, but probably slows the processes of healing and repair and may increase susceptibility to infection. Extensive or unusually severe sunburn may have to be treated as a second degree burn.

SKIN CANCER

Repeated sun exposure over a period of many years produces degenerative changes which commonly lead to cancer in the skin of individuals who are not darkly pigmented. These changes are cosmetically unattractive and demand vigilance in order to detect tumors when they are small and can be easily treated. (Most skin cancers do not have the lethal potential of cancer in other organs, partially because they are more easily detectable.) Degenerative skin changes are particularly prone to occur in persons who work out of doors such as farmers. Tanning probably provides some protection because dark skinned individuals can tolerate prolonged sunlight exposure without developing such changes, but the protection is minor and clearly incomplete.

Individuals who spend much of their time in sunlight can probably reduce the severity of such changes by conscientiously applying sunscreens whenever they are exposed, regardless of the risk of sunburn. Light skinned persons who are frequently on ski slopes, mountains, or water must be particularly careful to use such protection.

SNOW BLINDNESS

The surface of the eye (cornea and conjunctiva) absorbs ultraviolet radiation just like the skin. Excessive exposure can result in sunburn of these tissues, producing snow blindness (photophthalmia). Any source of ultraviolet radiation, including the sun, ultraviolet lamps, and electric welding equipment, may produce photophthalmia. During the period of exposure no sensation other than the brightness of the light serves to warn the victim. Symptoms may not develop until as much as eight to twelve hours later. The eyes initially feel simply irritated or dry, but as symptoms progress, they feel as though they are full of sand. Moving or blinking the eyes becomes extremely painful. Even exposure to light may cause pain. Swelling of the eyelids, redness of the eyes, and excessive tearing may occur. A severe case of snow blindness may be completely disabling for several days and may even lead to ulceration of the cornea, permanently damaging the eye.

Prevention

Snow blindness can and should be completely prevented by the consistent use of proper goggles or sunglasses. Any lens transmitting less than ten percent of the erythemal band of sunlight (below 320 nm) is satisfactory. Glasses should be large and curved or have side covers to block most of the reflected light coming from below and from the sides. Under severe radiation conditions, such as a concave high altitude snowfield, goggles are safer, even though they may be less comfortable and tend to fog. If only glasses are available, a sunscreen should be applied to the eyelids to prevent burning. Spare goggles or glasses should be carried, but emergency lenses can be made of cardboard with a thin slit or pin hole to see through. The eyes may be covered alternately so that only one eye at a time is exposed to the sunlight.

Eye protection is just as necessary on a cloudy or overcast day as it is in full sunlight. Snow blindness can even be produced during a snowstorm if the cloud cover is thin.

Treatment

Snow blindness heals spontaneously in a few days. The pain, which may be quite severe, may be relieved temporarily by cold compresses and a dark environment. Early and frequent (hourly) applications of an ophthalmic ointment or drops containing cortisone or some other anti-inflammatory steroid also help relieve the pain, lessen the inflammatory reaction, and shorten the course of the illness. The patient must not rub his eyes. Local anesthetics should not be employed because they rapidly lose their effectiveness and may lead to damage of the delicate corneal surface.

HEAT ILLNESS

The normal human body temperature is maintained in a relatively narrow range by sensitive control of the balance between heat produced or absorbed by the body and heat lost to the environment. Normal temperature is between 97° and 100° F (36° and 38° C). The widely accepted "normal" temperature of 98.6° F (37° C) is only an average; individual temperatures vary as much as 2° to 3° F (1° to 1.7° C) during each twenty-four hour period.

Heat illness results from the inability to dissipate heat produced within the body. (Some heat is absorbed from the atmosphere or from other sources in a hot climate, but the quantity is small compared to that produced by metabolism.) Most individuals generate between 2,000 to 5,000 kilocalories of heat per day, depending upon their size, physical activity, and state of nutrition, mostly through muscular activity. The body must get rid of this heat to prevent an increase in its temperature which, if severe, could have devastating effects. (If he did not lose any metabolic heat, in twenty-four hours an average sized individual [154 lbs or 70 kg] with an average metabolic rate [3,500 kilocalories per day] would increase his body temperature to approximately 190° F [88° C], the boiling temperature of water at 13,000 feet [4,000 m]!)

Humans lose heat largely through their skin. (Heat is also lost through the lungs, but only in small amounts in temperate or hot climates. At high altitudes more rapid, deep breathing of cold, relatively dry air can lead to significant heat loss which can contribute to hypothermia. The lungs are the principal route of heat loss [by panting] for many animals.)

The skin acts much like the radiator of a liquid cooled automobile engine. Blood is warmed as it passes through exercising muscles or other tissues in which heat generating metabolism takes place, just as the liquid circulating around the cylinders of an engine is warmed. When the warmed blood circulates through the skin, heat is lost to the surrounding atmosphere just as heat is lost from the radiator of an automobile engine. The thermostat on the engine increases the flow of coolant through the radiator when the engine is hot, and comparable mechanisms dilate the cutaneous blood vessels when heat must be lost, increasing blood flow to the skin and elevating the rate of heat loss.

However, a typical automobile radiator is cooled only by air passing over it.

Skin also loses heat this way (convection), and some heat may be lost by conduction if the individual is in contact with water, snow, or rock. However, by far the largest avenue of heat loss from the skin in a hot climate is through the evaporation of perspiration.

Perspiration greatly cools the skin as it evaporates because such a large amount of heat is required to change water from a liquid to a vapor. The evaporation of one cubic centimeter (1 cc) of perspiration requires about 580 calories, enough to reduce the temperature of approximately 1,000 cc of blood 1 ° F (or 580 cc of blood 1 ° C). Most of this heat is extracted from the skin (or respiratory passages.) In practical terms, the evaporation of 500 cc of water in the form of perspiration can remove a bit over 200 kilocalories of heat, which is about two-thirds the amount of heat produced during one hour of moderate exercise.

The maximal sweating rate for individuals not acclimatized to heat is about 1,500 cc per hour. Acclimatization takes about one week, results in an increased tolerance for exercise in a hot environment, and is produced by mechanisms that increase the maximum sweating rate but reduce salt loss. Water deprivation does not accelerate or contribute to the acclimatization process.

Preventing Heat Illness

Almost all heat injuries can be prevented by two measures: consuming adequate (generous) quantities of water and salt; and recognizing conditions (high humidity and temperature) in which heat can not be dissipated and sharply curtailing physical activity in those conditions.

An active climber produces heat at the rate of several hundred kilocalories or more per hour. If he is in a hot environment, he may also be absorbing heat. In such circumstances the only possible avenue of heat loss is through the evaporation of moisture from the body surface. Staggering amounts of water and salt can be lost through perspiration under severe conditions. Sustained maximal exercise such as distance running can generate as much as 1,000 kilocalories per hour, which is equivalent to the heat lost through evaporation of 1,500 to 2,000 cc of perspiration. Fluid and electrolyte replacement is vitally important under such conditions. The only alternative is dehydration and an increase in body temperature (both of which commonly occur in distance runners).

The magnitude of the fluid and salt requirements under such severe conditions is illustrated by the precautions taken during military exercises. During U.S. Army maneuvers in the deserts of southern California in which temperatures of 100 ° to 110° F (38 ° to 43 ° C) were expected, participants were required to drink eight liters of water and to take three to five grams of extra salt every day. Israeli soldiers operating in the Sinai Desert during the battles with Egypt were alloted ten liters of water a day.

Thirst or hunger for salt alone do not provide an adequate intake. A conscious effort to consume the needed quantities is essential. During desert operations, military personnel in command positions are held responsible for ensuring their men meet the daily intake requirements.

If the atmosphere is hot and humidity so high that evaporation is greatly retarded, heat loss is slow or nonexistent. In the southeastern United States, where such conditions are common in the summer, experienced residents know that a man dripping with perspiration is in danger of heat illness. If the perspiration were evaporating and cooling him, it would not accumulate in such quantities on his body surface. In such conditions, the only way to avoid heat illness is to get out of the sun and stop all vigorous physical activity. The image of the languid Southerner, although inaccurate, clearly has a basis in physiologic necessity.

Wearing plastic or rubberized suits while exercising in a hot climate in order to lose weight is a hazardous practice. Such suits increase body temperature during physical activity because they do not allow perspiration to evaporate. Fortunately, this danger has become more generally recognized in recent years.

Other factors also increase the risk of heat injury. More susceptible to heat illness are elderly or very young persons and individuals with skin diseases that interfere with heat loss or sweating, hyperthyroidism, cardiovascular disorders, chronic diseases such as diabetes, or fever produced by infections. Drugs such as amphetamines and LSD as well as a number of agents that are not commonly abused have been implicated in heat stroke deaths.

Causes of Hyperthermia

An elevated body temperature (hyperthermia) can result from many conditions. Most common is the fever that accompanies infections and some other disorders. This form of hyperthermia results from a biochemical change in the body's temperature control mechanism which sets the "thermostat" at a higher level. A fever can be controlled quite well with drugs such as aspirin, but the best treatment is that needed for the underlying condition.

The inability to dissipate heat leads to hyperthermia that has been labelled "heat illness." Strenuous exercise increases the body temperature whenever heat production exceeds heat loss. Distance runners commonly develop temperatures as high as $104\,°F\,(40\,°C)$ during a race. If they are well hydrated and acclimatized to heat, their temperature usually returns to normal shortly after the race and no illness develops, but heat illness is common in distance runners. When exercise is carried to an extreme, or when moderate exercise is carried out in an extreme environment (hot and humid), particularly by individuals who have not maintained their fluid and salt balance and are not acclimatized to the heat, heat illness results. This type of heat illness is called "exertional hyperthermia."

The most frequent causes of exertional hyperthermia in the United States have been distance running (including jogging) and football practice in late summer, which combines vigorous physical activity, a uniform that inhibits evaporation of sweat, and a hot, often humid environment. Fatigue and lack of sleep also are significant factors predisposing to the development of heat illness.

Another type of heat illness occurs in some individuals, particularly the elderly, debilitated, or chronically ill, as the result of defective temperature regulation. Typically such patients have inadequate or absent sweating mechanisms, although dehydration commonly plays a contributing role. As a result, they are not able to dissipate the heat generated by their metabolism, meager though it may be.

Drugs such as aspirin are not effective for the treatment of heat illness and should not be administered because they increase the bleeding tendency which is a common complication of heat stroke.

TYPES OF HEAT ILLNESS

Heat illnesses of different severity form a spectrum, ranging from very mild to lethal injuries. Typical patterns of illness have been given specific names, but the various types of heat injury merge imperceptibly with each other and all must be recognized as different manifestations of the same basic disorder. Mild heat illnesses always have the potential for becoming severe and must be carefully treated.

Heat Syncope and Heat Exhaustion

Heat syncope and heat exhaustion are two similar, relatively mild forms of heat illness which result from physical exertion in a hot environment. Dehydration resulting from inadequate fluid replacement contributes significantly. In an effort to increase heat loss the blood vessels in the skin dilate to such an extent that the blood supply for the brain is reduced. A reduction in blood volume due to dehydration contributes to the diminished cerebral blood flow. The result is a disorder very similar to fainting. The victim feels faint and is usually aware of a rapid heart rate. Nausea, vomiting, headache, dizziness, restlessness, or even brief loss of consciousness are not uncommon. The presence of sweating and the skin color are variable.

These two disorders have been separated on the basis of body temperature, which is normal with syncope but elevated to 102° to 104° F (39° to 40° C) with heat exhaustion. (No sharp division between heat exhaustion and heat stroke is possible, and some physicians would consider anyone with an elevated temperature, particularly when associated with signs of brain dysfunction such as dizziness or brief unconsciousness, to have heat stroke.)

Heat syncope should be treated just like fainting. If the individual recognizes preliminary symptoms such as dizziness or weakness, he should lie down, or at least sit down, to avoid injury. His feet should be elevated. He should try to get to a cooler environment and should at least be protected from direct sunlight. He should be given fluids, particularly fluids containing salt, and should not engage in vigorous activity for at least the rest of that day. Only after he has completely restored his body fluids and salt and has a normal urinary output should he cautiously resume exercise in a hot environment.

An individual with heat exhaustion should be treated in the same way but in addition must have his body temperature closely monitored. If his temperature goes above 104° F (40° C) he should be actively cooled as described for heat stroke. Victims of heat exhaustion probably have an even greater fluid and salt deficit, which must be corrected. Such persons must be very careful about resuming physical activity and probably should be examined by a physician beforehand.

Heat Stroke

Heat stroke (also called "sunstroke") is a more severe form of heat illness. Fatalities sometimes occur, and permanent residual disability is relatively common. Young, previously healthy victims most commonly have been exercising in a hot, humid atmosphere. Older victims with chronic diseases may not have been exercising.

The onset typically is very rapid and is characterized by changes in mental function. Confusion and irrational behavior are most frequent, but incoordination, delirium, and unconsciousness often follow. Convulsions occur rather commonly. The pupils may be dilated and unresponsive to light. Some investigators think any alteration or loss of consciousness under conditions of heat stress should be considered heat stroke.

The rectal temperature is almost always above 104° F (40° C) and is commonly above 107° (42° C). The skin feels hot. (If the temperature is not measured for some time after the onset of the illness, it may have fallen. A rectal thermometer reading to 113° F (45° C) is usually needed to measure such temperatures and rarely would be carried by climbers unless severe heat stress had been anticipated, in which case effective preventive measures should have been employed.)

If the victim has been actively exercising, he is often covered with perspiration. The hot, dry skin long associated with heat stroke is more typical of individuals with deranged temperature regulation than those with exertional heat illness. However, sweating does decrease with time during exercise and can fall to quite small volumes, particularly when exercise has been prolonged and the individual has become dehydrated and salt depleted. Young victims of exertional heat stroke may have dry skin.

Both pulse and respiratory rates are increased. The faster pulse may represent an effort to pump more blood to the skin to increase heat loss, and faster breathing may be an effort to increase heat loss through the lungs. Shock is usually present.

The treatment for heat stroke should be instituted as rapidly as possible. **Heat stroke is one of the few true medical emergencies.** Any delay often increases the residual disability. If the patient is unconscious, an open airway must be maintained. Shock should be treated by elevating the feet and any other methods that are feasible.

Efforts to lower the body temperature should be started immediately. The victim should be moved to a cooler spot as rapidly as possible, or he should at least be shaded from bright sunlight. His clothing should be removed and his body fanned to increase air circulation and evaporation. If possible, the extremities and trunk should be covered with cool, wet cloths or towels. Immersion in cool (but not icy) water is also useful. Any reasonable method for cooling the victim should be employed.

Ice packs or ice cold water tend to make the blood vessels in the skin constrict and may actually delay cooling. They also can cause cold injuries. Water that is cool but not cold is more effective. Sponging with alcohol should be limited. Alcohol, particularly isopropyl alcohol, may be absorbed through the skin, especially by children.

During cooling, the extremities should be massaged vigorously to help propel the cooled blood back into the organs of the body and head. Oxygen should be administered if available.

After the temperature has been reduced to 102° F (39° C), active cooling should be slowed to avoid hypothermia, but the patient must be closely monitored to ensure his temperature does not climb back to higher levels. Rebound is particularly common three to four hours after cooling. Aspirin is not effective, may aggravate complications, and should not be administered.

As soon as possible the victim should be evacuated to a hospital, particularly if he has been unconscious for more than a few minutes. The complications of heat stroke are numerous, are often severe, and include kidney failure, liver failure, blood clotting abnormalities, gastrointestinal ulceration with bleeding, heart damage, biochemical alterations, and extensive brain damage. Unconsciousness of more than two hours duration is a poor prognostic sign which is usually followed by permanent disability.

Muscle Cramps

Muscle cramps are severe, spasmodic contractions of one or more muscles, most commonly the leg muscles. Cramps may last up to fifteen minutes or even longer, and the muscles are usually painful for several days afterward.

Cramps usually can be stopped almost immediately by stretching the muscle. For example, the calf muscle can be stretched by extending the leg and pulling the foot upward toward the body. Kneading or pounding the muscle is less effective and probably contributes to the residual soreness.

Cramps usually appear in the most heavily worked muscles and may be produced, in part, by an excessive water intake without accompanying salt, resulting in dilution of the salt in the extracellular fluid. Cramps are more common in circumstances that tend to cause salt depletion and can be prevented to a large extent by consuming large quantities of salt and water.

ADDITIONAL READING
1. McElroy CR. Update on heat illness. *Topics Emer Med* 1980;2:1-18.

CHAPTER FIFTEEN

Animal Bites and Stings

The danger of infection following the bite of any animal is very great. The mouths of all animals — including humans — contain numerous bacteria which are introduced into the wound at the time the bite is inflicted. Human bites tend to produce particularly virulent infections.

All bite wounds should be treated as contaminated soft tissue injuries. The wound should be washed with copious quantities of soap and water, after which an antimicrobial agent such as povidone-iodine (Betadine and others) or aqueous benzalkonium chloride (Zephiran) should be poured into the wound, particularly if the bite was inflicted by a possibly rabid animal. Under no circumstances should the wound be sutured. It must be left open and a sterile dressing should be applied. The patient must be watched closely for evidence of infection.

RABIES

Rabies is a viral infection transmitted by infected animals. The catastrophic effects result from infection of the brain (encephalitis). Rabies has been known and deservedly feared since antiquity. Until recently, not a single human patient with proven rabies had ever survived. Within recent years, a few people have survived fully developed rabies infections, but they have had severe residual brain damage.

Within the United States, human rabies has been controlled to a large extent by vaccinating domestic animals. Dog rabies diminished from over 5,000 cases in 1946 to just 180 in 1973. Human rabies has concomitantly declined from more than twenty cases a year in the 1940s to less than two cases a year in the 1970s. Now almost all confirmed animal rabies is in wildlife, primarily skunks, foxes, bats, and raccoons.

Rabies occurs in few rodents. Bites by rats, mice, chipmunks, squirrels, rabbits, or other rodents have rarely been proven to produce human rabies. However, bat rabies is endemic in all areas of the continental United States, both urban and rural, and poses a threat to cavers.

Outside the United States, Canada, and Western Europe, particularly in underdeveloped countries, vaccination of domestic animals for rabies is almost nonexistent. The risk of contracting rabies from pets or other animals in these areas is much higher.

Essentially all carnivorous animals are susceptible to rabies and capable of transmitting the infection. The virus appears to travel along nerves at a relatively constant speed to reach the brain. Bites at the ends of the extremities allow more time for obtaining treatment than bites about the face, which are particularly dangerous and must be treated urgently.

In an infected animal, the virus involves the salivary glands and is present in the saliva. Transmission of the infection occurs when a wound is contaminated with the saliva of the rabid animal. The virus can not penetrate intact skin but can pass through an intact mucous membrane such as the lining of the mouth, nose, or eyelids. The infection can be transmitted by licking without a bite having been inflicted. Infection has been transmitted by breathing aerosolized rabies virus in a medical laboratory and probably can be transmitted by breathing the air in caves inhabited by rabid bats.

Diagnosis

If rabies is to be prevented, it must be recognized (or assumed to be present) in the attacking animal so the human victim can be immunized before symptoms develop. Treatment begun after the victim begins to show signs of rabies is almost always ineffective.

One of the most reliable ways to diagnose rabies in an attacking animal is to confine it under observation for ten days following the bite. If the animal is healthy at the end of that time, it almost certainly did not have transmissible rabies at the time the bite was inflicted. If the animal can not be captured alive and is killed or dies in captivity, the diagnosis of rabies is usually made by shipping the head (under refrigeration) to an appropriate laboratory, where the brain is examined to determine whether the rabies virus is present. Within the United States, public health services generally are responsible for transporting the head to a central, reliable laboratory. Facilities in underdeveloped countries may not be so dependable.

If the animal can not be killed or captured, it should be assumed to be rabid, except in those few areas where rabies does not occur. (Hawaii, as an example, is considered to be free of all forms of wildlife rabies. All animals brought into the islands are quarantined for prolonged periods, regardless of their vaccination history, to prevent the introduction of this infection.)

Within the continental United States almost all small wild animal bites should be considered to have been inflicted by a rabid animal, particularly if the animal was behaving in an unusual manner, such as acting friendly instead of fleeing. In contrast, for bites by normally behaving pet dogs or cats that have been previously vaccinated and that can be captured after the bite has been inflicted, treatment can be withheld safely while the animal is held in captivity for a period of ten days.

Rabies in animals follows a highly variable course. The well known "mad dog" foaming at the mouth is almost never seen. Unprovoked attacks are the most common indication of rabies. (Bites incurred while feeding an unknown animal are considered provoked.) Occasionally the only outward sign of rabies is a lack of fear of man, which may even appear to be a show of friendliness. Animals such as skunks, which usually scurry away from any threatening situation, may actually pursue a supposed attacker.

Treatment

Treatment of the bite wound is a vital part of the care for patients exposed to rabies. The severity and speed of onset of any infection is dependent to a certain extent upon the number of organisms (viruses or bacteria) introduced. Washing saliva out of the wound helps to reduce the number of viruses that can enter the tissues.

The wound should be thoroughly washed with large quantities of soap and water. After thoroughly rinsing away the soap, the wound should be flushed with povidone-iodine or an aqueous solution of benzalkonium chloride, which can actually kill some of the viruses. Immediate washing is of such urgency that it should be instituted without delay. If soap and water are not available, anything on hand — including a favorite whiskey — should be used.

Because the mouths of animals contain so many bacteria, treatment for tetanus (toxoid injection) should be administered if the individual has not had a recent booster.

Specific treatment for rabies consists of administering vaccine to build up immunity to the rabies virus during the incubation period between the bite and the appearance of signs of the disease. (See Chapter Twenty-Four, "Allergies.") In most circumstances, serum from an individual already immune to rabies — rabies immune globulin — is also administered. The accompanying algorithm, adopted from recommendations of the Viral Diseases Division, Bureau of Epidemiology, Centers for Disease Control, Public Health Service, U.S. Department of Health and Human Services, depicts the type of therapy that should be administered following different types of rabies exposure.

If immune serum of human origin is available, twenty international units (20IU) per kilogram of body weight should be administered. (2.2 pounds = 1 kilogram.) If the immune serum is of animal (equine) origin, the dose is 40 IU per kilogram. One-half of the serum should be infiltrated around the wound, and the remainder should be injected intramuscularly in another extremity.

One milliliter (1 cc) of human diploid cell rabies vaccine should be injected intramuscularly on the day of the bite (day zero) and on days three, seven, fourteen, and twenty-eight. (The rabies vaccine currently available in the United States is prepared from viruses grown on human diploid cell cultures and is largely free of the serious side effects that were common with older vaccines.)

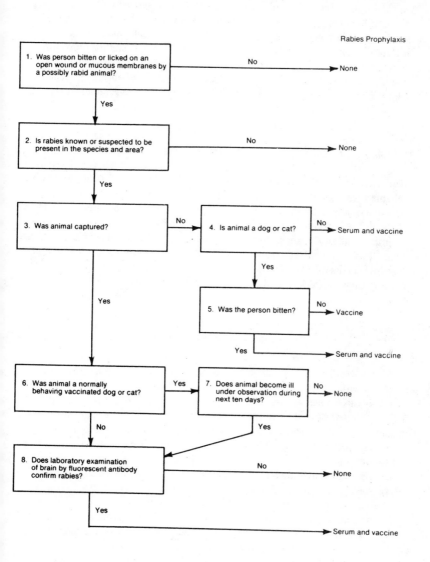

Figure 40. Postexposure rabies prophylaxis algorithm. (From J.A.M.A., April 21, 1975, vol. 232, no. 3. Used by permission.)

Vaccination

The human diploid cell culture vaccine has proven safe and effective for vaccinating humans against rabies. Preexposure vaccination is recommended for veterinarians, animal handlers, and laboratory workers who have a higher risk of infection. In view of the wide distribution of rabies in bats and the possibility of contracting the infection from the air in caves they inhabit, cavers and others frequently exposed to this source of infection should probably be vaccinated. Climbers visiting countries in which rabies is a significant danger may also be well advised to obtain preexposure vaccination.

Obtaining Treatment Outside the United States

U.S. citizens who are exposed to rabies while visiting other countries, particularly underdeveloped countries, may have considerable difficulty obtaining reliable treatment from local physicians or institutions. These individuals may have the best possible intentions, but the essential vaccines may not be available to them. The best course is to go immediately to the nearest American, Canadian, or British embassy. Many of these embassies have English speaking physicians on their staffs, and all have means for obtaining reliable vaccines essentially anywhere in the world within twenty-four hours or less. The embassies of all three countries have always welcomed the opportunity to assist citizens of any of the three nations in an emergency.

POISONOUS SNAKE BITE

About no other medical subject has so much has been written when so little has been known!

Poisonous snake bites are unquestionably serious, potentially deadly accidents. Nonetheless, the danger from a single bite has been greatly exaggerated, particularly in the United States, where an average of less than fifteen people die each year as the result of bites by poisonous snakes. Less than one percent of poisonous snake bites in this country are lethal. In other parts of the world poisonous snake bites are a more serious problem. Many of the snakes in those areas have a much more toxic venom, treatment is less successful, and sophisticated medical care is less available.

Unfortunately, the treatment of poisonous snake bites remains a subject of controversy and confusion. (Even the material used to treat snake bites is variously referred to in the English literature as antivenom, antivenin, or antivenene.) The authoritative publication of untested personal opinions or the results of poorly designed and inadequately controlled animal experiments, aided by an uninformed, sometimes sensationalist press, have produced widespread misinformation. The problem has been compounded by the failure to distinguish between appropriate treatment for urban situations, where hospitals are only minutes away, and remote wilderness areas — or between "first aid" and hospital care.

Poisonous Snakes of the World

The world's poisonous snakes have been divided into three families. Within the family *Elapidae* are the North American coral snakes (eastern, western, and Sonoran); the Indian krait, found in India and Pakistan; the tiger snake of Australia; the death adder of Australia and New Guinea; the Indian cobra, which occurs in most of Southeast Asia, including Indonesia and Formosa (and which reportedly is responsible for more deaths than any other species); the mamba of East Africa; and the ringhals of South Africa.

The *Viperinae* include the puff adder found in most of Africa and southern Arabia, the saw scaled viper which occurs from northern and western Africa to northern India and Ceylon, the Palestine viper of the Middle East, and the Russell's viper which is found from West Pakistan to Formosa.

The *Crotalinae* are of major importance in North America. They include all of the North American rattlesnakes as well as the copperheads and cottonmouth moccasins, the fer-de-lance and neotropical rattlesnakes which are found from Mexico to Argentina, the jararaca of tropical South America, and the habu which occurs in the Ryukyu Islands of Japan with closely related species in Formosa and the southeastern part of the People's Republic of China.

Identification of Poisonous Snakes

The poisonous snakes of the United States are the many species of rattlesnakes, the various species of copperheads and cottonmouth or water moccasin, and the coral snakes. All United States poisonous snakes except the coral snakes are pit vipers and have a characteristic triangular head and a heavy body. The body markings are rarely sufficiently unique for species identification by inexperienced individuals.

These snakes are called "pit vipers" because they have a small pit located between the eye and the nostril, a feature found only in these poisonous species. The pit vipers are also characterized by single scales reaching across the undersurface of the body posterior to the anus. Most other snakes have double scales. If fangs are present, the snake is undoubtedly poisonous, but searching for fangs is dangerous. The fangs may be folded back against the roof of the mouth, making them difficult to identify. One or both fangs may be broken off; three or four are occasionally found. The presence of rattles is of obvious significance; the absence of rattles may not be because the rattles can get broken off. The Catalina Island rattlesnake sheds his rattles with his skin and never has more than one rattle.

The coral snakes are small, thin, brightly colored snakes with small heads, quite different from the pit vipers. They can be identified by the adjacent red and yellow bands. The nonpoisonous king snakes and other harmless species with

HARMLESS

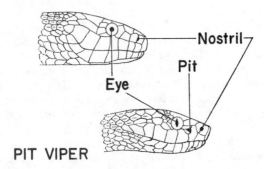

PIT VIPER

Figure 41. Comparison of the heads of pit vipers and nonpoisonous snakes.

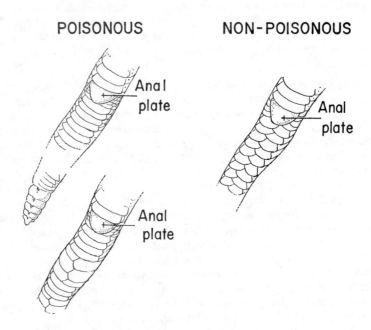

Figure 42. Comparison of the scales on the undersurface of tails of poisonous and non-poisonous snakes.

similar coloration have adjacent red and black bands. A helpful mnemonic is:

"Red and yellow — kill a fellow;

Red and black — venom lack."

Poisonous snakes from other parts of the world do not closely resemble their American counterparts. The vipers do have rather large heads and heavy bodies and tend to resemble the pit vipers, although they lack pits. The elapids have small heads and thin bodies like the coral snakes. However, few have the coloring of the coral snakes. Except for a few species with distinctive hoods (mostly cobras), they have an appearance similar to many nonpoisonous snakes. Travellers who are not knowledgeable herpetologists should avoid all snakes when in areas inhabited by these reptiles.

The poisonous snakes of Australia, including the innocent sounding brown snake and the more appropriately named death adder and tiger snake, are elapids; many of the poisonous snakes of Africa, including the notorious black mamba, are elapids. To individuals accustomed to the heavy bodied American crotalids or pit vipers these snakes appear harmless, but their venoms are vicious. Herpetology texts should be consulted for more detailed information about the identification of these species.

Snake Venoms

The venoms of all poisonous snakes contain similar toxins. Some of these components affect blood and the blood vessels and some affect the nervous system, but to classify snakes according to a single target for their toxin is misleading and can result in inadequate medical therapy. Vascular toxins damage the walls of blood vessels; others inhibit blood clotting; the combination of the two results in bleeding into the tissues at the site of the bite as well as spontaneous bleeding from the gums, nose, or gastrointestinal tract. The damaged blood vessels allow proteins and fluid to leak into the tissues, which produces swelling at the point where the bite occurs. Such fluid loss in combination with the destruction of red blood cells and blood proteins reduces the circulating blood volume and leads to shock, a constant occurrence with severe poisoning by snakes of all species.

The ultimate effect of the neurotoxins is paralysis, most importantly respiratory paralysis. However, abnormal sensations such as tingling or prickly feelings and partial paralysis of the eyelids are more common. Although pit vipers have been described as having predominantly hemolytic toxins, one of the characteristic early symptoms following the bites of some rattlesnakes is numbness and tingling of the lips and a metallic taste, both of which result from the effects of the toxin on neural tissues.

Crotalid venoms do tend to have higher percentages of hemolytic toxins; elapid and viperine toxins tend to have higher percentages of neurotoxins. However, more than a dozen different venom components have been identified. Different species within the same family have venoms of different composition. Venom concentrations also vary; some, like that of the copperhead, are rather weak, while others, like that of the Mojave rattlesnake, are concentrated and quite potent. Additionally, larger snakes are able to inject a larger volume of venom than smaller snakes. The concentration of the venom, the concentrations of its individual components, and its total volume are different in the same snake at different times of the year.

Because the venom of a copperhead is so mild, persons bitten by these snakes require little more than supportive therapy. Antivenom is almost never needed for full size adults bitten by a single snake. In a compilation of over 400 copperhead bites occurring in eastern North Carolina, only two deaths could be found. In both instances, the victims had been bitten simultaneously by three or more snakes.

In contrast, the eastern diamondback rattlesnake, a large species which is more aggressive than most snakes, produces a venom that is only moderately toxic, but the volume is so great that bites by this snake require vigorous treatment. In the United States this species is responsible for more poisonous snake bite deaths than any other. (Most of the bites by this snake occur in Florida, which is the site of very limited mountaineering activity.)

The Mojave rattlesnake is small but has a very potent venom with a high concentration of toxins that affect the nervous system. The effects of envenomation by this species tend to be delayed, appearing some twelve to sixteen hours after the bite and commonly becoming much more severe than would be expected from the initial reaction to the bite. Bites by this species must be treated aggressively from the outset.

Diagnosis of Envenomation

Following a bite by any snake, the offending reptile should be precisely identified if possible. Every year a number of people are injured from unnecessary treatment following the bite of nonpoisonous snakes. More significantly, a deadly bite by a snake such as a Mojave rattlesnake may produce very little reaction in the hours immediately after it occurs when treatment is most effective. Only if the species of snake is known can optimal therapy be started without delay. Preferably the snake should be killed and brought to a medical center with the patient so the exact species can be determined.

The two antivenoms used for treating snake bites within the United States are a polyvalent preparation effective for the bites of all pit vipers, and a specific antivenom for coral snake bites. In other countries, however, broad spectrum antiserum is not available (in some cases, not possible) and specific antiserum for the offending snake must be used. If the snake can not be precisely identified, effective specific therapy may be impossible.

After determining that the snake is poisonous, the bite should be inspected. Typically the fangs of a pit viper produce two small puncture marks, which are a reliable indication that the snake was a member of this family. However, such characteristic fang marks are distinctly uncommon. The victim is usually moving and the snake's strike is rarely so accurate. Only one fang may strike the victim, or the fangs may only graze or scratch the skin. The snake may have had one fang broken off; occasional snakes have three or even four fangs. The fang marks may be hidden among the marks from the other teeth if the pit viper has embedded his fangs so deeply that the other teeth have also penetrated the skin. When only the fangs have entered the skin, a U-shaped row of teeth marks from the bottom jaw may be present.

Even when an attacking snake can be positively identified as poisonous, the subject of its attack does not require specific treatment unless venom has been injected (envenomation). Poisonous snakes attack humans out of fear, not for food. Sometimes the snake strikes without even opening its mouth or extending its fangs. Occasionally its venom is only sprayed on the surface of the skin. Even when the fangs pierce the skin, no venom or only a very small quantity may be injected.

Approximately twenty percent of the patients with rattlesnake bites actually transported to the University of Southern California—Los Angeles County Medical Center over a period of years had not been envenomated. For about two-thirds of these nonenvenomated patients, the fangs had only scratched the skin or had penetrated too superficially for venom to be injected. In the remaining one-third, the fangs had penetrated deeply but no venom had been injected. About fifty percent of cobra bites are not associated with envenomation; for sea snake bites the incidence of nonenvenomation is about eighty percent.

If the victim has been bitten but not envenomated, the bite should be treated like any other animal bite. It must be thoroughly cleaned, and since the wound is a puncture wound, bleeding should be encouraged and tetanus prophylaxis should be administered.

Crotalid Envenomation

The reaction following the bite of a crotalid (pit viper) is one of the best indications that the snake was poisonous and is the only indication that envenomation has occurred and that treatment is needed. This reaction begins within minutes after the bite, is typically severe following an eastern diamondback rattlesnake bite, but is usually less marked after other pit viper bites. The reaction may be deceptively mild following the bite of a Mojave rattlesnake and almost nonexistent after a massagua or pygmy rattlesnake bite. The onset is characterized by pain or burning at the site of the bite, although some victims experience relatively little pain. Shortly afterward the area begins to swell as fluid and blood pour out into the tissues. The blood usually produces a purple or green discoloration, but this change may take several hours to appear. Numbness or a tingling sensation about the mouth or tongue — sometimes extending into the scalp or involving the fingers and toes, and often associated with a metallic or rubbery taste — commonly follows the bite of eastern diamondback and some western rattlesnakes.

Additional changes that may occur later include spread of the swelling and discoloration further from the site of the bite, the appearance of large blisters or bullae that contain either clear or bloody fluid, the appearance of enlarged and tender regional lymph nodes, particularly in the armpit or the inguinal crease, and the development of a systemic reaction. The victim usually becomes weak and dizzy, his skin becomes cold and clammy, and his pulse becomes weak and thready. Other signs typical of shock also may be present.

Prehospital Care for Urban Crotalid Snake Bite

Most of the poisonous snake bites within the United States occur in situations where the victim can be hospitalized within two hours or less. The average interval between a bite and hospitalization has been reported to be about thirty-five minutes. In situations where the victim can be taken to a hospital within two hours or less, the only treatment needed is to limit the spread of the snake venom and to immobilize the bitten extremity. No other measures, including incision and suction, should be attempted.

Tourniquets have been recommended to help reduce spread of the venom but are rarely used correctly. They commonly do more harm than good. Tourniquets that obstruct the flow of arterial blood to an extremity temporarily prevent spread of the venom, but they are too painful to be tolerated by a conscious patient for more than a few minutes. Furthermore, arterial tourniquets must be released for thirty to sixty seconds every ten minutes to allow arterial blood flow to the limb and prevent gangrene. Venom can escape into the rest of the body during that interval.

Tourniquets that only obstruct the flow of venous blood also produce discomfort after a period of time and can increase bleeding or extravasation of blood at the site of the bite. Properly applied, the tourniquet should only obstruct lymphatic flow. The tourniquet should be made from a band at least one inch wide and should not be so tight a finger can not be inserted beneath it without difficulty. Such tourniquets can easily be applied too loosely or become too tight as swelling spreads up the limb. Because it seems almost impossible to apply such tourniquets correctly, some individuals have recommended that they not be applied at all.

A recently devised method for inhibiting the spread of venom, which has been proven effective in experimental studies and by clinical use, is to wrap the bitten extremity snugly with fabric and immobilize it with a splint. Any kind of fabric, including an elastic bandage, is satisfactory. The fabric should apply firm pressure to the bitten tissues, almost as if holding the venom in place. With most snake bites, venom is injected into the subcutaneous (superficial) tissue, not into the underlying muscle. A snug fabric wrapping that compresses the subcutaneous veins and lymphatics eliminates most blood and lymph flow from those tissues and thereby effectively immobilizes the venom without compromising blood flow to the limb. The wrap is not tight enough to interfere with arterial flow, and although it compresses the superficial veins, venous blood can still return through the deep veins.

An inflatable splint can be useful for this purpose because this device can both splint the extremity and apply pressure. The pressure in the splint must be rather high, approximately 50 to 60 mm Hg. Any available splint can be used and does not have to be as carefully applied as a splint for a fracture.

The immobilized extremity should be kept at the same level as the heart, and the victim should be transported to a hospital with as little effort on his part as possible. Movement by the victim, even just walking, increases the circulation of blood and speeds the movement of venom away from the bite to the rest of the body. However, the effects of activity are frequently worse than would be expected from this consideration alone. The victim must be kept quiet, lying still if possible. No drugs, including alcohol, should be administered; no other treatment should be attempted.

After the victim reaches the hospital, the wrapping should not be removed from the extremity until preparations have been made to administer antivenom. If significant envenomation is known to have occurred, antivenom should be started before the wrapping is removed.

Wilderness Crotalid Snake Bite Therapy

Few poisonous snake bites occur in truly remote wilderness situations for reasons that are unknown. Perhaps backpackers and climbers are more aware of the habits and habitats of poisonous snakes and are better able to avoid them. Hiking boots that cover the ankles undoubtedly prevent some bites. Snakes, like all cold blooded animals, can not control their body temperature very well and must avoid extremes of heat or cold. Snakes are much less common at altitudes where temperatures can drop to low levels at night.

The prehospital care for snake bite in a remote area is basically the same as that for an urban environment: compression of the bitten extremity, immobilization, and transportation (by litter if possible) to the nearest medical facility. However, if evacuation requires more than three hours and the victim has been envenomated by a pit viper, incision and suction may be considered. This form of therapy must be undertaken only with the full realization that it is a relatively ineffectual, stopgap measure useful only for pit viper bites. Under ideal conditions, incision and suction removes less than twenty percent of the venom. The risk of infection or damage to underlying tissues is considerable. However, after severe envenomation, particularly of a child or elderly adult, even that small benefit may be significant.

The following conditions must be met before incision and suction is attempted:

1. The victim is three hours or more from the nearest medical facility, and the use of incision and suction must not delay evacuation.
2. The snake has been clearly identified as a pit viper, and significant envenomation must be manifested by severe pain and swelling.
3. Incision and suction can be initiated no less than ten minutes after the bite, preferably sooner.
4. The necessary personnel and equipment are available. (A solitary individual should not attempt incision and suction if he does not have suction cups and can not reach the site of the bite to apply suction orally.)
5. Someone in the party knows how to perform incision and suction properly, particularly how to apply a tourniquet that does not obstruct arterial blood flow.

The following procedure should be carried out:

1. A tourniquet should be applied, using a handkerchief or similar broad band that restricts lymphatic flow only.
2. The skin should be washed and swabbed with an antiseptic. (Such obvious measures to reduce contamination are frequently neglected, resulting in infections which are responsible for a large part of the residual damage from snake bites. The bacteria that cause tetanus and gas gangrene have both been isolated from the mouths of poisonous snakes.)
3. Incisions parallel to the long axis of the limb, one-quarter to one-half inch (six to thirteen millimeters) long and one-eighth inch (three millimeters) deep, should be made with a scalpel or razor blade, preferably sterile, through the fang marks. No other incisions should be made. In view of the ineffectiveness of incision and suction, incisions should probably not be made on the hands or feet unless severe envenomation has obviously occurred.
4. Suction should be applied, preferably with suction cups, but orally if necessary. (The person applying suction must have no open wounds or sores in his mouth, no history of peptic ulcer, and should not swallow the venom.) Suction should be applied for thirty minutes for adults; up to an hour for children.
5. After suction has been discontinued, the limb should be wrapped in fabric and splinted.

A person by himself in a remote area has no choice but to walk out, perhaps after attempting incision and suction. He must not exert himself any more than absolutely necessary. If a companion is present, the companion should make sure the victim is warm and comfortable, perhaps perform incision and suction, wrap the limb, and then go for help, preferably a helicopter. If the party is large enough, the victim can be carried out. Even jostling on a makeshift stretcher probably stimulates blood flow and venom absorption less than attempting to walk out.

Antivenom Therapy

Antivenom against the venom of the attacking snake is the only specific treatment for poisonous snake bite. However, the antivenom currently available is prepared in horses, and many individuals are allergic to horse serum. As a result, the administration of antivenom can be hazardous and should not be attempted by anyone other than a physician, and even then only in situations such as hospital emergency rooms where potentially lethal allergic reactions can be treated. Some recent investigations have disclosed that allergic reactions of some type, mostly mild but occasionally severe, occur in seventy percent of antivenom recipients who were not previously allergic to horse serum.

A few individuals carry single vials of antivenom when travelling in snake infested areas so they can be prepared to treat themselves should they be bitten. This practice is futile and dangerous for the following reasons:

1. A poisonous snake bite victim in the United States who needs the Wyeth crotalid antivenom needs five to fifteen vials — sometimes as many as forty — not one.
2. Carrying antivenom could impart a false sense of security which could cause the individual not to take adequate precautions to avoid poisonous snakes.
3. If the antivenom were administered and a major allergic reaction occurred, the individual would not be able to take care of himself effectively and could die from the reaction.

The antivenom most widely available in the United States is a polyvalent or general purpose crotalid antivenom made by Wyeth Laboratories which is effective against all North American pit vipers. A specific *Micrurus fulvius* antivenom, which should be used for bites by coral snakes, is made by the same company. Antivenoms for bites by other species are discussed under Elapid and Viperine Bites.

Cold Therapy

Packing an extremity bitten by a poisonous snake in ice or snow probably would not be possible in most wilderness situations because snakes do not inhabit areas where ice and snow are available. However, such therapy for poisonous snake bite has been recommended in the past. The basis of such therapy was the assumption that the active components of snake venom were enzymes, the activity of which would be reduced by cooling. However, subsequent studies have determined that most of the toxins in snake venom are peptides, which are not in-activated by cooling. Additionally, since snakes are cold blooded animals, their enzymes remain active at temperatures at which a warm blooded human's defenses are immobilized. Furthermore, some enzymes are driven deeper into warmer tissues by cooling the skin.

Few physicians still advocate local cold therapy; even fewer would deny that its use outside of a hospital as a technique for emergency care has caused the loss of many limbs.

Coral Snake Bites

The coral snakes are the only elapids native to the United States. These snakes have a range largely restricted to the coastal states from southern North Carolina to Texas. The eastern coral snake inhabits this area from Mississippi eastward; the western coral snake is found in Louisiana and Texas. The Sonoran coral snake is found in a limited portion of southern Arizona.

These North American elapids are shy and rarely seen; bites are even less com-mon. Reportedly, children may play with these snakes for hours without being bitten. Envenomation appears to occur in less than forty percent of the bites that are inflicted. Coral snake bites make up less than two percent of all U.S. snake bites.

In striking contrast, elapids in other countries are among the most aggressive and have the most potent venoms of all poisonous snakes. The black mamba of Africa commonly attacks after minimal provocation. Its bite is often lethal even when specific therapy is administered immediately. Cobras are elapids with well deserved notoriety; the death adder of Australia is an appropriately named elapid.

Fatalities from coral snake bites apparently have not occurred since the development of specific *Micrurus fulvius* antivenom. This antivenom is effective for bites of the eastern coral snake, *Micrurus fulvius fulvius,* and the western cor-al snake, *Micrurus fulvius tenere.* It is of little value for bites by the Sonoran coral snake, *Micruroides euryxanthus,* but these bites are usually even less severe.

Elapid bites are rarely associated with the local reaction — severe pain and swelling — typical of crotalid bites. The puncture marks from the fangs may be difficult to identify, particularly if the victim was intoxicated and can not provide a reliable account of the bite. Some pain may be present and may radiate up the limb. Often the first sign of elapid envenomation is painful enlargement of the regional lymph nodes. With severe envenomations numbness and weakness of the limb appear within one to two hours, sometimes less. Later signs and symp-toms include drowsiness, apprehension, weakness, tremors of the tongue or other muscles, difficulty swallowing, nausea, and vomiting. Pronounced weakness of the eye or eyelid muscles may occur; pupils may be pinpoint in size; breathing may be labored. Convulsions may occur. Eventually, in inadequately treated patients, unconsciousness and paralysis are followed by death in shock from respiratory and cardiac failure.

Antivenom is the only effective therapy for elapid bites. The limb should be wrapped as previously described to immobilize the venom, and should be splinted. The patient should be rapidly transported to a hospital with as little effort on his part as possible. Incision and suction, cooling, or other forms of nonhospital treatment are of no proven value. All coral snake bite victims with identifiable fang marks should be observed in a medical facility for at least six hours, even if envenomation does not appear to have occurred. The onset of symptoms of envenomation may be delayed for hours.

Bites by Exotic Poisonous Snakes

Bites by snakes that are not native to the United States occasionally occur among collectors, amateur and professional herpetologists, and exhibitors. Such bites also occur in urban and wilderness areas in other countries. The treatment for such bites is essentially identical to that for coral snake bites: immobilization of the venom by wrapping the limb, splinting, and transportation to a medical center. Incision and suction or cooling have no value in treating such bites.

Within the United States, antivenoms for bites by exotic species of snakes, as well as the names of consultant physicians experienced in treating such bites, may be available through local zoos. Local poison control centers and herpetologists on the faculty of local univerisities also can be valuable sources of information and assistance. The Antivenin Index in Oklahoma City (405-271-5454) maintains a twenty-four hour service to assist in locating antivenoms and provide advice about the treatment for snake bites. Another source of information is the Poisondex central office in Denver (800-332-3073).

In other countries, such information and antivenoms may not be so easy to obtain. Several of the manufacturers or distributors of antivenoms in countries containing popular climbing areas are listed. Communication with these companies from a remote location would no doubt be difficult. The nearest hospital would probably be the most reliable source of information and assistance, particularly in areas where snake bites are common.

SOUTH AMERICA

Instituto Butantan
Ciaxa Postal 65
Sao Paulo, Brazil

Instituto Nacional de Higiene
Lima, Peru

Instituto Nacional de Salud
Ave. Eldorado con Carrera
Zona G
Bogota, D.E., Colombia

EUROPE

Institut Pasteur
Annexe de Garches
92 (Haust-de-Seine)
Paris, France

Behring Institut
Behringwerke AG D3550
Marburg/Lahn
Germany

AFRICA

The South African Institute for
Medical Research,
P.O. Box 1038
Johannesburg 2000
Republic of South Africa

ASIA

Central Research Institute
Kasauli (Simla Hills)
(H.P.) India

Haffkine BioPharmaceutical Corporation, Ltd.
Parel, Bombay
India

AUSTRALIA

Commonwealth Serum Laboratories
45 Poplar Road
Parkville, Victoria 3052

Other Considerations

If a victim of a poisonous snake bite in a wilderness area can not be evacuated for several days (after which evacuation may not be needed), antibiotics may be needed to combat wound infection. A barbiturate or similar medication every four to six hours may help keep the victim quiet and allay anxiety but must not be given to an unconscious patient. Pain should be controlled with aspirin and codeine; morphine or meperidine may have harmful effects and should not be administered. Alcohol increases absorption of the venom. Physical activity by the victim must be avoided.

Most snake bite fatalities result from shock, regardless of the species of snake or whether the venom is primarily hemolytic or neurotoxic. This complication should be anticipated and treated.

Every patient with a poisonous snake bite is different and the treatment for each must be individualized. Children and elderly persons tolerate poisonous snake bites poorly and require more vigorous treatment. Bites occurring in the spring, when the snake has just emerged from hibernation and its venom is more concentrated, are more severe than bites occurring at other times of the year. Bites about the head or trunk are more dangerous than bites on the extremities and require more aggressive treatment. Obviously such sites can not be splinted, and immobilization of the venom is difficult.

Avoiding Poisonous Snakes

Poisonous snakes and their bites are best avoided, not treated. Several simple measures would prevent almost half of all envenomations:

1. Poisonous snakes should not be teased or handled, even after they are dead. Reflex strikes with envenomation can occur for several hours after death.
2. Unprotected hands should not be inserted under logs or stones or into cracks or crevices that have not first been visually inspected.
3. Snakes are nocturnal animals. After dark special care must be taken to avoid them. Walking barefoot or collecting firewood after dark are two of the more frequent contributors to poisonous snake bites.
4. Snakes rarely strike higher than the ankle. Wearing loose fitting pants and hiking boots that cover the ankles would prevent many bites.

SPIDER BITES

Almost all spiders produce toxic venoms, but either their fangs are too weak and small to penetrate the skin or the venom is too weak or its volume too small to pose a significant threat for humans. The black widow, *Latrodectus mactans,* is the only spider found in the United States that is capable of routinely producing serious illness by its bite. The "tarantula" native to the Southwest bites only after extreme provocation. Its weak and ineffective fangs can only penetrate the thin skin on the sides of the fingers; the effects of the bite are no worse than an insect sting.

Other parts of the world are inhabited by a number of spiders that can cause severe, even fatal poisoning in humans. Other species of *Latrodectus* produce effects similar to the black widow. The bites of large, hairy tarantulas found in areas such as Brazil or Peru can have similar results. The Sydney funnel web spider, reportedly limited in distribution to the area within 100 miles of the center of Sydney, Australia, is capable of inflicting a bite that can be lethal for healthy young adults.

Some spiders, such as the brown or violin spider, *Lososceles reclusa,* inflict bites that cause fairly extensive damage at the site but usually have less severe generalized effects. The jumping spider Phidippus is the most common biting spider in the United States. This spider, trapdoor spiders, orbweavers, and spiders of the *Chiracanthium* species such as the garden spider are capable of producing mild local reactions with occasional systemic symptoms. However, they almost never produce disorders requiring hospitalization. Anyone suspecting that they have been bitten by one of these spiders should bring the spider in to be identified. Capturing the spider is usually easy because it typically clings to the site of the bite. In fact, if the spider can not be found, some other arachnid such as a bedbug should be suspected.

Rarely an individual may be bitten repeatedly by a relatively harmless spider or insect and develop an allergy to the toxin produced by that species. Subsequent bites can produce severe, even fatal allergic reactions. Fortunately, such events are rare. The treatment for such reactions would be identical to the treatment for allergic reactions to insect stings.

Black Widow Spider Bites

The female black widow typically is coal black and has a prominent, spherical abdomen. The body may be as large as one-half inch (1.25 cm) in length, not including the legs. On the undersurface of the abdomen is a red or orange figure which usually resembles an hourglass, but may be round, broken into two figures, or have some other configuration. Markings of the same color but in varying patterns are sometimes present on the back, although only the undersurface markings are considered characteristic. In some southwestern states black widow spiders have irregular white patches on their abdomens. Different species of *Latrodectus* in other countries have a similar appearance. (The male is smaller, has a brown color, and is harmless.)

The black widow weaves a coarse, crudely constructed web in dark corners, both indoors and out. Almost half the black widow bites reported in the medical literature in the first four decades of this century were inflicted on the male genitalia by spiders lurking underneath the seats of outdoor toilets. However, this spider is timid and would rather run than attack an intruder.

About thirty years ago some five to ten deaths a year resulted from black widow spider bites, although they were limited almost entirely to small children or elderly individuals in relatively poor health. Recognition and treatment of such bites has improved so much that any deaths at all are now rare within the United States. (Bites in children weighing thirty pounds or less would still have a mortality of about fifty percent if untreated.) In healthy adults, black widow spider bites cause painful muscle spasms and prostration for two to four days, but complete recovery essentially always follows. Antivenom treatment is not recommended for healthy adults.

At the time the bite is inflicted the victim may feel a slight pain similar to a pin prick, slight burning, or nothing at all. Small puncture wounds, slight redness, or no visible marks at all may be found at the site of the bite. Within about fifteen minutes painful muscle cramps develop at the point of the bite and rapidly spread to involve the entire body. The characteristic pattern of spread is by continuity. From a bite on the forearm the cramps would spread to the elbow, then to the shoulder, and then over the chest to involve the rest of the body, including the legs. The abdominal muscles are characteristically rigid and hard, although actual abdominal tenderness is not present. Weakness and tremors are also present.

The typical victim is anxious and restless. A feeble pulse and cold, clammy skin suggest shock; labored breathing, slurred speech, impaired coordination, light stupor, and rarely convulsions (in children) suggest a disease involving the brain. The victims are often covered with perspiration; dizziness, nausea, and vomiting are common. If the spider or its bite have not been observed, the signs and symptoms may lead to an erroneous diagnosis of an acute abdominal emergency.

Symptoms typically increase in severity for several hours, occasionally as long as twenty-four hours, and then gradually subside. After two to three days essentially all symptoms have disappeared, although a few minor residua may persist for weeks or months.

Treatment consists of antivenom and efforts to relieve the painful muscle spasms. No treatment at all should be directed to the site of the bite, with the possible exception of applying an ice cube to relieve pain. Incision and suction is damaging and useless and should never be performed.

The patient should be hospitalized if possible; small children must have such care. Antivenom, produced in the United States by Merck Sharp & Dohme, or the drugs to control spasms would rarely be available anywhere else. The antivenom is prepared in horses and should not be given to persons allergic to horse serum. It is usually not administered at all to healthy adults between the ages of sixteen and sixty, and only to individuals of small body size with severe symptoms who are twelve to fifteen years old. Instructions with the vial of antiserum should be followed.

Muscle spasms may be aided by periodic injections of 10 cc of a ten percent calcium gluconate solution or 10 cc of methocarbamol, but these would almost never be available outside of a hospital. Diazepam (Valium) may help relieve less severe muscle spasms; hot baths are occasionally helpful. Analgesics such as morphine are helpful but rarely provide complete pain relief.

Brown Spider Bites

The brown or violin spider, *Lososceles reclusa,* incorrectly labelled the "brown recluse spider," has received attention as the cause of "necrotic arachnidism."

Following the bite of this spider a blister surrounded by an area of intense inflammation about one-half inch (1.25 cm) in diameter appears. Pain is mild at first but may become quite severe within about eight hours. Over the next ten to fourteen days the blister ruptures and the involved skin turns dark brown or black. Eventually the black, dead tissue drops away, leaving a crater which heals with some scarring. Rarely the area of skin loss is so large that skin grafting is required to cover the defect. Some children have lost considerable portions of their faces. However, much smaller wounds are far more common.

Generalized symptoms may appear over the next thirty-six hours and can include chills and fever, nausea and vomiting, joint pain, and a skin rash or hives. With severe reactions, red blood cells are broken down (hemolysis) and platelets are destroyed (thrombocytopenia), which can result in a significant anemia and bleeding tendency. Rare fatalities have occurred, mostly in children.

Essentially nothing can be done for such bites in a wilderness situation. If the victim can be hospitalized within less than eight hours, the site of the bite can be surgically excised. Such therapy should be reserved for bites from spiders clearly identifiable as *L. reclusa,* so the spider should be captured as intact as possible and should be brought to the hospital to be identified. After eight hours the area involved is usually too large to be excised. Corticosteroids may also be administered. Dexamethasone, 4 mg administered intramuscularly every six hours until the reaction starts to subside, and then given in gradually tapered doses, is one recommended program.

SCORPION STINGS

Scorpions are found throughout most of the United States, but the species lethal for man, *Centruroides sculpturatus* Ewing, is limited to Arizona, New Mexico, Texas, southern California, and northern Mexico. In this area scorpions are a serious problem. Sixty-nine deaths resulted from scorpion stings in Arizona between 1929 and 1954. Only twenty deaths resulted from poisonous snake bites during the same period. With improved techniques for the medical management of the complications of scorpion stings, no deaths have occurred from that cause in Arizona for over ten years.

Scorpions are eight legged arachnids which range in length from three to eight inches (7.5 to 20 cm) and have a rather plump body, thin tail, and large pinchers. They are found in dry climates under rocks and logs, buried in the sand, in collections of lumber, bricks, or brush, and in the attics, walls, or understructures of houses or deserted buildings. The problems created by scorpions in Arizona are undoubtedly related to their tendency to dwell in the vicinity of human habitation where children are frequently playing.

Scorpion stings can usually be avoided by exercising care when picking up objects such as stones or logs under which they like to hide during the day. Since scorpions are nocturnal, walking barefoot after dark is inadvisable. Shoes and clothing should be shaken vigorously before dressing in the morning, particularly when camping outdoors.

The lethal species of scorpions are often found under loose bark or around old tree stumps. They have a yellow to greenish yellow color and can be distinguished from other species by a small knoblike projection at the base of their stingers. Adults measure three inches (7.5 cm) in length and three-eighths inch (1 cm) in width. One subspecies has two irregular dark stripes down its back.

The sting of a nonlethal scorpion is similar to that of a wasp or hornet, although usually somewhat more severe, and should be treated in an identical manner. Lethal scorpion stings are much more painful, but fatalities have been limited almost entirely to small children.

Initially the sting of a scorpion of one of the lethal species usually produces only a pricking sensation and may not be noticed. Usually nothing can be seen at the site of the sting. (Swelling and red or purple discoloration are indications that the sting has been inflicted by a nonlethal species.) Pain usually follows in five to sixty minutes and may be quite severe. The area is usually quite sensitive to touch, and tapping it lightly may produce a tingling or prickly feeling which travels up the extremity toward the body. This area is the last part of the body to recover from the sting. Sensitivity may persist as long as ten days, although other symptoms have usually disappeared within ten hours.

Victims typically are extremely restless and jittery. Young children characteristically are writhing, jerking, or flailing about. The movements are completely involuntary. However, in spite of his constantly moving body, the child can talk. Although he appears to be writhing in pain, he usually states that he does not hurt. Convulsions have been described, but the true nature of these events is somewhat questionable. Visual disturbances such as roving eye movements or a fluttering type of movement known as nystagmus are common. Occasionally a child complains that he can not see, but nothing abnormal can be found when examining his eyes, and sight returns spontaneously in a few minutes. Children under six years of age may develop respiratory problems such as wheezing and stridor, and a few may need assisted respiration.

Victims typically have an elevated blood pressure, which may be an important diagnostic sign since hypertension is rare in children. The blood pressure usually returns to normal within four to six hours and becomes life threatening only in infants.

Victims of a sting by one of the lethal scorpion species should be taken to a hospital at once. Only a medical facility of that sophistication would have the equipment and supplies necessary to deal with the complications of such stings. An ice cube applied to the site of the sting may help reduce pain, but no other therapy is possible outside of a hospital. Goat antiserum (which avoids the problem of sensitivity to horse serum) is available in Arizona but has not been extensively tested and is not needed by adults. Treatment with barbiturates has significant disadvantages and is generally unnecessary.

Other countries have species of lethal scorpions much more deadly than those in the southwestern United States. Mexico reportedly has had as many as 76,000 scorpion stings resulting in 1,500 deaths in a single year. The stings of such scorpions must be treated with antivenom, which is rarely obtainable outside of a hospital, particularly by someone who does not speak the country's language. Death from the stings of such scorpions is usually the result of sudden, very severe high blood pressure. Adrenergic blocking agents such as propanolol may be an effective method for treating such stings and perhaps should be carried by visitors to the countries where such lethal species of scorpions exist.

INSECT STINGS

Between fifty and one hundred deaths occur in the United States each year as the result of hypersensitivity (allergic) reactions to the stings of bees, wasps, hornets, and fire ants *(Hymenoptera),* many more than all the deaths from rabies, poisonous snakes, spiders, and scorpions combined. Approximately one of every two hundred people in the U.S. population has experienced a severe reaction to such stings. Fatal reactions now can be prevented or successfully treated in individuals known to have such allergies, but many deaths still occur in persons whose allergic status had not been previously recognized. The problem of allergies and the severe, lethal allergic reactions known as "anaphylactic shock" are discussed in Chapter Twenty-Four, "Allergies."

An individual allergic to insect stings usually experiences milder allergic reactions following such stings before having a fatal or potentially fatal reaction. Two types of relatively severe but nonlethal reactions occur: large local reactions and systemic reactions.

Large local reactions are characterized by severe swelling limited to the limb or portion of the limb that is the site of the insect sting. Almost all insect stings are associated with some swelling, but the swelling is usually limited to an area about three inches (7.5 cm) or less in diameter. The swelling that occurs with severe local reactions involves a major portion of an extremity such as the entire forearm. The swollen area may also be painful, may be associated with some itching, and may be mildly discolored.

Systemic reactions occur in areas of the body some distance from the site of the sting. Probably most typical are hives over large parts of the body, but generalized itching or reddening of the skin also occur. Persons with more severe reactions may have hypotension (low blood pressure) and difficulty breathing. (Clearly the last two reactions could be fatal if severe.)

Investigators of insect hypersensitivity reactions now recommend that individuals who have had a systemic reaction to an insect sting undergo skin testing with *Hymenoptera* venoms. (If the results of skin tests are inconclusive, more sophisticated measurement of venom specific IgE antibodies by the radioallergosorbent procedure should be carried out.) About half of the people who have had a systemic reaction and also have a positive skin test would have a severe, possibly fatal reaction if stung again. Therefore, desensitization with purified insect venoms — not whole body extracts — is recommended for these individuals.

Desensitization can be a drawn out, uncomfortable procedure but also can be life saving. Starting with very small quantities, increasingly larger amounts of the insect venoms are injected subcutaneously until the allergic reaction is "overwhelmed" or "neutralized." The individual is still allergic to the *Hymenoptera* venoms, but the antibodies responsible for producing the allergic reactions are "used up" by the repeated injections of the material with which they react. Generally, even after successful desensitization, injections must be continued at approximately monthly intervals for years or indefinitely. If the desensitization injections are stopped, the former allergic condition usually reappears promptly.

Desensitization must be carried out under the close supervision of a physician experienced with the procedure. Severe, life threatening allergic reactions to the desensitization injections can occur, and a physician must be on hand to deal with such reactions. However, a physician who is standing by watching for a reaction can treat it effectively. Allergic reactions to insect stings in a wilderness environment without a physician in attendance are a far greater threat.

Desensitization, or even skin testing, is not recommended for individuals who have large local reactions because these are rarely followed by systemic reactions. However, carrying epinephrine (adrenaline) is recommended for individuals who have had either type of reaction. Epinephrine is commercially available in small kits but only with a physician's prescription. One such kit contains two 0.3 cc doses of a 1:1,000 dilution of epinephrine in a preloaded syringe, packaged under nitrogen to prevent deterioration. Specific directions for their use accompany the kits, but a hypersensitive individual should develop his own strategy for using the kit with the physician who writes the prescription for its purchase. Generally speaking, one 0.3 cc dose should be injected subcutaneously as soon as the person is stung. The second dose should be held in reserve in case it is needed subsequently. The sting victim should make every effort to get to a hospital or a physician's care as rapidly as possible even though the epinephrine has been administered and the allergic reaction appears to have been controlled.

Rock climbers who have systemic allergic reactions to insect stings have a uniquely high danger of fatal reactions because they are subject to stings in locations such as rock walls where they can not be immediately treated by others and only with great difficulty by themselves. Such persons should undergo desensitization now that purified venom preparations, which make that procedure so much more reliable, are available.

ADDITIONAL READING

1. Russell FE: *Snake Venom Poisoning.* Great Neck, N.Y., Scholium International Inc., 1983.

SECTION FOUR
NONTRAUMATIC DISEASES

CHAPTER SIXTEEN

Diseases of the Respiratory System

The respiratory system moves air in and out of the lungs to provide oxygen for the body and to eliminate carbon dioxide. The components of this system are:

1. The nose and mouth, trachea, bronchi, and bronchioles, which form the passages through which air moves;
2. The mucous membranes lining the air passages, which remove foreign material, saturate the air with water, and raise or lower its temperature to that of the body;
3. The alveoli, or air cells, which make up the major portion of the lung tissue and in which oxygen and carbon dioxide are exchanged between blood and air;
4. The thin, membranous pleura, which covers the lungs, lines the inner surface of the chest wall, and facilitates the movement of the lungs within the chest;
5. The chest wall and diaphragm, which act like a bellows to move air in and out of the lungs;
6. Sensing cells that detect chemical changes in the circulating blood (chemoreceptors); other sensing cells that detect movements of the chest wall, diaphragm, and lungs (neuroreceptors); and the network of nerves that carries information from these receptors to the brain, which controls the rate and depth of respiration.

The rate and depth of respiration are controlled by a complex system of receptors throughout the body. Chemical receptors respond to oxygen deficiency, accumulation of carbon dioxide, or a change in the acidity of the blood (which normally is maintained at a slightly alkaline pH of 7.4) to bring about faster, deeper breathing.

Under ordinary resting conditions approximately a half liter of air is inspired with each breath. The normal respiratory rate is ten to twelve breaths per minute, and the corresponding normal respiratory volume is five to six liters per minute. The respiratory volume is decreased as much as twenty to thirty percent during sleep (which further decreases oxygenation of the blood at high altitude and thereby aggravates the symptoms of altitude sickness). Exertion increases the need for oxygen and also increases the production of lactic acid and carbon dioxide, which stimulate the respiratory center in the brain to increase the respiratory volume, occasionally to as much as 150 liters per minute during vigorous exercise. Even at very rapid respiratory rates, oxygen is taken up by the blood and carbon dioxide given off with extraordinary efficiency.

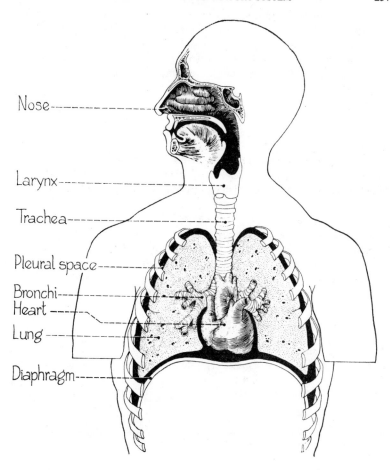

Figure 43. Anatomy of the respiratory system.

Widely varying disorders centered at a number of different locations can affect the function of the respiratory system. Breathing is usually slowed or stopped by head injuries or diseases of the brain, but occasionally it is increased. Airway obstruction in the throat, which is usually sudden and often traumatic, may completely stop effective breathing. Injury, with or without fracture, can impair the bellows action of the chest wall and diaphragm. Air, blood, or fluid in the chest cavity can compress a lung and prevent expansion during inspiration. (An injury that damages the lung in such a way that inhaled air continuously leaks into the space between the lung and chest wall but can not be exhaled (tension pneumothorax) is potentially life threatening. Collections of fluid in the alveoli due to edema or infection can block the exchange of gases between inhaled air and blood.

SYMPTOMS

The principal symptoms produced by diseases of the lungs are pain, cough, shortness of breath, and fever. Details which must be clarified about each of these symptoms in order to diagnose the disorder which has caused them are:

PAIN

Exact location — any change or radiation;
Severity;
Nature — stabbing, sharp, dull, crushing, continuous, or intermittent;
Onset — sudden or gradual;
Relation to respiration, movement, and exertion;
Relation to onset of other symptoms.

COUGH

Dry or productive (sputum is coughed up);
Color and consistency of material produced (purulent material [pus] or blood).

SHORTNESS OF BREATH

Relation to position;
Factors that cause aggravation or provide relief;
Time and nature of onset.

FEVER

Daily range (recorded every four hours);
Accompanied by chills or sweating.

Pain caused by diseases of the lung or pleura or injuries of the chest wall varies with respiratory movements; deep inspiration typically causes sharp, stabbing pain. An irritating, dry, frequent cough is very common at high altitude due to drying and irritation of the throat. Such a cough may not be an indication of lung disease, but recent studies suggest that many, perhaps most, high altitude coughs are due to accumulation of fluid and may be a warning of early high altitude pulmonary edema. The sputum is usually thin, watery, and pink or bloody with this disorder. (See Chapter Twelve, "Medical Problems of High Altitude.") The cough due to infections of the lung is deeper and usually produces sputum that is green, yellow, or rust colored, and thick and stringy. With pulmonary embolism (see below) the sputum is usually bloody. Chest pain, shortness of breath, and watery, pink sputum may be symptoms of heart disease or heart failure. (See Chapter Seventeen, "Diseases of the Heart and Blood Vessels.")

PHYSICAL EXAMINATION

The entire patient must be examined even though the principal site of disease appears to be in the lungs. An elevated pulse rate and fever are indicative of significant disease. Fever is usually a sign of infection but may be seen with other disorders such as pulmonary embolism or high altitude pulmonary edema.

When examining the chest, it should be inspected visually first. Obvious breathing difficulty, irregularities of respiratory rhythm, and differences in the movements of the two sides of the chest during respiration should be sought. Signs of respiratory difficulty include forced or labored breathing, rapid respirations, shallow or irregular breathing, noisy breathing, cyanosis (blue or purple color) of the lips, nails, or skin, or even the complete absence of respiration. Flaring of the nostrils and tensing of the neck muscles are signs of severe respiratory difficulty. The respiratory rhythm can be observed while measuring the respiratory rate. Minor changes of rhythm are of no significance; important irregularities are unmistakable. In contrast, differences in the movements of the two sides of the chest may be very subtle and should be sought during quiet respiration and during deep breathing.

Auscultation consists of listening to the sounds made by air passing in and out of the lung. A stethoscope makes the sounds somewhat easier to hear and is more convenient, but the sounds can be heard by pressing the unaided ear closely against the chest. Quiet breathing in normal lungs produces sounds so faint that they are barely audible. Therefore, the patient must breathe fairly deeply through his mouth during the examination so that these sounds may be heard. All portions of the lungs should be examined to be sure no abnormalities are missed and the extent of the diseased area is recognized.

Many diseases of the lung cause fluid to collect in the small bronchi and alveoli, producing bubbling or crackling sounds known as rales. Such fluid accumulation is typical of infection or pulmonary edema. Wheezing is more indicative of asthma or some other form of small airway obstruction. Wheezing that can be cleared by a single cough is rarely significant. With severe pneumonia or pulmonary embolism a portion of the lung is often consolidated due to fluid and infection in the alveolar sacs. Over these areas, the breath sounds heard may be quite different — harsher and louder — than over normal lung. Infection or an embolus often produces inflammation of the pleura overlying the involved lung, which makes the pleural surface rough. Since the pleura no longer slides smoothly over itself, movement of the lung within the chest during respiration produces a squeaking sound like two pieces of leather being rubbed together. This sound is referred to as a "friction rub" or simply a "rub."

If no sounds whatever are heard over a portion of the chest, there is probably fluid or air in the space between the lung and the chest wall. Rarely the absence of breath sounds may be due to obstruction of a large airway leading to that portion of the lung.

Auscultation of the lung, although it requires practice and experience, is not too difficult to learn and can be a valuable diagnostic aid, particularly in a remote, wilderness situation.

CHRONIC LUNG DISEASE

Chronic lung disease can be the result of long standing infection (such as tuberculosis), slowly growing tumors, small airway infection, or chronic obstructive disease. Emphysema, a disorder characterized by destruction of the walls of alveoli and the formation of numerous cystlike areas, is the result of chronic lung disease, most often involving the smallest air passages, the bronchioles. Both obstructive disease and emphysema can result from long exposure to air pollution, particularly cigarette smoking. Asthma also may lead to emphysema if severe and present for many years.

Most individuals with chronic lung disease are aware of the problem and are not likely to venture into the mountains. However, the early stages of these diseases may not be detectable except during strenuous exertion or at altitude. The first sign of chronic obstructive lung disease or of emphysema may be a decrease in the respiratory reserve. This reserve is the extra breathing capacity that is called on at high altitudes, during exertion, or whenever infection of the lungs, shock, or loss of blood decreases the availability of oxygen to the rest of the body. Persons who know they have impaired respiratory reserve should be cautious about altitude, particularly about exertion at altitude.

DISORDERS OF RHYTHM

Cheyne-Stokes Respiration

Above 13,000 feet (4,000 m) almost everyone has Cheyne-Stokes (periodic) breathing; it is not rare as low as 8,000 feet (2,400 m), particularly in children. The typical pattern of respiration begins with a few shallow breaths, increases in depth to very deep, sighing respirations, and then falls off rapidly. Respirations can cease entirely for a few seconds. (An observer may fear that the person is dead.) Then the shallow breaths resume and the pattern is repeated. (In healthy persons the Cheyne-Stokes respiratory pattern is often not fully developed and consists only of alternating periods of relatively slower, shallow breathing and somewhat faster, deeper breathing.)

This type of irregular breathing is so common at high altitudes that it should not be considered abnormal. Cheyne-Stokes breathing may be present on some occasions and not on others. It may be a sign of a serious disorder if it occurs for the first time during an illness or after an injury, particularly a head injury.

A.

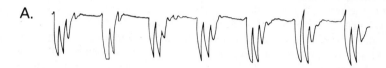

B.

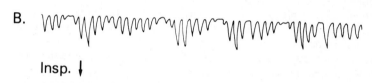

Insp. ↓

Figure 44. Actual tracings of Cheyne-Stokes respirations. A, increasing and decreasing depth of respirations. B, two to three deep inspirations followed by total cessation of respiration for about twelve seconds.

Some persons have intermittent upper airway obstruction (manifested by irregular snoring) at sea level, which may be worse and cause unpleasant morning headache and lethargy at any increased altitude. This disorder tends to be familial and is thought to be responsible for some cases of "crib death" in infants.

During the period when breathing has stopped, the person often becomes restless and sleep may be broken. Occasionally the individual awakens with a rather distressing sense of suffocation. Acetazolamide at bedtime may help intermittent upper airway obstruction as well as the periodic breathing seen at altitude. Sedatives are potentially harmful in such situations and should be avoided. An aminophyllin rectal suppository at bedtime may be beneficial if respiratory irregularity prevents adequate rest.

HYPERVENTILATION SYNDROME

The hyperventilation syndrome is characterized by "overbreathing." The victim is breathing rapidly and deeply and appears to be suffering from serious pulmonary disease. However, this syndrome is almost entirely emotional in origin. Individuals who hyperventilate are usually nervous, tense, and apprehensive, although the disorder can occur in apparently stable persons. Among beginning climbers, apprehension about climbing or fear of exposure might initiate such a reaction. Knowledge of the patient's emotional status, particularly unusual anxiety, helps establish the diagnosis.

As the victim breathes rapidly and deeply, an abnormally large amount of carbon dioxide is lost through the lungs, altering the acid base balance, increasing the pH of the blood, and producing the characteristic symptoms.

The first symptom to appear and the most prominent overall is shortness of breath accompanied by a rapid pulse, dizziness, faintness, sweating, apprehension, and a sense of suffocation. The victim often complains "the air doesn't go down far enough." He, or more frequently she, breathes in gasps or takes frequent deep sighs. As the blood becomes more alkaline, numbness or tingling around the mouth and in the fingers appears. These symptoms may subsequently increase to painful cramps or spasms of the fingers, hands, and forearms, which are particularly frightening to the victim.

The shortness of breath is puzzling since respiratory regulatory mechanisms would be expected to correct the hyperventilation. However, in this condition, these mechanisms are overridden.

Even though the hyperventilation syndrome is suspected, the patient should be examined to ensure no other problem is present. If not, reassurance and explanation usually are sufficient to reverse the disorder. The patient should be instructed to deliberately slow or stop his breathing. He can breathe gently in and out of a bag held over the mouth and nose, which permits carbon dioxide to accumulate in the lungs and blood and usually relieves the symptoms promptly. If these measures are not effective, a mild tranquilizer may be necessary. Once he has recovered, the patient may feel weak and shaky and may have a headache. The mechanism of the disorder should be explained in some detail to help prevent recurrences.

INFECTIOUS DISORDERS

Tracheitis

The trachea is the large airway leading from the throat to the middle of the chest where it divides into the two main bronchi. This structure sometimes becomes inflamed and occasionally infected. Usually the patient has pain in his throat below the tonsils or beneath his sternum, which becomes worse with breathing. Coughing may cause pain in the same area and may produce thick sputum. The treatment of tracheitis is the same as that for bronchitis.

Bronchitis

Bronchitis, or more properly tracheobronchitis, is an infection of the major air passages to the lungs. Such infections are rarely disabling but can progress to pneumonia. This disease frequently comes on during or after a cold, resulting in a "chest cold." However, a cold is a viral infection. Although the trachea and bronchi may be infected by the same virus, bronchitis is usually a bacterial infection which supervenes during the viral infection. Bronchitis can also occur without a preceding viral infection.

Some individuals with asthma have a strong tendency to develop tracheobronchitis following a cold. Prevention of such infections, particularly on a mountaineering outing, would be one of the few good reasons to administer antibiotics to a patient with a cold. Such individuals should confer with their physicians to determine the type of antimicrobial therapy that would be preferable for them to prevent this type of infection.

The predominant symptom of bronchitis is a persistent, irritating cough which may be dry but frequently becomes productive after one or two days. The sputum is usually green or yellow and is thick and tenacious. Slight pain may be associated with the coughing and the victim may notice easy fatigability, particularly at high altitudes. However, he usually does not appear severely ill, and has only a slight fever or none at all. If the infection involves the larynx (voice box), he may be hoarse (laryngitis). A few wheezes and rales may be heard throughout the chest, but these tend to disappear with coughing.

The treatment for tracheitis or bronchitis begins with adequate hydration. The patient must drink lots of fluids, particularly warm liquids. If possible, he should inhale steam from a boiling kettle or pot to moisten and "loosen" or liquefy the material in his bronchi so it can be coughed up more easily.

Many physicians advocate administering a broad spectrum antibiotic if laboratory facilities are not available, but others prefer to withhold antibiotics except for severe infections. At high altitudes, where progression of the infection to pneumonia could be disastrous, antibiotics probably should be administered. For individuals not allergic to penicillin, ampicillin is more broadly effective. For patients allergic to penicillin, tetracycline or erythromycin would be the drugs of choice. Newer broad spectrum antibiotics are more expensive and probably are not needed except for laboratory diagnosed specific infections or in extreme situations when other measures seem ineffective.

Rest, warmth, and aspirin are helpful. The patient does not need to go to bed but should refrain from strenuous exercise. If the condition persists for more than two or three days, descent to a lower altitude may be necessary.

Pleurisy

Pleurisy is an inflammation of the thin membranes that cover the lungs and inner chest wall. The inflammation most commonly originates in the lung as part of some other process, often pneumonia, but occasionally a virus infection of the pleura itself, an injury of the chest wall, or irritation due to pulmonary embolism can produce similar symptoms. Viruses occasionally cause infections limited solely to the pleura. These disorders are of short duration and are not severely disabling. They are rather uncomfortable, particularly at high altitudes where the victim is required to breathe more rapidly and deeper than at sea level.

The principal symptom, usually the only symptom, is pain with respiration. The pain is usually sharp and stabbing and is limited to a rather small area in one side of the chest. Deep inspiration elicits a particularly severe twinge.

Physical signs are slight or absent. Motion of the affected side may be somewhat limited and a few wheezes or rales may be heard over the involved area. Sometimes a leathery, rough, rubbing sound can be heard over the area where pain is worst. This "friction rub" is diagnostic of pleurisy but does not indicate its origin. The patient may be more comfortable when lying on the affected side, limiting the motion of that part of the chest. The general appearance of the patient is important. If pleurisy alone is present the patient rarely appears seriously ill. If the fever is high, the pulse rapid, or the patient seems quite sick, some underlying condition such as pneumonia or embolism should be suspected.

Pleurisy unaccompanied by another disease, although painful, usually clears in three or four days and requires little treatment other than rest. Antibiotics should be given only if pneumonia is suspected. The patient should be taken to a lower altitude if an underlying disease is suspected.

The pain of pleurisy can be alleviated by splinting the chest with adhesive tape. Wide strips of tape should be placed from a point one to two inches beyond the vertebral column to beyond the sternum over the painful area. (It is helpful to paint the skin with tincture of benzoin before applying the tape.) The tape should be removed after three days but can be replaced if necessary. Taping or splinting the chest increases the risk of pneumonia, but if the pain of pleurisy (or broken ribs) is very severe, temporary splinting may be unavoidable. Under no circumstances should both sides of the chest be splinted at the same time.

Pneumonia

Bacterial and viral pneumonia are infections of the lung tissue, notably the alveoli. Persons weakened by fatigue, exposure, or disease elsewhere in the body are particularly susceptible. The alveoli fill with infected fluid, impairing the exchange of carbon dioxide and oxygen. Fever increases the body's need for oxygen as the infection itself decreases the supply. If a large amount of lung is involved, hypoxia combined with toxic substances released from the bacteria may cause death. Pneumonia should always be taken seriously; descent to lower elevations and evacuation to medical facilities should be carried out as rapidly as possible.

The symptoms of pneumonia vary with the causative organisms and the severity of the infection. All pneumonias usually cause a fever of more than 102° F orally

(39° C), a rapid pulse, and an increased respiratory rate. Bacterial pneumonias are often ushered in by one or more shaking chills, followed by a high fever. The patient appears quite sick and may be very weak.

Coughing is a prominent symptom of all lung infections. The cough may be dry at first but usually becomes productive after one or two days. The sputum, which is usually green or yellow, but sometimes has a rusty color, is thick and mucoid and frequently resembles pus.

Some bacteria tend to localize in a single segment of the lung, producing consolidation of the involved tissues. The signs of disease are limited to that area of the lung. The overlying pleura is often involved by the infection and stabbing pain with breathing may be severe. Not infrequently, pleuritic pain is an early, sometimes the first, indication of underlying infection. Since the pain varies with the depth of respiration, the chest is often splinted by involuntary muscle spasm and respiratory movement on that side is reduced.

Lobar pneumonia, usually caused by the pneumococcus and limited to one or two lobes of the lung, has become much less frequent in recent years for reasons not completely understood. At the same time, other infections have become more common. Viruses, fungi, yeasts, and other microorganisms are identified as the cause of pulmonary infections more frequently now than several decades ago. Each of these infecting organisms produces a somewhat different type of disease with different signs and symptoms. Most of them cause poorly localized, widely scattered small areas of infection, which rarely produce signs of consolidation or pleurisy. These infections, called bronchopneumonia, viral pneumonia, or diffuse pneumonitis, often begin rather insidiously and become severe only after a longer period than the lobar or bacterial pneumonias. Consequently they are harder to diagnose and often are unsuspected. So called "walking pneumonia" is generally due to a virus. It creeps up on an individual, is difficult to treat and resistant to most antibiotics, and usually disables the patient for longer periods of time. If this type of insidiously developing pneumonia is suspected, the patient should be taken to a lower altitude. Pneumonias due to the rarer organisms are more difficult to diagnose and usually require special tests in a well equipped hospital.

"Legionnaire's disease" has received much publicity in recent years, but has been around for a long time. It is caused by a specific organism that produces signs and symptoms resembling the viral pneumonias. The mortality rate is high. If this disease is suspected, erythromycin should be administered at once and evacuation begun.

If a patient is suspected to have pneumonia or bronchitis and appears seriously ill, the onset has been rapid, and signs suggesting lobar pneumonia are present, antibiotics should be started immediately. The choice of antibiotics depends upon several considerations. If the patient is not allergic to penicillin, then penicillin or ampicillin is preferred and should be given four to six times a day, usually after a "loading dose" of twice the usual dose. If the patient is allergic to penicillin, then erythromycin or tetracycline is preferred. Treatment should consist of a loading dose followed by a regular dose every four hours. Whatever medication is given should be continued for at least seven and preferably ten days. Stopping therapy after a shorter period of time can lead to a relapse of the infection with organisms that have become resistant to the antibiotic.

The antibiotic may prevent the identification of some less common infective organisms once the patient has reached a hospital. Consequently, some physicians urge that no treatment be given until the organism has been identified. However, if hospitalization must be delayed for more than two or three days, or the patient is quite ill, treatment should be started before the organism is known.

A patient with any type of pneumonia is oxygen deficient at altitudes above 8,000 feet (2,400 m). When oxygen is available, it should be given freely while transportation is arranged. The combination of fever and infection increases the demand for oxygen at a time impaired lung function decreases the supply. Patients should be evacuated to a lower altitude as soon as possible whenever pneumonia is suspected.

Recovery depends on the severity of the infection and the organism. Rarely can a person who has had pneumonia resume climbing in less than two to three weeks.

OTHER PULMONARY DISORDERS

High Altitude Pulmonary Edema

Although high altitude pulmonary edema was clearly described over seventy years ago, only in the last twenty years has it been recognized as a major problem for mountaineers. Cases that occurred prior to 1960 were usually diagnosed as pneumonia, and acute pulmonary edema and pneumonia do have similarities. This important and serious mountaineering problem can occur and has been lethal as low as 9,000 feet (2,700 m), although it is unusual below 12,000 feet (3,700 m). It is more fully described in Chapter Twelve, "Medical Problems of High Altitude."

Asthma

Asthma is a disease of the bronchi caused by allergy. Contact with the substance to which the individual is allergic (the allergen) increases the secretion of mucus into the bronchi. Simultaneously, the muscles in the walls of the bronchi go into spasm, constricting these air passages. The narrowed bronchi filled with excess mucus obstruct the passage of air and cause respiratory difficulty.

Asthma may be very mild, severe, or even fatal (fortunately, very rarely). A first attack may occur at any time and any place, although most frequently the patient is aware of his asthma long before he takes up mountaineering.

Asthma is a recurring disease; a climber with this disorder would usually have suffered a number of previous attacks. He should be under the care of a physician from whom he should obtain the medications necessary to care for himself during an asthmatic attack. However, individuals with mild asthma are not particularly limited in the extent to which they can partake in mountaineering.

The most significant sign of asthma is difficulty in breathing, particularly during expiration. The expiratory phase of respiration, which normally requires less time than inspiration, is considerably prolonged and may require conscious effort on the part of the patient.

An incessant, irritating cough is often present. Toward the end of an asthmatic attack the patient may cough up considerable quantities of very thick mucus. Fever is usually absent, but the pulse rate may be moderately increased. The respiratory rate is usually faster than normal in spite of the difficulty in breathing.

When the patient is examined, the chest may appear more expanded than normal at the end of expiration. Loud wheezes and some bubbling and crackling sounds are usually audible throughout all parts of the lung.

The keystone of asthma treatment is adequate fluid intake. Regardless of the medication used, tripling the intake of liquids benefits the patient. Steam inhalations are also helpful. Mild asthma responds well to one of the oral theophylline preparations. Attacks of moderate severity can often be controlled with an orally administered isoproterenol solution. Severe attacks require subcutaneous injections of 0.3 cc of a 1:1,000 solution of adrenalin, which can be repeated every five to ten minutes for several doses. The pulse rate rises, often to an uncomfortably high level, following adrenalin. If more than a few injections are given, or if the series is repeated after several hours, pulse and blood pressure should be recorded ten minutes after each injection. Aminophyllin by rectal suppository is often beneficial but requires twenty to thirty minutes to take effect. Inhalation of nebulized medication has become popular in recent years. When nebulizers are used only occasionally and only for severe attacks, they can be dramatically effective. However, nebulizers should not be used more frequently than every one or two hours and should rarely be used for more than one day. Many asthmatics carry a nebulizer or a least know which one is effective.

Since asthma further limits the amount of oxygen obtainable by the body, oxygen inhalation is usually helpful at high altitudes, but any mucus blocking the airways must be coughed up or the oxygen is less effective. The best way to ensure such obstructions are eliminated is to provide plenty of liquids and the most appropriate medication.

Prevention of asthmatic attacks is important. Patients with allergies that cause severe asthma should be aware of their susceptibility and avoid the allergens whenever possible.

Severe asthmatics should obtain detailed instructions and all medications required for their care from their personal physicians before embarking on mountaineering outings. Since persons who have long standing severe asthma tend to have chronic obstructive pulmonary disease as well, they may be unwise to venture above 8,000 feet (2,400 m). Some physicians have the impression that persons with asthma tend to be more susceptible to high altitude pulmonary edema, but this predisposition can not be proven or disproven.

Persons with asthma are well advised to be more cautious with altitude and to allow more time for acclimatization. However, above snowline the allergens causing asthma are rarely encountered, and mild asthmatics may have no difficulty with snow and ice climbing.

Pneumothorax

Occasionally lung tissue may rupture spontaneously, allowing air to leak into the chest cavity. Lacerations of the lung can also occur with penetrating injuries of the chest, or nonpenetrating injuries which fracture and displace ribs. The lung on the side of the air leak tends to retract, due to its inherent elasticity, and does not expand well during inspiration. As a result, pulmonary function is compromised. This condition is known as pneumothorax, meaning "air in the chest."

Rarely the tear in the lung behaves like a valve, allowing air into the pleural space but not allowing it to leave, which causes the pressure within the space to build rapidly. The pressure collapses the adjacent lung and can even apply pressure on the opposite lung, drastically interfering with pulmonary function. If untreated, this disorder is usually lethal, particularly in the hypoxic conditions of higher elevations. This condition is labelled "tension pneumothorax" because the air is under increased pressure.

Pneumothorax should be suspected when unexplained shortness of breath appears suddenly in an otherwise healthy, active person. Sometimes the onset is associated with sudden pain of mild to moderate severity. The diagnosis is confirmed by the absence of breath sounds over the entire lung on the affected side. A tension pneumothorax should be suspected when shortness of breath is severe and the patient is fighting for air. His lips and fingernails are usually purple. Sometimes the trachea just above the sternum is shifted to the side away from the pneumothorax; the point where the heart is felt may also be shifted in the same direction.

No treatment is needed unless a tension pneumothorax develops. Then the pressure must be relieved by inserting a tube into that side of the chest, a simple procedure that may be life saving, but one that should be done only by a physician except in desperate circumstances. This procedure is discussed in greater detail in Chapter Ten, "Chest Injuries," and in Appendix B, "Therapeutic Procedures."

Patients with a spontaneous pneumothorax need to rest for a week or longer until the "leak" in the lung tissue has healed, as it usually does. In mountaineering circumstances, the patient should be moved to a location where a physician's help can be obtained should a tension pneumothorax develop unless the move would require undue exertion. Persons who have had one episode of spontaneous pneumothorax are more vulnerable to successive episodes. They may want to consider surgical therapy to try to eliminate the condition, and they certainly should learn, or have their climbing partners learn, how to recognize and treat tension pneumothorax if it should develop.

THROMBOPHLEBITIS AND PULMONARY EMBOLISM

Clotting of the blood in the veins of the legs (or rarely the arms) is not uncommon in mountaineers. Thrombophlebitis, as the presence of such clots is called, was seldom recognized in climbers before 1950 but is now known to occur with some frequency. Complications also are common.

The major danger from thrombophlebitis lies in the tendency for the blood clots to break off and be carried back through the heart into the lungs, a development known as pulmonary embolism. The clots (or emboli) obstruct the pulmonary arteries, reducing pulmonary blood flow and the oxygenation of blood in the lungs. Extensive embolism or obstruction of a major pulmonary artery such as the artery to an entire lung is usually fatal.

An increased tendency of the blood to clot (increased coagulability), and slowing or even cessation of blood flow in the veins (stasis) favor the development of thrombophlebitis. Factors increasing the coagulability of blood are:

1. Dehydration, which causes the blood to become thicker and more viscous;
2. Increase in the number of red blood cells due to high altitude, a normal mechanism of acclimatization which also increases the viscosity of blood;
3. Stress, from climbing and a hostile environment, which causes the secretion into the blood of substances that cause the blood to clot more readily;
4. Hypoxia, which causes blood to clot more readily at higher elevations by mechanisms that are not understood.

Factors predisposing to stasis are:

1. Prolonged immobility, such as being storm bound for days in a small tent, immobile, and resting in cramped, awkward positions;
2. Low temperature, which produces constriction of the arteries in the extremites to conserve heat, thereby reducing the blood flow to the limbs and the volume of blood being returned to the heart through the veins;
3. Heavy packs, which increase stasis in the legs, or standing immobile for long periods of time on complicated and difficult climbs, which is even more dangerous;
4. Tight clothing, which easily constricts and obstructs veins because they have thin walls and the pressure within them is low.

Oral contraceptive drugs also promote the development of thrombophlebitis and pulmonary embolism. Women taking such drugs should discontinue them several weeks in advance of any mountaineering outing during which a stay of more than two or three days at altitudes higher than 10,000 feet (3,000 m) is anticipated, particularly when cold or other conditions may lead to circumstances predisposing to thrombophlebitis.

Diagnosis of Thrombophlebitis

The most common symptom of thrombophlebitis is a deep, aching pain in the calf, inner side of the thigh, or back of the knee, which frequently comes on suddenly and is aggravated by walking. When the thrombosed vein is located in the calf, as it most frequently is, the overlying muscles are tender. Flexing the foot upward also causes pain in the calf.

Rarely clots form in the legs or pelvis without causing inflammation, a condition known as phlebothrombosis. In the absence of inflammation, these clots produce no symptoms, and they also are more loosely attached to the vessel walls and more likely to be detached and carried to the lungs. Consequently, if a patient is in pulmonary distress and other pulmonary disorders do not appear to be present, pulmonary embolism must be suspected even though signs of thrombophlebitis are absent.

Red, tender, slightly swollen streaks along the arms or legs can be indicative of thrombophlebitis, but embolism rarely results from involvement of these superficial veins.

Swelling of the affected leg usually occurs and can be most easily detected by measuring the circumference of both legs at identical five inch intervals from the ankle to upper thigh. Differences in circumferences of one-half inch are frequent and are of no significance; greater differences are cause for concern. The limb may be pale, is sometimes cyanotic, and may have diminished arterial pulsations. Fever of 100° to 102° F (38° to 39° C) is sometimes present and persists an average of seven to ten days.

Diagnosis of Pulmonary Embolism

The typical symptoms of pulmonary embolism are the sudden onset of chest pain accompanied or followed shortly by cough, shortness of breath, and a rapid pulse. Later, the pain becomes pleuritic and is aggravated by respiration, particularly deep breathing. White, frothy material is coughed up at first, but the sputum becomes obviously bloody within a few hours. The respiratory and pulse rates are moderately increased and a slight fever is frequently present. Signs of consolidation (increased or absent breath sounds and dullness to percussion) may appear over the involved area a day or so after onset.

However, these easily recognized signs and symptoms are characteristic of a relatively large embolus. Symptoms of smaller emboli are more subtle, but their recognition is vital if larger emboli are to be avoided. Instead of pain, the patient may feel only pressure, or may have no symptoms related to his lungs at all. He may have only a sense of oppression, a sense of heaviness and obstruction, accompanied by panic or feelings of impending death. Some shortness of breath is usually present but may appear to be emotional in origin. Coughing, signs of consolidation, and other signs of embolism are commonly absent.

If a massive embolus obstructs a large artery, the patient commonly collapses and dies immediately. Such emboli, for reasons that are not understood, are frequently accompanied by a sensation of the need to defecate. Experienced physicians know that the patient who dies suddenly while on a bedpan usually has suffered a large pulmonary embolus. If the patient does not die, the initial symptom may be the sudden onset of a sense of suffocation rather than pain. More severe shortness of breath, cyanosis, distention of neck veins, and signs of shock follow shortly. Patients who do not die immediately could be expected to commonly develop fatal hypoxia at high elevations.

Prevention

Prevention is important but difficult. Climbers confined to a tent by a storm should be careful to exercise their feet and legs for a few minutes every hour or two and to avoid tight, constricting clothing. Maintenance of an adequate fluid intake is absolutely essential. Persons with varicose veins should either avoid high altitude climbing, obtain instructions on how to deal with their problem, or have the condition surgically corrected.

Treatment

Aspirin has a tendency to decrease blood coagulability, particularly at high altitude. Therefore, aspirin should be administered when thrombophlebitis or pulmonary embolism is first suspected. Stronger anticoagulant therapy is routinely given for thrombophlebitis with or without embolism within a hospital, but the consequences of an overdose are too dangerous for such treatment to be used without laboratory control.

Once thrombophlebitis develops, the patient must be completely confined to bed. Walking or any other movement may cause the clots to break off and embolize. The feet should be elevated slightly, the clothing kept loose, and awkward positions avoided. Aspirin and codeine may be given for pain if needed, but no other medications are necessary. Immobilization should be continued until all signs of thrombosis have been absent for four or five days.

Table Eight. Diagnostic Features of Various Severe Pulmonary Diseases

	Pneumonia	High Altitude Pulmonary Edema	Heart Failure	Pulmonary Embolism
ONSET	Gradual, 24 to 36 hours	Gradual, 12 to 36 hours after ascent	Gradual	Sudden
CHILLS	Frequent at onset	Absent	Absent	Absent
FEVER	Usual; often high	Absent or low	Absent or low	Moderate; may be absent
SPUTUM	Thick, stringy, green, yellow, or rusty	Frothy; white or pink	Frothy; white or pink	Frothy; later bloody
PAIN	Pleuritic; may be absent	None	Uncommon	Pleuritic
FLUID (EDEMA)	Localized or diffuse, often slight	Usually diffuse	Legs; lower portions of lungs	Localized if present
PHYSICAL FINDINGS	Crackling rales; rub; loud, harsh breath sounds	Crackling rales; bubbling	Rales and bubbling at lung bases	Rub; harsh or absent breath sounds
OTHER FEATURES	May follow a cold or bronchitis	No history of heart disease; rapid ascent to above 9,000 feet (2,700 m)	History of heart disease	Signs of thrombo-phlebitis

Because so much fluid is lost through breathing and insensible perspiration at altitude, dehydration is very common and very dangerous. All climbers, particularly those confined to camp by storms and those who already have thrombophlebitis, must force themselves to consume large quantities of fluids.

Elastic bandages wrapped snugly (but not tightly enough to obstruct circulation) around both legs are desirable. Such bandages collapse the superficial veins and increase blood flow in the deep veins of the legs and therefore are a good means for preventing thrombophlebitis for patients immobilized by frostbite or injury at high elevations. Frostbite does predispose the victim to thrombophlebitis and may lead to pulmonary embolism.

A party with a member who has thrombophlebitis on a mountain expedition is faced with a difficult decision. It is desirable to keep the victim quiet, his leg bandaged, and to hydrate him carefully, but it is often difficult to stay for very long in a mountain camp and the temptation to transport the patient is strong. The dilemma is far greater once pulmonary embolism has occurred and life is threatened by subsequent emboli. Evacuation is essential, but the patient should be carried as much as possible. If climbing is unavoidable, the affected limb should be carefully bandaged, particularly if embolism has occurred. Not to evacuate such patients to hospital care is too risky, but every precaution must be taken to ensure that minimum activity and stress result.

CHAPTER SEVENTEEN

Diseases of the Heart and Blood Vessels

The heart and blood vessels circulate blood, which transports oxygen and nutrients to the body tissues, and carries away carbon dioxide and "wastes." The heart consists of a four chambered pump: right atrium, right ventricle, left atrium, and left ventricle. Blood is pumped from the left ventricle into the aorta, the body's main artery. This vessel repeatedly branches into smaller and smaller arteries and finally into capillaries barely large enough to permit passage of single red blood cells. In the capillaries, oxygen and nutrients diffuse into the tissues, carbon dioxide and wastes diffuse back into the blood, and other substances move back and forth between blood and tissue. From the capillaries, blood flows into larger and larger veins and returns through the right atrium into the right ventricle. Blood is then pumped from the right ventricle to the lungs, where it replaces the oxygen it has lost and gives off carbon dioxide. It returns through the left atrium to the left ventricle.

Four valves permit the heart to function as an efficient pump. The tricuspid and mitral valves in the right and left ventricles close during cardiac contraction (systole), preventing reflux of blood into the atria. Also during systole, the pulmonic and aortic valves open, permitting blood to be pumped into the pulmonary artery and aorta. After systole has been completed, the pulmonic and aortic valves close, preventing reflux of blood into the ventricles. When the heart chambers are relaxed (diastole), the tricuspid and mitral valves open, allowing the ventricles to fill.

Valves are also located in veins. Compression of peripheral veins by contracting muscles, and the low pressure within the chest produced by inspiration, produce a pressure gradient which moves blood from the extremities toward the heart. Venous valves permit blood to flow toward the heart but prevent backflow when pressures change.

Delicate receptors sense blood volume and oxygen and carbon dioxide content and dictate cardiac output (heart rate and the volume of each stroke) and the amount of blood supplied to different areas of the body.

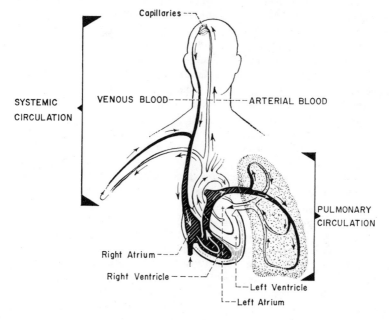

Figure 45. Diagram of the circulation of the blood.

PHYSICAL EXAMINATION OF THE CARDIOVASCULAR SYSTEM

Simple methods for examining the functions of the heart and circulatory system can provide highly significant information, even for inexperienced examiners. The examination should include: (1) determining heart rate and rhythm; (2) judging arterial and venous pressure; (3) evaluating the peripheral circulation; and (4) listening to the heart and lungs.

Heart Rate and Rhythm

The heart rate is most conveniently measured by carefully palpating the outer edge of the wrist at the base of the thumb, where the pulsations in the radial artery can be felt. Gentle pressure should be applied so the artery is not occluded. The pulsations are usually counted for fifteen, twenty, or thirty seconds and multiplied by four, three, or two to obtain the rate per minute. (Longer counts, sometimes as long as two to three minutes, may be needed for individuals with irregular rhythms.)

In some subjects, particularly victims of shock, the radial artery pulsations may be too weak to count, and the carotid or femoral pulse must be sought. The carotid pulse can be found on either side of the neck in the groove between the thyroid cartilage (Adam's apple) and the prominent strap muscle that extends from behind the ear to the top of the sternum (breastbone.) The femoral pulse can be found in the fold where the leg meets the abdomen about midway between the center of the pubic area and the lateral bony edge of the hip. Clothing must be removed from the area before the femoral pulse can be palpated.

If shock is so severe no pulses can be felt, the heart rate can be determined by listening with a stethoscope placed on the chest between the left nipple and the sternum. Each heartbeat is accompanied by two heart sounds of slightly different tone (lub-dup, lub-dup). Although heart sounds in normal subjects can be heard with the unaided ear pressed against the chest, the heart sounds are usually faint in shock and a stethoscope is often needed. A little prior practice by the examiner — even listening to his own heart — is useful.

The normal resting heart rate ranges from fifty to ninety beats per minute. A few well conditioned individuals may have rates as low as forty per minute. The heart rate is slower during sleep. At high altitude the resting heart rate may be as high as 100 per minute during the first few days of acclimatization.

Normally the heart rhythm is regular. In teenagers the heart rate may change with respiration — increasing during inspiration and slowing during expiration. This variation is normal but can be positively identified by having the subject hold his breath, which causes the rhythm to become completely regular.

Arterial and Venous Pressure

When the pulse is barely palpable, the blood pressure is usually low. Strong, "bounding" pulses usually indicate a normal blood pressure and normal heart action.

Arterial pulses are usually equal in both wrists, both sides of the neck, and both sides of the groin. Absence of a pulse on one side may indicate arterial obstruction or injury.

When healthy persons are lying flat, the partially or fully filled neck veins can be seen extending from the middle of the clavicle (collar bone) to just below the lower edge of the jaw. When the subject is sitting upright or even partially upright (semirecumbent) filled neck veins should not be visible above the clavicle. Visible, distended neck veins in these positions are abnormal, and usually indicate heart failure or obstruction of venous blood flow to the heart.

Accurate measurement of blood pressure requires a blood pressure cuff (sphygmomanometer) and stethoscope. The cuff should be wrapped smoothly and snugly (but not tightly) around the patient's upper arm, well above the elbow, and should be inflated with its bulb to a pressure of about 180 mm (Hg) or until the radial pulse disappears. The stethoscope cup should be placed over the elbow fold of the patient's extended arm and the cuff pressure allowed to fall slowly by carefully releasing the valve located on or near the bulb. As the cuff pressure drops, a thumping sound synchronous with the pulse can be heard. The indicated pressure at which the sound first appears is the systolic blood pressure. As the cuff pressure continues to fall, the pressure at which the sound completely disappears is the diastolic blood pressure. If the radial pulse can be felt and a stethoscope is not available, the systolic blood pressure can be approximated by inflating the cuff and allowing the pressure to fall until the radial pulse first appears. This pressure is 10 to 20 mm lower than the pressure determined by a stethoscope, but the method is reliable in an emergency. Normal blood pressure ranges from 105 to 140 mm systolic and 60 to 80 mm diastolic.

Peripheral Circulation

The lips, tongue, and fingernails (nail beds) are normally pink, but when the oxygen concentration in the blood is low, they become blue or purple. This discoloration (cyanosis) is commonly noted at high altitude and is usually severe with high altitude pulmonary edema. At lower elevations cyanosis usually indicates inadequate oxygenation of the blood by the lungs and is caused by disorders such as airway obstruction, pneumonia, or chest injuries.

When the blood pressure is low and blood flow to the extremities is decreased, the nail beds may be cyanotic, and the lips and tongue may have a blue gray color. This type of cyanosis is due to decreased blood flow and may occur even though oxygenation of the blood in the lungs is normal. It is commonly seen in shock.

Edema is a general medical term for the accumulation of excess water in the tissues. It is not uncommon in women during the first few days at high altitude due to retention of salt and water. The face is usually puffy in the morning, the feet or ankles may be mildly swollen, and body weight may increase four to twelve pounds. More severe degrees of edema, particularly if progressive, may be indicative of a high altitude disorder; progressive edema lasting for more than a week suggests heart failure or kidney disease and should be investigated.

Individuals who become short of breath with mild exertion, or who experience shortness of breath when lying flat that is relieved by sitting up, usually have fluid accumulations in the lungs (pulmonary edema). At high elevations, high altitude pulmonary edema should be suspected, but at lower elevations heart failure is a more common cause. When listening to the chest of a patient with pulmonary edema from either disorder, crackling or gurgling sounds can usually be heard with each breath. (Asthma usually produces squeaking or groaning sounds, particularly during expiration. Auscultation of the lungs is discussed further in Chapter Sixteen, "Diseases of the Respiratory System.")

Records are particularly important in the care of anyone suspected to have heart disease. All observations, including the time of the observations, must be noted. Examinations should be repeated at frequent, regular intervals, such as every two to four hours. Such records are needed by the physicians when the patient is evacuated and may make possible a prompt, accurate diagnosis by radio.

CLIMBERS WITH HEART DISEASE

Heart disease is very common and many patients live long, active, useful lives after the onset of their disorder. Modern management of heart disease encourages physical activity within specified limits, particularly among older people, and many of these patients climb and backpack.

A patient with heart disease who climbs without consulting his physician not only risks his own health; he imposes upon his companions an unjustifiable responsibility for his care which they may not have sufficient preparation to provide. The patient must follow his physician's instructions and obtain for himself any prescribed medications. The outing leader should be familiar with the treatment the patient is receiving and must be alert for complications that require additional care or evacuation (but the patient's physician, not the trip leader, is responsible for the patient's medical management). For longer trips or expeditions, the leader should be supplied with a letter from the physician detailing the nature of the patient's condition, restrictions on activity that should be observed, medications to be taken, and any signs or symptoms that require additional therapy or evacuation.

In general, heart attacks, heart failure, or other cardiac emergencies are rare among climbers who maintain their physical fitness by regular exercise. Acute heart problems are much more common in individuals who only occasionally participate in vigorous activity. Many hunters or fishermen are largely sedentary most of the year and participate in their sport only when it is in season. Then they engage in strenuous outdoor activity such as hiking or climbing through heavy underbrush, carrying a deer, or carrying a heavy pack. During such activities for which they are not physically conditioned, heart attacks are much more likely to occur.

THE HEART AND ALTITUDE

High altitude climbing poses no threat for the hearts of normal individuals. During severe exertion at sea level, cardiac output can be increased to a maximum in an effort to supply oxygen to the tissues. Highly motivated individuals can even temporarily increase their activity beyond the level at which tissues are fully supplied with oxygen, exercising "anaerobically" and allowing lactic acid and other unoxidized metabolites to accumulate in the blood and tissues. However, their level of activity is essentially limited by their tissue oxygen supply, which in turn is limited by their cardiac output. In an effort to increase the tissue oxygen, the heart gets pushed to work at a maximum level.

At high elevations, the oxygen supply to the tissues is limited by the reduced availability of oxygen from the atmosphere, not by cardiac output. As a result, the heart does not get pushed to work at a maximum level. During maximal exercise at high altitude the heart rate, which is a rough guide to the work being performed by the heart, is lower than at sea level. If cardiac performance during exercise is normal at sea level, it is normal at high altitude.

MAJOR HEART DISEASES

Angina Pectoris

Angina pectoris is a type of chest pain or discomfort caused by narrowing of the coronary arteries that supply the heart muscle with blood. The narrowing is the result of arteriosclerosis ("hardening of the arteries") and consists largely of deposits of cholesterol and other fats in the inner lining of the arteries. Rupture of one of these fat deposits, or clotting of blood within an artery narrowed by such deposits, further impairs the cardiac blood supply and may cause the onset of angina (chest pain), an increase in the severity of preexisting angina, or an acute myocardial infarction (heart attack).

The discomfort of angina pectoris is typically described as a sensation of pressure or deep seated pain beneath the sternum, which characteristically appears during exercise and disappears after a few minutes of rest. The discomfort may be described as crushing, a sensation of being squeezed, a feeling of weight on the chest, feeling as if a band were around the heart, or a deep burning sensation. It may be felt in the neck, jaws, or arms as well as in the chest. If exercise is continued, the discomfort increases. Angina pectoris frequently is accompanied by shortness of breath, which subsides as the discomfort eases.

Patients with mild angina pectoris may be permitted by their physicians to take part in mildly strenuous hikes or climbs provided they follow instructions, do not exert themselves, and carry nitroglycerine tablets to relieve more severe episodes of pain. Such patients probably would not be able to take part in long trips or outings above 8,000 feet (2,400 m).

Individuals who develop angina for the first time, or who experience unusually frequent or severe attacks of angina, should be forced to lie down and rest completely and should be given nitroglycerine, if it is available, to relieve the discomfort. Nitroglycerine tablets should be held under the tongue until they have dissolved. Several tablets may be necessary to obtain relief. (Nitroglycerine tablets should be kept in their original brown bottle and should not be kept longer than six months after purchase. Cotton wads should not be kept in the bottle, which should be tightly capped to prevent loss of potency by the tablets.) Absolute rest with sedation should be continued for at least six to eight hours, or until the patient has no further episodes of angina. The patient then should be evacuated with as little exertion as possible, preferably transported by some means. Angina is an indication of severe heart disease and may be a prelude to a more serious heart attack.

Myocardial Infarction

Myocardial infarction, a common cause of sudden death, is a major medical emergency. Chest pain is the most common initial symptom and may appear at rest or during exercise. The pain resembles angina pectoris but is usually more severe, may last one to six hours, and usually is not relieved by nitroglycerine. Other symptoms and signs that frequently are present include nausea, vomiting, difficulty breathing, weakness, sweating, pallor, cyanosis, and cold extremities. The blood pressure may be low; the heart rate may be slow and occasionally irregular.

Myocardial infarction typically is caused by complete obstruction of a coronary artery, usually by a blood clot (coronary thrombosis) which results in death (necrosis or infarction) of the heart muscle supplied by that artery. Recovery requires weeks or months.

The patient should be made to lie down immediately and rest completely. Nitroglycerine to relieve pain should be tried, although it usually is ineffective. If the pain is not relieved in ten to fifteen minutes, meperidine or morphine should be given every two hours until the pain is relieved. If the patient is agitated, a sedative should be given. If oxygen is available, it should be administered at a flow rate of four to six liters per minute with a face mask. If the patient is coughing, short of breath, and can breathe more easily in that position, he should be permitted to sit up, preferably supported by some type of back rest. Administration of oxygen should be continued. Prompt evacuation, preferably by helicopter, is essential. A physician or advanced emergency medical technician should accompany the helicopter since cardiac resuscitation may be necessary at any moment.

Cardiac Dyspnea

Cardiac dyspnea is undue shortness of breath with exercise due to heart disease. Dyspnea may occasionally occur at night. The patient awakens with a sense of suffocation and feels compelled to sit up or move out into fresh air to obtain relief. He is usually anxious and has rapid heart and respiratory rates. Rales or crackling sounds indicating the presence of fluid in the lungs may be heard when listening to the chest. If the patient has a history of heart disease, a heart murmur, or treatment of heart failure, cardiac dyspnea should be diagnosed. Complete rest, sedation, and the administration of a diuretic (furosemide or acetazolamide) are required. The patient should be evacuated after twelve to twenty-four hours of rest with as little effort on his part as possible. If the dyspnea is severe, oxygen and meperidine or morphine should be given.

At high elevations, high altitude pulmonary edema should be considered, particularly if the subject has no history of heart disease and has recently ascended to that elevation. If high altitude pulmonary edema is suspected, rest, oxygen, and assisted evacuation to a lower altitude are necessary.

Valvular Heart Disease

Many patients have deformities of heart valves that cause heart murmurs and yet are capable of strenuous physical effort without difficulty. However, such activity may produce complications such as cardiac dyspnea, cardiac pulmonary edema, atrial fibrillation, or stroke for patients with some varieties of valvular heart disease. Any individual with a heart murmur or valvular heart disease should consult a physician to determine whether or not he should take part in climbing activities. Other members of an outing must be informed of that person's activity limits, medications to be taken, and complications that might be expected.

NONCARDIAC CHEST PAIN

Chest pain for most individuals is not a sign of heart disease, although an unfortunate number fear it is. Several common types of chest pain not related to heart disease are:

1. Aching and soreness due to muscular effort. After unaccustomed physical work involving the arms and shoulders such as climbing, cross country skiing, carrying a heavy pack, or cutting wood, pain may be present in the upper chest muscles for two to three days. The ache is usually constant, may be aggravated by motion, and the muscles may be tender. Aspirin and rest is effective treatment.
2. Chest discomfort due to anxiety. Nervous, anxious, or fearful individuals may notice a sensation of pressure across the chest associated with a sense of suffocation, trembling, dizziness, and occasionally numbness of the lips and fingers. The heart rate may be increased. Reassurance, rest, and mild sedation are the measures usually needed. (See Hyperventilation Syndrome in Chapter Sixteen, "Diseases of the Respiratory System.")
3. Aching or pricking pain over the heart. After heavy climbing or hiking some individuals note aching or a sharp pricking pain over the left nipple. The pain may be constant or intermittent, and is often worse at night. Reassurance, rest, and aspirin are all that is usually needed.
4. Heartburn. A burning pain below the end of the breast bone, sometimes extending upward into the throat or jaw, may be noted after a meal, excessive consumption of spicy foods, coffee, tea, or alcohol, or the use of carbonated beverages. The discomfort is not related to effort and may last for one to three hours. Heartburn should not be mistaken for angina. Antacids or milk, rest, and reassurance are the most appropriate management.

DISORDERS OF CARDIAC RHYTHM

Paroxysmal Tachycardia

This term is used for a disorder characterized by a very rapid heart rate, sudden in onset, which is associated with the symptoms of pounding in the chest, weakness, dizziness, and shortness of breath. The heart rate is very rapid (150 to 220 or more per minute) and completely regular. The pulses may be so weak that listening to the heart with a stethoscope is necessary to determine the rate. (When beating so rapidly, the heart does not have time to fill between contractions and the amount of blood pumped out decreases.) Victims may have experienced similar attacks previously.

Preferably, the patient should rest and let the episode stop spontaneously. However, if the tachycardia does not stop within ten to fifteen minutes, a few simple maneuvers may be tried. The patient can try forcefully blowing up a paper bag or an air mattress. He can try holding his breath as long as possible. Inserting a tongue blade or a spoon handle in the back of the throat and making him gag may stop the attack. Immersing his face in a bowl or bucket of water for as long as he can hold his breath sometimes works. A sharp blow over the heart with the edge of the hand (a Karate chop) may help. (The patient obviously should be warned in advance, and the blow must not be heavy enough to fracture ribs.) In some instances helping the patient stand on his head has terminated episodes of tachycardia.

If these measures fail, the right carotid artery can be massaged, gently at first, but firmly if necessary. The patient usually is immediately aware that the attack has ended. Since episodes of tachycardia tend to recur, the patient may need to be evacuated if the attack is his first and control has been difficult. However, paroxysmal tachycardia is almost never a sign of imminently threatening cardiac disease.

Atrial Fibrillation

Atrial fibrillation is a rapid, but irregular heart beat. The heart rate may be 100 to 180 per minute, and the onset may be sudden and resemble paroxysmal tachycardia. The important difference is the totally irregular rhythm of atrial fibrillation. Careful palpation of the pulse and listening to the heart may be necessary to be sure of the irregularity. With rates exceeding 160 per minute, irregularities are difficult to detect. Bed rest and sedation should be instituted; frequently normal heart action returns spontaneously after a few hours. Maneuvers employed to stop paroxysmal tachycardia are of no value for atrial fibrillation. If the attack does not respond to rest and sedation within twelve to twenty-four hours, the patient should be evacuated. Atrial fibrillation is a more significant disorder that may be a sign of serious heart disease.

Digitalis

Digitalis may be advisable if someone experienced with its administration is available and if evacuation of a patient with either of the above rhythm disturbances is difficult or unavoidably delayed. If the attack has not stopped within twelve to twenty-four hours, digoxin 0.25 mg may be given every two hours until a total dose of 1.5 mg (six 0.25 mg tablets) has been administered. (The patient must not have taken digitalis during the previous week.) If irregularities persist, digoxin 0.25 mg may be given daily. The patient must rest and should be sedated if necessary. Adequate fluids must be given to prevent the formation of clots, which could cause embolism or a stroke, in the irregularly beating heart. If nausea or vomiting appear, or the heart rate slows to below sixty per minute, digoxin should be stopped since these are signs of an overdose.

Cardiac Syncope

Cardiac syncope is loss of consciousness caused by heart disease. Two general forms are recognized: exertional syncope and arrhythmic syncope. With exertional syncope, loss of consciousness, fainting, or a "blackout spell" occurs during a burst of heavy effort such as running uphill. Unconsciousness may occur suddenly or may be preceded by a "gray out" sensation, severe dizziness, or weakness. Convulsive movements may occur. Exertional syncope most frequently occurs in patients with aortic stenosis (narrowing of the outlet valve from the left ventricle) but is occasionally seen in patients with arteriosclerotic coronary artery disease. The care for any unconscious patient must be administered. The blood pressure should be measured, the heart rate should be determined, and the rhythm should be evaluated.

Arrhythmic syncope occurs as the result of either a sudden abnormal increase in heart rate (tachycardia) or a marked slowing or temporary cessation of the heartbeat (heart block). The episode may occur suddenly, without warning, and the patient may fall and be injured. Convulsive movements may occur. General care for unconscious patients should be instituted. The blood pressure should be measured, the heart rate should be determined, and the rhythm should be evaluated. If a very slow heart rate persists after recovery, Isuprel glossets, if available, should be administered every hour.

Cardiac syncope can usually be distinguished from simple fainting, for which a cause, such as an emotional shock, an overheated room, or prolonged standing, is usually obvious. Fainting usually has a more gradual onset, does not occur during effort, and the heart rhythm is regular with a rate above sixty per minute.

Any individual with evident or suspected cardiac syncope should rest, with sedation if needed, for six to twelve hours and then be evacuated. A physician's care is needed as cardiac syncope may be an early warning of heart disease that can cause sudden death.

MINOR DISTURBANCES OF CARDIAC RHYTHM

Sinus Tachycardia

Anxious individuals, after heavy exertion or at high altitude, may be aware of a pounding sensation in their chests caused by a rapid, forceful heart beat, and may be fearful of heart disease. If the heart rate does not exceed 140 per minute and gradually slows with rest and sedation, a diagnosis of harmless sinus (normal) tachycardia may be made. No specific treatment except rest and reassurance is necessary.

Extrasystoles Or "Skipped Beats"

Normal individuals may notice occasional irregular thumping or "fluttering" sensations in their chests, especially at rest or during the night. They may feel their pulse and notice occasional pauses between beats. Such irregular beats are called extrasystoles and are of no significance unless the patient clearly has a heart disease such as angina, myocardial infarction, or cardiac dyspnea. Rest and reassurance are usually the only measures needed. Avoiding stimulants such as coffee and tea or tobacco may entirely eliminate the extrasystoles.

Cardiac Arrhythmias

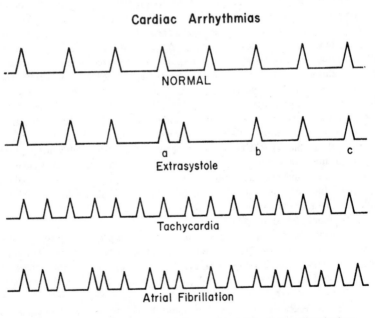

Figure 46. Diagrammatic comparison of normal and abnormal cardiac rhythms. (Note: interval ab = interval bc.)

If a bothersome irregularity of the heartbeat persists, if the skipped beats occur more than five times per minute, or if such irregularities have never been experienced before, evacuation to a physician's care is desirable.

HIGH BLOOD PRESSURE

Ten to twenty percent of the over-forty population of the United States has an elevated blood pressure, and many individuals with high blood pressure must be climbers. For such individuals to climb safely, the following guidelines should be observed:

1. Individuals with mild or drug controlled high blood pressure should climb only after consulting a physician. Such patients must supply their own medications and follow their physician's recommendations carefully. Fluid intake should be adequate and their diet should be low in salt and protein.
2. Individuals with severe, uncontrolled high blood pressure, or complications of high blood pressure, should not climb. The complications of high blood pressure include strokes, heart failure, coronary artery disease (angina), decreased visual acuity, and kidney failure.

Individuals with moderate high blood pressure may experience complications in the mountains with which outing leaders should be familiar. These complications include cardiac dyspnea, angina pectoris, stroke, and severe headache, any of which is an indication for prompt evacuation.

Some patients with only moderately high blood pressure have episodes of severe blood pressure elevation. Such episodes are typically associated with severe headache, confusion, forgetfulness, visual impairment, slurred speech, and other neurologic signs and symptoms. The blood pressure should be measured if such symptoms appear and the patient should be forced to rest, with sedation if needed. If the systolic pressure exceeds 200 mm, nitroglycerine should be given every hour to reduce the pressure. Evacuation should be arranged after six to twelve hours of rest and treatment.

Some high blood pressure patients experience an increase in pressure at high altitude. The rise in pressure, which may not be detectable unless the blood pressure is measured, is usually evident within one to two days at even moderate altitudes such as 6,000 feet (1,800 m). If a patient has a significant rise in pressure at such moderate altitudes, he should consult his physician, who may advise him to increase his medications when he is at high altitudes or may advise him not to go to high elevations at all.

Patients taking certain types of medication for their high blood pressure (such as propranolol, a beta blocker) may not experience the usual increase in heart rate at high altitude. Some patients taking drugs to lower their blood pressure develop a fall in pressure associated with dizziness or fainting when they stand up (orthostatic hypotension). They may feel weak and dizzy when walking, particularly at high altitude or during hot weather. Measuring the blood pressure with the patient lying down and again after two to three minutes of quietly standing erect, may disclose a fall in pressure during standing. A fall in systolic pressure of more than 20 mm is abnormal. Patients with orthostatic hypotension should decrease their medications for a few days and increase their intake of salt and fluid.

VASCULAR DISEASE

Claudication

Older individuals with arteriosclerosis of the arteries in their legs may experience pain or cramps in their calves, hips, buttocks, or thighs while walking uphill, particularly when carrying a heavy load. The pain occurs during effort, becomes more severe as effort is continued, and is relieved by rest. The medical term for this condition is claudication. When severe, it can appear while strolling on a level surface.

Claudication should be distinguished from common leg cramps, which typically occur at rest or during the night, are accompanied by painful contraction of the muscles, and usually involve the calf or foot.

If claudication is mild, a slower pace and a lighter load may permit the individual to continue climbing. Smoking increases the severity of claudication and should be avoided. If claudication is severe or appears suddenly, the patient should be evacuated with minimal effort on his part.

Varicose Veins

The veins of the extremities have numerous small valves within them to ensure that blood flows only in the direction of the heart. The blood pressure in veins is so low that the increase in intrathoracic or intraabdominal pressure associated with straining or strenuous exercise would reverse the direction of the venous blood flow if these valves were not present.

In some individuals the valves in the leg veins become incompetent, the direction of blood flow is no longer controlled, and the veins become dilated and tortuous (varicose). The return of venous blood from the limb to the heart may be impaired, causing persons with varicose veins to complain of aching in their legs, particularly after they have been on their feet for a prolonged period. The condition should be corrected surgically (by excising or ligating the affected veins) because it can lead to ulceration of the skin and other complications. The results are more satisfactory when surgical therapy is instituted early.

The greatest significance of varicose veins for mountaineers lies in the tendency for this disorder to increase the fatigability of the legs and limit endurance. A second problem is the greater tendency for veins in the legs to thrombose, which results from stasis associated with the reduced venous blood flow typically found with varicose veins. A less common problem is caused by the presence of greatly enlarged blood vessels just beneath the skin. Relatively minor injuries, which might go unnoticed, can penetrate one of these veins and produce relatively severe bleeding. Although the hemorrhage can be easily controlled, a person with varicose veins should be aware of this danger.

Patients with varicose veins should consult a physician about proper management of their condition during a climb. Elastic stockings may be prescribed. A patient with painful varicose veins should be encouraged to elevate his legs on pillows or a soft pad, which decreases the pressure within the veins, during rest stops. Relief may be obtained with a smooth elastic bandage or elastic stocking, which should applied when the patient is lying down and the veins are collapsed. The bandages or stockings should be removed at night. If one or more of the enlarged veins becomes hard, inflamed, and tender, the blood in the vein has clotted. Thrombosis of such superficial veins is rarely a problem except for the discomfort. However, swelling of the foot or leg beyond the area where clotting has occurred is indicative of clotting of the deeper veins. To avoid pulmonary embolism, the patient should be treated as described in Thrombophlebitis and Pulmonary Embolism in Chapter Sixteen, "Diseases of the Respiratory System."

ACKNOWLEDGMENT

Howard B. Burchell, M.D., provided valuable advice and suggestions in the preparation of this chapter.

ADDITIONAL READING

Selzer A: *The Heart: Its Function in Health and Disease.* Berkeley, University of California Press, 1966.

CHAPTER EIGHTEEN

Gastrointestinal Diseases

The gastrointestinal tract consists of the mouth and throat, esophagus, stomach, small and large intestines, liver, gallbladder, and pancreas. This system ingests food, converts it into forms that can be used by the body, and finally excretes the residual waste material.

The esophagus aids in swallowing and propels the food rapidly into the stomach, where it remains thirty to ninety minutes while being digested by enzymes and hydrochloric acid. The food next passes into the upper part of the small intestine (duodenum) where enzymes secreted by the intestinal mucosa and the pancreas further modify the partially digested food, preparing it for absorption. Bile salts, which are produced by the liver and stored in the gallbladder, help emulsify fats so they can be absorbed. Absorption takes place in the middle and lower segments of the small intestine (jejunum and ileum). In the large intestine, water is extracted from the residual wastes which are then excreted. Before travelling to the rest of the body, all of the blood from the small intestine goes to the liver where an array of complex biochemical reactions converts the absorbed nutrients to substances needed by the other tissues and organs.

Diseases of many organs produce symptoms referable to the alimentary tract, particularly nausea and vomiting. In addition, most gastrointestinal illnesses can not be exactly diagnosed in the field. Even when the cause of a disorder is known, no specific therapy may be available. Therefore, the treatment for most gastrointestinal diseases is directed towards eliminating or alleviating the patient's symptoms.

The most common signs and symptoms produced by diseases of the gastrointestinal system are nausea and vomiting, diarrhea, constipation, bleeding, jaundice, and pain. Pain that comes on suddenly and unexpectedly is such an eminent problem that it is discussed separately in Chapter Nineteen, "Acute Abdominal Pain." The physical examination of the abdomen is also described in that chapter.

VOMITING

The causes of vomiting are innumerable. A partial list includes such widely differing disorders as acute gastroenteritis, motion sickness, head injury, metabolic disorders, bacterial and viral infections, pregnancy, environmental heat, strenuous exertion, and appendicitis.

If the patient is stuporous or unconscious, a single bout of vomiting can be disastrous. The vomitus can be aspirated into the lungs, resulting in a severe, often fatal pneumonia. Respiratory obstruction can be lethal if the volume of aspirated material is large. At the first sign of vomiting, an unconscious patient's head must be lowered and turned to the side. He may be lifted by the waist about twelve to eighteen inches if he has not been involved in an accident that could have produced a fractured spine. (If a blow to the head is responsible for the unconsciousness, he should be assumed to have a broken neck.) The head down position must be maintained until vomiting has ceased and the vomitus cleared from his mouth. **The patient must not be allowed to aspirate the vomited material.**

Protracted vomiting sometimes ruptures the small blood vessels in the lining of the stomach, resulting in a small to moderate amount of bleeding. When vomiting is the result of excessive alcohol consumption such bleeding is fairly common but usually subsides promptly when the vomiting ceases.

Vomiting caused by minor disorders usually stops without any treatment. After the first bout the individual often feels better and is able to resume limited activity. If vomiting does not stop within a few hours, a serious underlying disease must be considered. Vomiting may be an important sign of brain injury, an acute abdominal disorder such as intestinal obstruction or appendicitis, drug overdose, or some other disease. If a patient had one of these disorders, control of vomiting with medications could delay diagnosis and definitive treatment.

When no underlying disease can be identified, vomiting can be treated symptomatically. If medications taken by mouth can be kept down, prochlorperazine (Compazine) can be given. Therapy should continue until the patient has been asymptomatic for at least four hours. If drugs given by mouth can not be retained, Compazine rectal suppositories can be inserted every four to six hours until medications taken by mouth can be kept down. Treatment for more than twenty-four hours should be avoided if possible. While under treatment the patient must not take part in any activities in which drowsiness, a common side effect of all drugs used to treat vomiting, could result in injury.

Following recovery, the patient should eat bland food, preferably liquid, for about twenty-four hours. Fluids that have been lost should be replaced as soon as possible to correct dehydration.

If vomiting is prolonged, the body becomes depleted of fluid and salt. On rare occasions, medications alone can not stop the vomiting until the fluid and salt are replaced, and treating such intractable vomiting requires intravenous fluids. If the proper fluids for intravenous therapy are not available, the patient must be evacuated.

MOTION SICKNESS

Symptoms of motion sickness can sometimes be reduced by lying down with the eyes open. Limiting the motion that causes the symptoms, for example by moving from the back to the front seat of a car, sitting over the wing of an airplane, or moving to the center of a ship, is the best form of therapy.

Treatment with drugs is most effective if started one hour before the motion is encountered. Dimenhydrinate (Dramamine) can be obtained without prescription. It should be taken sixty minutes before motion begins but must be taken every four hours thereafter until the abnormal motion ceases. Meclizine (Bonine and Antivert) is more effective for some individuals, is also available without prescription, and needs to be taken only once every twenty-four hours. Cyclizine (Marezine) has recently become available without prescription and is more effective for the control of motion sickness for some people. It should be taken every four to six hours as needed. Drowsiness is a common side effect of all of these drugs and may preclude driving automobiles and similar activities.

DIARRHEA

Of the many causes for diarrhea, the most common is a change in food or surroundings. Most other causes are equally benign, although a few diseases characterized by diarrhea can be life threatening.

The most common causes of diarrhea are listed in Table Nine according to the potential severity of the underlying disease and not the severity of the diarrhea.

Any of the diseases in the moderately severe and severe groups may produce only mild symptoms in any single individual. Indeed, amebiasis initially produces only mild symptoms in most patients but is included in the severe group because fatal complications can result from untreated infestations.

ACUTE GASTROENTERITIS

Acute gastroenteritis ("stomach flu") is characterized by rapidly developing generalized abdominal distress culminating in waves of cramps and diarrhea. During spasms of pain the patient typically draws his knees up against his abdomen for relief. However, the periods between spasms are relatively free of pain. Nausea is common and may be accompanied by vomiting. Sometimes nausea and vomiting are the dominant features of the illness.

Mild, generalized abdominal tenderness is commonly present, particularly in the lower part of the abdomen, and the bowel sounds are usually much louder than normal. Mild chills and fever may be present in severe cases but usually are absent.

Table Nine Common Causes of Diarrhea

MILD
    Acute (Acute Gastroenteritis)
        Staphylococcal Enteritis
        Food Allergy
        Viral Enteritis
        Traveller's Diarrhea
    Chronic
        Irritable Colon Syndrome
        Change of Food or Water
        Diseases of Other Organs

SEVERE
    Acute
        Cholera
        Invasive Bacterial Infections
    Subacute
        Typhoid Fever
    Chronic
        Amebiasis
        Inflammatory Bowel Disease

MODERATELY SEVERE
    Giardiasis
    Noninvasive Bacterial Infections

The diarrhea is frequently explosive in onset and is characterized by copious, watery, foul smelling stools. The number of stools varies from three or four to as many as twenty — sometimes more. Mucus is occasionally present in the stool, but blood and mucus are usually absent. The disorders with a more rapid onset are usually more severe but are of much shorter duration. Four specific types of acute gastroenteritis — staphylococcal enteritis, food allergy, viral enteritis, and traveller's diarrhea — usually can be recognized.

Staphylococcal Enteritis

Staphylococcal enteritis is caused by the ingestion of a toxin produced by staphylococcal bacteria. These organisms are present on the hands of about half of the population, and contamination of food is common. Any food may be contaminated, but meat, sweets such as cream pies, salads made with mayonnaise, and milk are the most common sources of the toxin. Staphylococcal enteritis occurs when food is contaminated during preparation and then is allowed to stand unrefrigerated for several hours during which the organisms multiply and produce their heat resistant toxin. Subsequent reheating — even boiling — does not destroy the toxin and prevent illness. To prevent this disorder, food must be consumed immediately after it is prepared, or it must be refrigerated.

The incubation period for staphylococcal enteritis is one to six hours, averaging three hours, and the onset is frequently abrupt. However, the disorder rarely lasts more than five to six hours. Typically, more than one person develops the disease — usually most of the individuals who have eaten the contaminated food.

Food Allergy

Food allergy is a rare disorder that results from an allergic reaction to food that is completely uncontaminated and causes no symptoms in others. The onset is characteristically sudden — frequently explosive — and comes within a few minutes to three or four hours after ingestion of the offending product. Nausea and vomiting frequently predominate. The disease disappears within a few hours or as soon as the offending food is eliminated. Very rarely is more than one person affected. The affected individual sometimes has suffered previous episodes of intolerance for the same food. A reaction can be anticipated in two circumstances: after unknowing ingestion of a known offending food, or after consumption of a food to which the individual has not previously recognized an allergy.

Viral Enteritis

Viral enteritis is caused by a number of viruses that are transmitted primarily by fecal contamination of water or hands but may be spread by other means, including personal contact. Common symptoms are nausea, abdominal cramps, vomiting, diarrhea, headache, and generalized muscular aching. Acute symptoms usually last from one to three days. The illness is benign, self limited, and rarely requires any specific therapy. Symptomatic treatment for headache or fever with aspirin, or for nausea and vomiting with prochlorperazine may be appropriate. Diarrhea should be treated by increasing the intake of salty fluids by mouth.

Traveller's Diarrhea

Most acute gastroenteritis occurring in visitors to tropical areas is classified as "traveller's diarrhea." This group of disorders has been labelled with highly descriptive names such as the Aztec two step, the Delhi belly, Montezuma's revenge, or, more commonly, "turista." Recently, enteropathogenic *Escherichia coli* have been clearly implicated as the most common cause of this disorder, although it is also caused by other bacteria, viruses, and even *Giardia*. *E. coli* are normal bacterial inhabitants of the bowel in everyone. Each individual becomes resistant to the particular strains found in his living area, and in him these organisms do not cause disease. However, upon exposure to toxin producing strains to which the individual has not developed resistance, symptomatic illness occurs. Precise identification of the toxin producing *E. coli* requires sophisticated bacteriological laboratory facilities; such studies are rarely needed or possible.

Infection is usually spread by fecal contamination of water or food, and is more common in underdeveloped countries with improper sewage disposal and inadequate water purification. However, travellers from other countries coming to the United States sometimes develop turista. The illness may be contracted anywhere.

Traveller's diarrhea can be prevented in several ways, of which avoiding the infection is clearly the best. Avoiding unpeeled fruits, salads containing leafy vegetables, and undisinfected drinking water are essential. Ice prepared from unclean water is notoriously infectious. Iodine disinfection of all water used for food preparation and for drinking may be necessary. (Beer and bottled soft drinks are usually safe.) Unfortunately, such precautions are not universally effective and are difficult to continue for a substantial time.

Antimicrobial agents can effectively prevent traveller's diarrhea. Unabsorbed sulfonamides, neomycin sulfate, trimethaprim-sulfamethoxazol (Bactrim or Septra) and doxycycline have been found to decrease the incidence of turista for at least four week intervals. Although these drugs are effective, physicians are quite justifiably reluctant to recommend them for the millions of people travelling to high risk areas. Antibiotics induce drug resistance in bacteria, and their use always carries the risk of introducing more dangerous, drug insensitive organisms into the environment. In addition, the most common side effect of doxycycline is diarrhea; the drug itself may produce the disorder it is being taken to prevent. Other side effects, particularly the tendency to cause solar sensitization which can lead to unusually severe sunburn, make the use of this drug for prophylaxis against traveller's diarrhea a calculated risk.

Bismuth subsalicylate (Pepto-Bismol) also prevents traveller's diarrhea when taken in quantities of 60 ml four times a day for up to three weeks. Obviously, consumption of a 240 ml bottle daily is inconvenient. Simply transporting the five liters per person of Pepto-Bismol required for three weeks' prophylaxis would create substantial problems in the wilderness. The tablets are not effective. Furthermore, although Pepto-Bismol significantly reduces the incidence of turista, it does not completely prevent the disorder. However, this drug has no major toxic side effects and appears to be considerably safer for routine prophylaxis than antimicrobial agents.

The incubation period for this disease is short, usually twelve to forty-eight hours, and it usually lasts two to five days. General symptoms such as chills and fever are uncommon; abdominal cramps, a feeling of being unwell, and frequent loose stools which do not contain blood or mucus are the usual features.

The treatment of diarrhea is discussed below. Specifically for traveller's diarrhea, bismuth subsalicylate taken after the onset of diarrhea is reported to diminish the number of loose bowel movements and relieve abdominal cramps. Antibiotic treatment begun after symptoms have started probably does not shorten the course of diarrhea due to enterotoxogenic *E. coli*.

Treatment

The essential treatment for all types of acute gastroenteritis consists of fluid and salt replacement. (The relief of symptoms, although desirable, is of secondary importance.) These disorders are rarely so severe that they produce significant dehydration, but occasionally this does occur. The almost invariable dehydration occurring at high altitudes would definitely be aggravated by severe vomiting or substantial diarrhea. Measuring the urine volume is a reliable method to assess dehydration; small volumes (less than 500 cc daily) of concentrated, deep yellow or orange urine indicate substantial fluid depletion.

To replace fluids and salts, fruit juices and salty broths and soups should be administered in substantial amounts. Oral rehydration with sugar and salt may be somewhat more effective. Formulas for several oral water and salt replacement solutions are listed. These formulas contain glucose (or sucrose that is broken down into glucose and fructose) to promote the absorption of sodium, but too much glucose can produce an osmotic diarrhea, particularly in children.

Table Ten Formulas for Oral Rehydration Salt Solutions

World Health Organization Formula

Sodium	84 mEq/L
Potassium	10 mEq/L
Chloride	80 mEq/L
Bicarbonate	30 mEq/L
Glucose	2 %

Available from Jianas Brothers Packaging, 2533 S.W. Boulevard, Kansas City, MO, U.S.A. ($.25 per package in lots of 5,000,); KBI, Berlin; ALLPACK, Waiblingen, West Germany; Geymont Sud, Anagni, Italy; and others. Also available as *Oralite*—Beecham; *Elotrans*—Fresenius, Bad Homburg; *Oral Rehydration Salts*—Servipharm, Basel; *Salvadora*—LUSA, Lima.

U.S. Public Health Service Formula (Centers for Disease Control)

Glass # 1	Glass # 2
8 ounces fruit juice	1/2 teaspoon baking soda (bicarbonate)
1/2 teaspoon honey or corn syrup	8 ounces water (uncontaminated)
1 pinch table salt	

Equal amounts should be drunk from each glass, alternating between the two.

Oral Fluid Replacement Solution

Sodium Chloride	3.5 g/l	1/2 level teaspoon
Sodium Bicarbonate	2.5 g/l	1/2 level teaspoon
Potassium chloride	1.5 g/l	1/4 level teaspoon
Glucose	20 g/l	6 level teaspoons
	or	
Sucrose (Table sugar)	40 g/l	12 level teaspoons

The WHO Oral Rehydration Salts are prepackaged in the quantities needed to make one liter of solution and are available from the firms listed. The U.S. Public Health Service solutions can be made from fruit juice, honey or corn syrup, salt, and baking soda as needed. The oral fluid replacement solution formula can be prepackaged at home in foil or small waterproof plastic vials, or made up in the field, but larger containers of the salts may be too heavy and bulky for small groups. The rather crude measurements of the components (teaspoons) are sufficiently accurate for anyone with normally functioning heart and kidneys, which will retain what is needed and excrete the rest. Furthermore, diarrheal salt losses vary at least as much as such measures. The salts and glucose must be dissolved in disinfected water. Patients with moderate diarrhea (five to ten watery stools per day) should drink one to two liters of one of these solutions every twenty-four hours. Patients with more severe diarrhea (ten or more watery stools per day) should drink enough of the solutions to equal the volume of the estimated losses plus one and one-half to two additional liters per day.

Treatment of nausea and vomiting with prochlorperazine may be necessary in order for adequate amounts of oral fluids to be consumed.

Whether drugs should be used to lessen or control diarrhea is controversial. Some evidence suggests these agents may prolong the illness even though the frequency of bowel movements is decreased. Fever and toxicity may actually increase if the diarrheal stool is still produced but is retained within the large intestine, perhaps allowing toxic products to be absorbed. A compromise that appears reasonable is to administer medications only to control severe cramps or in circumstances where frequent bowel movements would be hazardous or substantially inconvenient and uncomfortable. Certainly the threat of hypothermia when leaving a tent five to ten times a night would justify the use of a medication to lessen the frequency of bowel movements. Paregoric (tincture of opium), codeine, diphenoxylate (Lomotil), and loperamide (Imodium) are all potentially habit forming and are available only by prescription. These drugs vary in their effectiveness for different individuals. If known, the most effective drug for the patient should be administered; if the initial drug is not effective, one of the others may be tried.

Patients with severe diarrhea (more than ten stools a day), blood and mucus in the stool, persistence of symptoms for more than a few days, or with general symptoms such as chills and fever, should seek out a physician for diagnostic studies and treatment. If such care is unavailable, the patient can be treated for five days with trimethaprim-sulfamethoxysol or with ampicillin. If this treatment is ineffective and symptoms suggest giardiasis, quinacrine (Atabrine) or metronidazole (Flagyl) should be considered.

The amount of rest required by the patient varies widely. Some victims are able to continue climbing; most should restrict physical activity until symptoms improve or resolve.

CHRONIC MILD DIARRHEA

A mild diarrhea, consisting only of soft stools and a moderately increased frequency of bowel movements, may have many different causes. A change in food, water, or surroundings is the most common. Excitement or anxiety frequently produces such symptoms. Diseases of other organs are often accompanied by a mild diarrhea.

These disorders are classified as chronic because they may last for days or even weeks. However, the diarrhea is only mildly bothersome, not incapacitating, and usually clears up without any therapy. Diphenoxylate (Lomotil) or a similar drug three or four times a day may help reduce the number of bowel movements and return the stools to normal consistency. Antibiotics or other medications are unnecessary and should be avoided.

Irritable Colon Syndrome

The irritable colon syndrome, which is also known as "mucus colitis" or "spastic colon," is a common disturbance of large intestinal function which may result in either diarrhea or constipation. The syndrome is at least partially psychological in origin, and its appearance is directly related to emotional stress. This type of dysfunction can be expected to appear during mountaineering outings.

Most patients have some abdominal pain, and the pain may suggest some other disorder. Pain is most common in the upper abdomen or the left lower quadrant. Some patients may have severe pain in the left flank which radiates to the chest over the heart, the left shoulder, and down the inner surface of the left arm, suggesting heart disease such as angina or myocardial infarction. (See Chapter Seventeen, "Diseases of the Heart and Blood Vessels.") The pain may be relieved by the passage of gas or feces.

Patients with irritable colons often have other symptoms induced by nervous tension. Loss of appetite, nausea, belching, and occasionally vomiting are the more common gastrointestinal symptoms. Headache, sweating, flushing, shortness of breath, sighing respirations, and hyperventilation may be observed (see Chapter Sixteen, "Diseases of the Respiratory System.")

The stools are usually thin and tapered (pencil shaped), whether the patient has diarrhea or constipation, and a considerable amount of mucus is usually present.

Treatment consists principally of recognizing the nature of the disorder and reassuring the patient. If treatment of diarrhea is desirable, an anticholinergic drug is usually most effective. Drugs such as paregoric or diphenoxylate are usually not effective and should not be used. However, drug therapy of any type is usually not required. The disorder disappears as soon as the source of the stress is eliminated, although repeated episodes with subsequent stress are characteristic.

MODERATELY SEVERE DIARRHEAS

Salmonellosis (Nontyphoidal)

Human infection with this group of bacteria most commonly produces an acute gastroenteritis; however, enteric (paratyphoid) fever, localized abscesses, or occasionally invasion of the blood stream by these bacteria may occur. These are serious illnesses, but transient asymptomatic infection of the intestinal tract also may occur. Salmonellae are widespread. Virtually all domestic and many wild animals harbor these organisms. The number of asymptomatic human carriers in the general population has been estimated at two persons per thousand.

Man almost always acquires this infection by the oral route. Any item of food or drink can be contaminated. The greatest single source of human disease is poultry products — both birds and eggs — and raw meat. Household pets, including dogs, cats, birds, and turtles, all harbor these bacteria.

Host resistance plays a major role in determining the response to this infection. Lack of hydrochloric acid in the stomach predisposes to gastroenteritis. Alteration of the normal microbial flora in the intestinal tract by antibiotics increases susceptibility to infection by these organisms.

Symptoms of salmonella grastoenteritis develop eight to forty-eight hours after ingestion of contaminated food. Nausea and vomiting occur initially; shortly thereafter abdominal cramps and persistent diarrhea appear, occasionally with mucus or blood. An initial chill is not unusual, and fever from 100.5° to 102° F (38° to 39° C) is common. Usually symptoms subside in two to five days and recovery is uneventful. Considerable variation in the severity of symptoms is observed among patients infected at the same meal. A small percentage of patients may have high fever and up to thirty to forty liquid stools per day. Abdominal pain may be sufficiently intense, localized, and associated with enough rebound tenderness to suggest an acute abdominal disorder requiring surgical therapy.

Less commonly, this group of organisms produces an illness clinically indistinguishable from typhoid fever, although the disorder is usually milder, of shorter duration, and has a lower mortality rate. Blood stream invasion produces a severe illness characterized by chills, prolonged intermittent fever, loss of appetite, and weight loss. With this form of infection, gastrointestinal symptoms are usually absent, but abscesses can form at almost any site.

The most important aspect of treatment for salmonella gastroenteritis is the prompt correction of dehydration and electrolyte (salt) abnormalities. One of the fluid preparations described in Table Ten should be administered. Drugs to relieve cramps or diarrhea probably cause the illness to persist for a longer period of time. (Diarrhea may play a significant role in eliminating bacteria or their toxins from the bowel.) No convincing evidence that antibiotics reduce the duration of the illness has been found. If drug therapy seems necessary for an unusually severe or complicated illness, the drug of choice is trimethoprim-sulfamethoxazole or, if that is ineffective, ampicillin or chloramphenicol. Fatalities are very rare in young, previously healthy adults, but complete recovery may require several weeks.

Giardiasis

Over the past few years the protozoal parasite *Giardia lamblia* has been found in waters all over the world. Animals such as beavers harbor and excrete the organisms, which probably accounts for its presence in mountain streams, but the organism has been found in the municipal water supplies for a number of large cities in the United States. Giardiasis is commonly transmitted by public water supplies in countries as diverse as Nepal and the Soviet Union.

In the last few years outdoor publications have contained many articles about giardiasis resulting in undue concern about this infestation among many of their readers. Gastroenterologists and epidemiologists agree that *Giardia* have essentially always been present in wilderness streams and in the water supplies for most cities but have not been detected because they are not isolated by routine bacterial culture techniques.

In man, the active parasite lives in the upper intestinal tract, where it forms large numbers of cysts, which are passed in the stool. The cysts do not produce active disease, but they are much more resistant to disinfectants and other agents in their environment and do transmit the infestation. Fecal contamination of water is the most common route of transmittal. Less common, but significant, is direct passage from the stool to the hands of a person preparing food and to the food itself. Presumably the organisms infesting animals also cause disease in man. Iodine in a concentration of eight parts per million effectively kills the cysts within ten minutes (twenty minutes if the water is cold — 32° to 40° F [0° to 5° C]).

Symptoms of giardiasis include abdominal pain, nausea, abdominal distention, intestinal gas, and frequent or recurrent diarrhea. Stools are bulky and foul smelling but do not contain blood or pus. Acutely, mild to moderate general symptoms of illness may be present, including weakness, loss of appetite, and chilly sensations. Chronic untreated infestations may cause malabsorption of nutrients, loss of weight, ulcerlike stomach pain, and other chronic disturbances.

A definitive diagnosis can be made by microscopic identification of the cysts in the stool in approximately fifty percent of infested people. Aspirating material from the upper part of the intestinal tract is a more reliable method of diagnosis but is far less comfortable. Since symptoms are fairly typical and do suggest this illness, a diagnosis in the field can be made with reasonable certainty. A therapeutic trial is probably justified for diarrhea lasting more than a week. Two drugs are equally effective. Metronidazole (Flagyl) for five to ten days is the usual therapy; good cure rates have also been obtained with a single large dose of this drug. Quinacrine (Atabrine) for one week is equally effective therapy, but this drug has a bitter taste and side effects of nausea and vomiting. Both drugs have about an eighty percent cure rate. In the event of failure with one drug, the dose can be repeated or the other can be tried. A few patients with longstanding diarrhea due to giardiasis have been successfully treated with both drugs at the same time. Alcohol should be avoided during and for twenty-four hours after the consumption of Flagyl.

Little is known about the number of *Giardia* necessary to establish an infestation. In one thoroughly studied epidemic, only eleven percent of a population exposed to heavy water contamination developed symptomatic disease, although forty-six percent had organisms in their stools. In the same study, eight and one-half percent of the population of a neighboring city was found to have totally asymptomatic *Giardia* infestations.

SEVERE DIARRHEAS

The severe diarrheas are all of infectious origin and are most frequently transmitted by fecal contamination of drinking water. In areas where these diseases exist all water must be carefully disinfected. Persons dwelling in cities where the public water supply is of uncertain cleanliness should drink bottled water or other bottled beverages. All foods should be thoroughly washed in a strong solution of chlorine or iodine and peeled if possible. Contamination of food during preparation must be avoided. Stool cultures to detect carriers of infectious diseases are desirable for the native personnel in large expedition parties, particularly those engaged in preparing meals, but are essentially impossible to obtain. Furthermore, modern concepts of sanitation are totally alien to many natives of mountainous countries. They must be monitored to ensure that they wash their hands after using the toilet and before preparing food.

Strict precautions are necessary to avoid spread of infection. A patient who has contracted one of these diseases should be isolated from the other members of the party as much as possible. The number of attendants should be limited to two or three, preferably party members who have been previously immunized against the patient's illness.

The attendants must take all possible measures to avoid spreading the infection. They should wear protective rubber or plastic gloves if they are available. They must scrub their hands vigorously, preferably with an antiseptic soap such as pHisoHex or Betadine, after any contact with the patient. All feces and vomitus should be mixed with an antiseptic such as one percent Cresol, and buried deeply in a spot where contamination of water is unlikely. All utensils and other instruments should be immersed in boiling water. Indispensable items, such as clothing or sleeping bags that can not be boiled, should be aired in bright sunlight for at least two or three days after the patient is recovering.

Cholera

Cholera, once a scourge throughout the world, is almost nonexistent where modern sanitation and water purification methods are practiced. When accurately diagnosed, it can be easily and effectively treated. However, cholera is still common in some areas. Epidemics that claim many lives still occur in many Southeast Asian countries, particularly during the early days of the monsoons when feces that has collected on the ground and in the streets is washed into streams and rivers.

Cholera is caused by a bacterial infection that is transmitted primarily through contaminated water. The infection may also be contracted from food, particularly items that are not cooked. A vaccine has been developed but only provides partial immunity for about six months. However, all persons entering or passing though areas in which cholera is known to exist probably should receive this vaccine beforehand and should be revaccinated every six months. (The principal value of cholera vaccination may be to facilitate travel through countries that require it for entry by individuals who have been visiting or living in an area where cholera is endemic.)

Fortunately, the cholera organism can not survive for long periods outside the human body. Therefore, most cases of cholera occur near areas of significant population and thus in areas where hospital care is available. However, some patients with cholera have mild symptoms suggestive of one of the mild diarrheas and go undiagnosed. Also, people who are carriers, although much rarer than in diseases such as typhoid fever, do appear occasionally. As a result, cases of cholera do occur at some distance from hospitals. The severity of the disease and its rapid onset may prevent evacuation of the patient, making treatment in the field necessary.

The incubation period for cholera is one to three days, during which the victim may notice mild diarrhea, depression, and lassitude. The onset at the end of the incubation period often is explosive. The patient has voluminous diarrhea, copious vomiting, and is prostrate. The disease can become overwhelming with amazing rapidity, leaving the patient severely dehydrated and in shock just from diarrheal fluid loss within one to three hours.

The gastrointestinal tract is quickly emptied and the stools lose their fecal character and are not foul smelling. The patient is constantly dribbling stools consisting almost entirely of water containing flecks of mucus. The name "rice water stools" has been given this material because the mucus looks like grains of rice floating in water. However, the stools rarely contain blood.

Frequently no warning of the need to defecate is felt, resulting in repeated, almost uncontrollable bowel movements. Similarly, vomiting may occur without antecedent nausea, although vomiting is rarely present after the onset of the illness. As the patient becomes dehydrated, fever and a high pulse rate appear. The features become gaunt, the eyes shrunken, and the skin shriveled and dry. The blood pressure frequently drops below normal and the pulse may be difficult to feel. Urinary output falls to less than 500 ml per day.

The treatment for cholera consists of fluid replacement. The entire volume of stool and vomitus must be replaced with oral or intravenous salt solutions. Stool volumes must be measured if replacement is to be accurate. Intravenous administration of fluids is often necessary during the early stages of the disease and may be lifesaving if the patient is severely dehydrated and in shock. Two to four liters of saline or Ringer's lactate may be required in the first hour, and as much as eight or more liters during the first day. However, after dehydration has been corrected and the patient is no longer in shock, he usually is able to take fluids orally. Fluid losses can be replaced orally with any of the solutions listed in Table Ten. Ordinary maintenance fluids — two liters of five to ten percent glucose and one-half liter of Ringer's lactate, or similar volumes of other liquids if taken orally — must also be administered in addition to the replacement fluids.

Victims of cholera are severely ill and obviously require bed rest. A canvas cot with a hole in the center through which the patient can defecate without having to move helps make him more comfortable and facilitates the collection and measuring of the stools during the first few days of the illness.

Tetracycline every six hours helps reduce the duration of diarrhea but is only an adjunct to therapy and must not be substituted for fluid and electrolyte replacement. Sedatives only make care of the patient more difficult and should be avoided.

Cholera is not very contagious and is spread principally through fecal contamination. Strict sanitary measures regarding the disposal of feces and vomitus must be enforced and all contaminated articles, including clothing, bedding, and utensils, should be cleaned to avoid further spread of the disease.

The acute phase of the disease rarely lasts more than three to five days. The patient usually is able to eat a bland diet by the third day. However, several weeks may be required for him to fully regain his strength.

Bacillary Dysentery

Bacillary dysentery (or "shigellosis") is caused by bacteria of the genus *Shigella* and occasionally by other organisms. These organisms are widespread, being found in temperate as well as tropical areas. However, the more severe cases of bacillary dysentery appear most frequently in tropical or semitropical climates. The infection is spread by contaminated water and food. Crowded living conditions and inadequate sewage disposal increase the likelihood of infection.

The incubation period varies from one to six days with an average of forty-eight hours. The onset is usually rather abrupt and is characterized by severe, intermittent abdominal cramps followed by copious diarrhea, which soon produces watery, foul stools. This infection typically is associated with fever and chilly feelings or frank, shaking chills. The patient is obviously ill and may be prostrate.

The stools contain large amounts of mucus and pus and occasionally moderate amounts of blood, particularly four to five hours after the onset. Nausea is common but vomiting frequently does not occur. Abdominal tenderness may be severe, is most marked in the lower portion of the abdomen, and is frequently accompanied by spasm of the abdominal muscles.

After six to eight hours the symptoms abate somewhat, but the disease may take seven to ten days to run its course.

Bacillary dysentery may be indistinguishable from acute gastroenteritis. However, with dysentery the symptoms are usually more severe, the patient is febrile and more obviously ill, pus and blood are present in the stools, and the disease runs a longer course.

The patient should be placed in bed and given fluids to prevent dehydration. Intravenous fluids may be necessary for more severe cases. A bland diet may be given if it can be tolerated. A hot water bottle or other source of warmth placed on the abdomen may reduce some of the pain and tenderness. Drugs to stop the diarrhea should not be given because these drugs tend to produce intestinal paralysis, which prevents the patient from taking fluids orally. They also may make the fever and overall disability worse.

These infections should be treated with antibacterial agents, of which trimethoprim-sulfamethoxazole is the drug of choice, particularly in Central and South America where bacterial strains resistant to other agents are common. Alternatively, ampicillin or chloramphenicol may be used. The drug should be given orally every six hours; the first dose should be twice as large as the usual dose. Antimicrobial therapy frequently produces marked improvement in twenty-four hours or less but should be continued for at least three or four days or until all symptoms have disappeared.

The victim of bacillary dysentery frequently requires seven to ten days to recover his strength after the symptoms of his disease have disappeared. Isolation and prevention of spread of the infection are essential.

Typhoid Fever

Typhoid fever is an infection caused by *Salmonella typhi*, which produces a generalized infection as well as diarrhea. After food or water contaminated by these bacteria has been ingested, the organisms invade the wall of the small bowel, multiply there, and then enter the blood stream.

Occasionally people who have recovered from typhoid fever continue to harbor the organisms in the gastrointestinal tract and excrete them in their stools (carriers). The bacteria can survive for weeks or months under natural conditions. Uncooked foods, salads, raw milk, and water contaminated by sewage are the most important sources of infection.

The incubation period is seven to fourteen days. The symptoms during the first week consist of fever, headache, and abdominal pain. The onset is usually insidious. Often there is no change in bowel habits during the initial ten days of illness. Near the end of the first week, enlargement of the spleen is detectable. A brief semidiagnostic rash can be seen in seventy percent of light skinned patients about seven to ten days after the onset of symptoms. The rash consists of "rose spots" which are deeply red, usually few in number, two to four millimeters in diameter, often present in clusters, blanch on pressure, and occur most often on the lower chest and upper abdominal wall. During the second week of illness, the fever becomes more continuous and many patients are clearly severely ill. The pulse rate is often slow in comparison to the severity of the fever (a pulse rate of eighty-five may accompany a temperature of 104° F [40° C]), an important diagnostic feature. Cough and nosebleeds may occur. In the third week, extreme toxicity, disordered thinking, and greenish peasoup diarrhea may occur. The latter may presage the dire complications of perforation of the intestine or intestinal hemorrhage. For survivors, the fourth week often brings improvement in their status. However, typhoid fever is one of the most longlasting and debilitating bacterial infections.

For the treatment of typhoid fever, rest and maintenance of fluid balance are important. Aspirin may lower the temperature but can also make the patient feel worse and should not be administered. Chloramphenicol is the antibiotic of choice, but the diagnosis of typhoid fever without laboratory facilities is unreliable, and chloramphenicol, a potent broad spectrum antibiotic, rarely causes a severe, often lethal blood disorder as a side effect of prolonged therapy. Ideally this drug should only be used when a definite diagnosis of typhoid has been established by bacteriologic cultures. If typhoid is strongly suspected in a situation where laboratory studies are not available, ampicillin is probably the drug of choice for persons not allergic to penicillin. If this therapy is not effective within three to five days or the patient is allergic to penicillin, the risk of chloramphenicol may have to be accepted.

Prior to travel to an area where typhoid may be encountered, immunization for typhoid and paratyphoid fever should be obtained. Although immunization does not completely prevent infection, it does reduce the severity of the disease and reduces the incidence of complications.

Sources of infection, particularly fecal contamination of food and water, and contamination of food by carriers, should be avoided.

Amebiasis

Amebiasis is caused by the protozoan *Endamoeba histolytica,* a larger and more complex organism than bacteria. Although generally thought of as a tropical disease, amebiasis is by no means limited to such areas.

These organisms invade the wall of the large intestine where the adult parasites form cysts that are passed in the feces of the host and are responsible for the spread of the infection. The cysts are most commonly ingested in contaminated water. Food that has been fertilized with human excreta, carelessness in food preparation, and insects — particularly flies — are other sources of infestation.

Chlorine, when used to disinfect drinking water, does not kill the cysts; boiling (at least at sea level) and iodine destroy them quite effectively.

Amebiasis is usually a very mild disorder in its early stages and symptoms may be entirely absent. More commonly, mild diarrhea with soft stools and a moderately increased number of bowel movements occurs. Occasional individuals develop constipation rather than diarrhea. A few patients have more severe symptoms suggestive of acute gastroenteritis, including numerous watery stools that contain mucus or even blood, and abdominal cramps. However, a period of mild gastrointestinal dysfunction usually precedes the onset of the more severe stage of amebiasis. Easy fatigability, a low fever, and vague pains in the muscles, back, or joints are frequently present. Nervousness, irritability, and dizziness occasionally develop. In a typical patient no abnormality can be found by physical examination, although slight tenderness in the right lower quadrant of the abdomen is sometimes present. The diagnosis is suggested by the chronicity and mildness of the diarrhea and a history of exposure to conditions in which infection is likely. Laboratory facilities are required to make a definitive diagnosis.

If amebiasis is suspected, metronidazole (Flagyl) should be given three times a day for five to ten days. Occasionally metronidazole may not completely eradicate the infection.

All persons visiting an area in which amebiasis is prevalent must be examined for this infestation upon their return. The amebae may lie quietly within the large intestine for years, producing no symptoms, and then spread to the liver, where they form abscesses and from which they occasionally even invade the lung. This form of the disease has a high mortality rate. Fortunately, it can be easily prevented by early diagnosis and treatment.

CONSTIPATION AND RECTAL PROBLEMS

Healthy adults rarely need to be concerned about constipation. The concept that normal individuals should have a bowel movement every day is a myth perpetrated on bowel conscious people by herb peddlers and overprotective mothers. Bowel rhythm can vary widely. For some individuals three stools a day is normal; others normally have one stool every three days.

The type of food consumed plays a large part in determining the character and frequency of stools. Foods that are almost completely absorbed, such as liquids or carbohydrates, can not be expected to produce a copious stool; the reverse is true for foods with a large unabsorbed residue such as bran or many leafy vegetables. Reduced food intake due to illness or dieting leads to smaller stool volume.

Constipation is more accurately defined as the passage of hard, dry stools rather than a specified frequency of bowel movements. Reduced intake of water or other fluids, dehydrated foods, and disruption of normal schedules with infrequent stops all tend to cause constipation. An adequate fluid intake — at least two quarts per day — and the inclusion in the diet of fruits and other foods that loosen the stools help to maintain normal bowel function.

In general, laxatives have very little prophylactic or therapeutic value. If, in an unusual situation, laxatives become necessary, the best and safest is magnesium sulfate, particularly in the form of milk of magnesia, one or two tablespoonfuls or two to four tablets at bedtime.

Fecal Impaction

Under conditions in which the urge to defecate is resisted, such as weather that confines climbers to their tents or, more commonly, during recovery from an injury or disease, the normal bowel reflexes may become insensitive and permit stool to accumulate in the rectum. Conditions producing dehydration, such as inadequate fluid intake or high fluid losses due to altitude, fever, or similar condi-

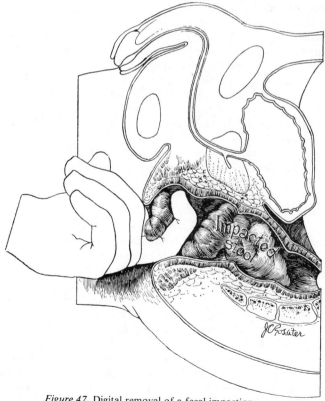

Figure 47. Digital removal of a fecal impaction.

tions, may cause the water in the stool to be reabsorbed with such avidity that a bulky, hard residue that can not be evacuated in a normal manner results.

The best way to determine whether impaction has occurred is to insert a moistened or lubricated and (if available) gloved index finger into the rectum. If a mass of hard stool is found, it must be extracted. The mass of stool should be broken up with the index finger and the fragments removed as gently as possible. Injury of the rectal and anal tissues must be avoided. Following manual removal of the impaction, an enema should be given and the causes of the impaction corrected.

Although breaking up and extracting a fecal impaction is esthetically unpleasant, no alternative exists. Enema fluids will not enter the solidified fecal mass; laxatives have no effect on the dilated, flaccid rectal wall. Paradoxically, fecal impaction may be accompanied by the passage of a number of small, watery stools — the only material that can get past the impacted mass.

Anal Fissure

With constipation the stool may become so hard and bulky that its passage causes a small tear (fissure) in the skin of the anus. Subsequent bowel movements are painful and may be associated with a small amount of bleeding.

Avoiding bowel movements, particularly bulky or hard stools, for a few days often permits the fissure to heal. The diet should be low in fiber and consist of foods that are almost totally absorbed, such as milk, soups, and carbohydrates. Straining at stool should be avoided indefinitely.

Mineral oil, one tablespoonful (15 cc) twice a day, lubricates the stool and reduces the pain with bowel movements. (Mineral oil is not a true laxative — only a lubricant.) A bland anesthetic such as dibucaine ointment may be applied to the anus if the pain is bothersome. The area should be cleaned gently after each bowel movement and wiping, scratching, and rubbing should be avoided.

Hemorrhoids

Hemorrhoids (or "piles"), which are abnormally dilated veins that protrude from the rectum or anus, are usually more annoying than disabling but can be a source of considerable irritation due to itching and pain and can cause severe pain and disability if they become prolapsed and thrombosed. Occasionally a small amount of bleeding follows the passage of a hard, bulky stool, but serious bleeding from hemorrhoids is rare. Climbers with hemorrhoids should have them treated surgically before a major expedition. Hemorrhoidectomy is an uncomfortable but minor operation requiring only limited hospitalization.

If hemorrhoids are bothersome, the stools should be loosened by the ingestion of large quantities of fluids and plenty of fruit. Mineral oil, one tablespoon twice a day, may be taken to lubricate the stool. Sitting in warm water for fifteen to thirty minutes three or four times a day helps relieve the burning and itching (but interferes with climbing). A bland anesthetic, such as dibucaine ointment applied to the anus, or hemorrhoidal suppositories, often relieves symptoms. However, allergy to local anesthetic creams can develop, resulting in a contact dermatitis in the anal skin. If symptoms worsen after use of dibucaine ointment, it should be discontinued. An alternative treatment would be the use of a one-quarter percent hydrocortisone ointment, which often provides symptomatic relief without the hazards of a local anesthetic ointment.

Thrombosed Hemorrhoid

Occasionally the blood within a hemorrhoid clots, producing moderate to severe pain. The pain may come on gradually or suddenly, and the victim usually has noted prior symptoms attributable to hemorrhoids. A swollen, tender, purple nodule can be seen protruding from the wall or opening of the anus.

Clots smaller than one-half inch (one cm) in diameter are best allowed to resolve spontaneously. Clots larger than one inch (two cm) should be surgically treated. The amount of pain should determine how clots between these two sizes should be treated.

After washing the area with soap and water, an incision can be made in the top of the thrombosed hemorrhoid and the clot evacuated. Relief of pain is frequently dramatic and many days of distress can be avoided if the thrombosed hemorrhoid is large. Aspirin and codeine can be given for pain prior to incision; a local anesthetic can be injected if available but is not essential. Sterile pads should be left in the intergluteal cleft for several days to reduce soiling of clothing and irritation of the incision site. Warm baths or packs help relieve pain and anal muscle spasm.

Rectal Abscess

Abscesses in the tissues surrounding the rectum and anus usually follow chronic anal disease, which should be corrected before a prolonged mountaineering outing is undertaken. Abscesses in this location are not basically different from abscesses elsewhere in the body.

The cardinal sign of rectal abscess is throbbing pain in the region of the anus. Malaise, fever, and chills are commonly present, and the patient may appear acutely ill. Examination usually reveals the characteristic signs of an abscess — redness, tenderness, increased heat, and swelling. The abscess may come to a point in the skin adjacent to the anus. A few rectal abscesses are located deeper beneath the skin and can only be detected as moderately firm, painful masses felt during digital examination of the rectum.

Rectal abscesses require the same treatment as abscesses anywhere — incision and drainage. If the abscess points in the skin about the anus, an incision should be made in the center of the fluctuant area. If a deeper abscess is felt, the patient should be evacuated, since drainage of such abscesses must be carried out by a physician. Serious complications can follow an abscess in this location if it is not properly treated. If the patient has a fever, ampicillin or tetracycline should be administered every six hours during evacuation.

PEPTIC ULCER AND RELATED PROBLEMS

A peptic ulcer is a crater in the lining of the stomach or intestine produced by the digestive action of the enzymes and acids in the stomach. The cause of peptic ulcers is not well understood, although emotional factors often appear to play a part in their development.

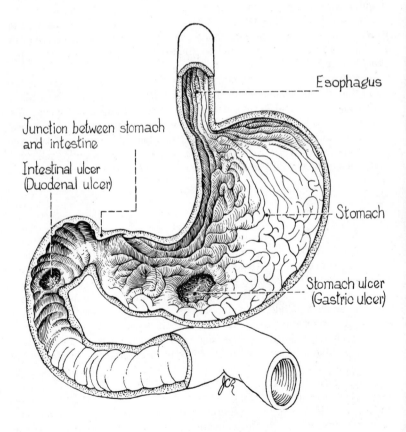

Figure 48. Gastric and duodenal ulcers.

An uncomplicated ulcer is not usually disabling, although the pain can be severe. However, an ulcer is dangerous because serious complications can occur, most importantly hemorrhage and perforation. These complications are disabling, life endangering conditions requiring immediate evacuation to a medical center. Perforation is discussed in Chapter Nineteen, "Acute Abdominal Pain."

The characteristic symptom of an ulcer is a gnawing or raw pain, usually located high in the upper portion of the abdomen near the midline. The pain typically comes on one to four hours after eating or between midnight and two o'clock in the morning. Bland food, milk, or an antacid usually relieves the pain fairly promptly.

The pain is thought to be caused by the effects of stomach acid on the ulcer. Food and antacids tend to neutralize the acid and thus relieve the pain. The characteristic times at which the pain occurs are the periods when there is no food in the stomach to counteract the acid. (No explanation for the absence of pain in the early morning when the stomach is clearly empty has been found.)

Treatment

Therapy for an ulcer is directed toward neutralizing stomach acidity and relieving emotional tension. An antacid should be taken every hour while awake. Since overdosage with these drugs is not a problem, more should be administered if the pain persists or the adequacy of dosage is questionable. Some antacids produce diarrhea as a side effect; others cause constipation. Judicious balancing of both types of antacid usually resolves either problem. (Delcid causes diarrhea; Amphogel causes constipation.) Some tablets are ineffective; preferred preparations include Alkets, Tetralac, or Robalate.

Antacid therapy has become less important since histamine receptor antagonists such as cimetidine (Tagamet) have become available. This drug is very effective for treating peptic ulcer disease. The usual dosage is one tablet four times a day, supplemented by enough antacid to relieve symptoms.

A bland diet with large quantities of mild cheese, puddings, and noncitrus fruit juices should be given in six meals scattered evenly over the waking hours. These foods tend to neutralize the stomach acids most effectively. Eating six meals a day tends to keep food in the stomach constantly and prolongs the acid neutralizing effect. Alcohol, coffee, tea, cola drinks, chocolate, vinegar, and citrus juices tend to increase gastric acid production and should be avoided.

A patient with an ulcer should avoid strenuous exertion and may need extra rest such as an afternoon nap. However, he does not need to be confined to bed. A sedative or a tranquilizer may be given four times daily to provide sedation and relieve the emotional tensions that play a large role in causing ulcers. Patients who do not respond to therapy within ten to fourteen days should be evacuated to a physician's care as the danger of complications increases with time.

Indigestion

Indigestion is a vague, poorly defined disorder that is often not associated with any demonstrable abnormality of the upper gastrointestinal system. However, the symptoms of indigestion may be confused with those of an ulcer. Since an ulcer poses a threat of severe complications but indigestion does not, the conditions should be distinguished.

The symptoms of an ulcer and indigestion characteristically differ in several respects. Usually the symptoms of indigestion are associated with eating rather than coming on one to four hours afterward. With indigestion a sense of fullness, excessive belching, or vomiting small amounts of food or sour stomach contents are more common than actual pain, although a burning sensation may be present beneath the breastbone (heartburn). Usually the symptoms of indigestion are related to only a single or an occasional meal, while ulcer symptoms are more consistent. The symptoms of indigestion may be relieved to some extent by antacids but are frequently aggravated by the ingestion of more food, contrary to ulcer symptoms. The symptoms of indigestion become less noticeable with time and the passage of food from the stomach, also the opposite of ulcer symptoms. If indigestion becomes so severe that treatment is necessary, it can be treated with antacids and antispasmodics just as an ulcer. Eating smaller quantities of food with each meal may also be beneficial.

Gastrointestinal Hemorrhage

One of the most serious problems that can occur far from medical facilities is massive hemorrhage from the stomach or intestines. Even with the expert treatment available in large medical centers, a rather large percentage of patients die as the result of this type of bleeding. Since blood transfusions are usually necessary, every effort must be made to get an affected climber to a hospital. **Hemorrhage is very likely to recur. Any delay may prove fatal!**

Except for the occasional individuals who bleed slightly after prolonged retching because small blood vessels in the esophagus or stomach are broken, essentially all gastrointestinal bleeding in otherwise healthy young adults (without liver disease) is due to peptic ulcer. On an expedition such bleeding should be assumed to be the result of an ulcer since other conditions causing bleeding can not be effectively treated in the field. Symptoms of an ulcer, although usually present prior to the hemorrhage, may be totally absent.

The signs and symptoms of serious gastrointestinal bleeding include:

1. Faintness or weakness, which is more prominent when erect than when lying down;
2. Vomiting obvious blood;
3. Vomiting "coffee ground" material (blood that has been partially digested in the stomach);
4. Rectal passage of obvious blood;

5. Rectal passage of liquid or solid "tarry black" material (stools containing digested blood);

6. Shock.

Aggressive ulcer treatment should be instituted immediately and should include cimetidine (Tagamet), liquid antacids hourly while awake (and during the night whenever the patient awakens spontaneously), and strict avoidance of foods containing acids, alcohol, or caffeine. The patient should be put to bed and forced to rest as much as possible. Treatment for shock should be instituted if signs of shock, particularly low blood pressure, are present.

A young person with a bleeding peptic ulcer usually stops hemorrhaging within twelve to twenty-four hours if he is kept quiet and given appropriate therapy. He should be treated in camp until the bleeding stops and for one to two days more prior to evacuation. Moving a patient with active gastrointestinal bleeding is likely to increase the severity of the bleeding.

The patient is usually very weak after such a bleeding episode and requires considerable rest and assistance during evacuation. He should by no means try to go on with his climb even though he feels quite well. **A small bleeding episode is often followed by a horrendous gush!**

DISEASES OF THE LIVER

Jaundice

Jaundice is produced by diseases of the liver. One of the numerous functions of the liver is to remove from the blood the pigment resulting from the normal destruction of old red blood cells. This pigment is excreted into the intestine through the bile ducts and, following further changes in the intestinal tract, imparts the normal brown color to the stool.

In diseases that severely damage the liver this pigment is not removed from the blood. As a result it accumulates in the body and imparts a yellow or bronze color to the whites of the eyes and later the skin. If the pigment is excreted into the intestine in smaller amounts or not at all, the stools become pale or "clay colored." The pigment is partially excreted by the kidneys, imparting a brown color to the urine and causing the foam produced by shaking to have a yellow color instead of the normal white appearance.

When jaundice is suspected, the patient should be examined in daylight. Flashlights and other artificial lights usually produce a yellowish color that can be confusing — either masking or simulating true jaundice.

Hepatitis

Hepatitis is a group of virus infections that selectively involve the liver. Hepatitis A is caused by an RNA virus that is spread principally by fecal contamination of water and food. Hepatitis B is caused by a DNA virus that is spread principally by body fluids through personal contact, particularly sexual contact (semen). Non-A,non-B hepatitis is probably caused by two or more viruses and became notorious because it is spread by blood transfusions. However, about ninety percent of cases of non-A,non-B hepatitis result from intravenous drug abuse or "travel to underdeveloped countries." Undoubtedly all types of hepatitis can be spread by all routes. These diseases are common, particularly where large numbers of people are living in crowded conditions with contaminated water supplies. The epidemiology and prevention are discussed in greater detail in Chapter Five, "Preventive Measures."

The vast majority — well over ninety percent — of hepatitis infections produce no symptoms. The patient is not even aware that he is ill. These infections almost all clear up, leaving no residual liver disease. However, some patients with hepatitis B or non-A,non-B hepatitis go on to develop chronic liver disease and about half of these patients progress to cirrhosis, which is usually fatal.

Hepatitis is the most important cause of painless jaundice likely to occur for the first time under mountaineering conditions. (Jaundice associated with pain is discussed in Chapter Nineteen, "Acute Abdominal Pain." Patients with previous attacks of jaundice should be evaluated by a physician and instructed in the treatment for their condition prior to undertaking an outing.) Untreated malaria and other conditions cause jaundice on rare occasions due to the excessive destruction of red blood cells. However, such disorders can usually be recognized from other findings.

The onset of hepatitis may be abrupt or insidious and follows an incubation period ranging from three weeks to six months. The earliest symptoms are loss of appetite, general malaise, and easy fatigability. Later a low fever and nausea and vomiting appear. Many patients have a peculiar loss of their taste for cigarettes. In patients with more severe infections the symptoms increase in severity. Light colored stools and dark urine may precede the appearance of jaundice by several days. Vague upper abdominal discomfort and tenderness may be present, particularly in the right upper quadrant, but severe pain is absent. After the appearance of jaundice, some patients experience ill-defined joint or muscular pains. A highly variable skin rash may be present and some patients have generalized itching.

The severity of the disease runs a full range from asymptomatic cases to the relatively rare fatalities. When jaundice does develop it often lasts three to six weeks; the malaise, easy fatigability, and loss of appetite may persist for several more months.

No specific treatment is available. A study of previously healthy young adults in the U.S. Army indicated that restriction of exercise had no effect on the course of the disease for that rather select group of patients. Most climbers would fall into the same group of previously healthy, relatively young adults. However, most patients do not feel capable of more than very mild exercise. A nourishing diet high in proteins and carbohydrates and supplemented with vitamins should be provided.

All drug therapy should be avoided if possible, including drugs to promote sleep. Most drugs are metabolized by the liver. When that organ's function is impaired by hepatitis, such metabolism may be much slower than normal. If the drugs are not completely metabolized between doses, they can accumulate in the blood and may rapidly reach toxic concentrations.

Most hepatitis patients should be evacuated. Recovery usually takes so long that delaying evacuation until the patient is well is impossible. In addition, complications that require a physician's care may develop.

ADDITIONAL READING

1. Grady GG, Keusch GT: Pathogenesis of bacterial diarrheas. *New Eng J Med* 1971;285:831, 891.
2. Gangrosa EJ, Barker WH: Cholera: Implications for the United States. *JAMA* 1974;227:170.

CHAPTER NINETEEN

Acute Abdominal Pain

An episode of acute abdominal pain can be frightening because successful management of some conditions causing such pain requires surgical therapy. However, the most common disorders producing pain in this location do not require any specific therapy; many others can be effectively treated without surgery.

In mountaineering situations, the major problem — almost the only problem — in caring for a person with acute abdominal pain is deciding whether he does require surgery. If any doubt exists, the patient must be evacuated. True abdominal emergencies that are not treated in the most effective manner can have a mortality rate approaching 100 percent. Disrupting a carefully planned expedition because a member has a bellyache requires mature judgment, but such decisions reflect mountaineering wisdom just as surely as does turning back within view of a summit when avalanche conditions are encountered.

During evacuation the patient almost always must be carried. A supine position with the head and knees moderately elevated is usually most comfortable. Continuous antibiotic therapy, analgesics, intravenous fluids, and nasogastric intubation may all be required.

SIGNS AND SYMPTOMS

The key to proper treatment is an accurate diagnosis which, in turn, requires a detailed history and a careful physical examination. An outline such as the following should be used to obtain a history of the disorder:

PAIN

Exact time of onset;
Nature of onset — gradual or sudden;
Location, change in location, radiation;
Nature of pain — sharp, stabbing, gnawing, cramping, constant,
  or intermittent;
Progression of pain since onset;
Factors relieving or aggravating pain — coughing, deep breathing, voiding,
  bowel movements, position of body.

OTHER SYMPTOMS

Nausea and vomiting — time of onset in relation to onset of pain
— vomiting blood;
Diarrhea or constipation — time of last bowel movement;
Chills or fever;
Blood in the urine;
Presence of a hernia — reducibility;
Other members of the party with a similar disorder.

PAST HISTORY

History of having eaten food not eaten by other members of the group;
Previous episodes of similar pain — diagnosis and treatment at that time;
History of pain relieved by milk, food, or antacids;
History of indigestion or pain following ingestion of fried or fatty foods;
History of jaundice;
History of previous abdominal operations;
Time of last menstrual period — any abnormalities.

If possible, the physical examination should be performed in a quiet, secluded spot where the patient can be warm and comfortable. He should be lying on his back with his hands at his sides and his entire abdomen from the nipple line to the crotch bared for examination.

The abdomen should be examined by observation, auscultation, and palpation. Spasms of pain, aggravation of pain by breathing, and the presence of scars from previous operations should be noted. The examiner should place his ear or a stethoscope against the patient's abdomen and listen for increased or absent bowel sounds. Increased bowel sounds can frequently be heard several feet from the patient. The absence of bowel sounds, which is indicative of intestinal paralysis (paralytic ileus), can only be diagnosed when no sounds are heard after listening for at least two or three minutes.

Palpation of the abdomen is a skill that requires years of practice and experience to perfect. However, valuable information can be gained from this examination by a beginner who has had a modicum of prior instruction and practice. The examiner must be gentle; his hands must be warm. He should place his hands on the patient's abdomen with the palms down and exert gentle pressure with the pads of the fingers. Jabbing with the finger tips causes the patient to contract his abdominal muscles so that no information can be gained from the examination.

Areas of tenderness must be accurately located. Spasm of the abdominal muscles over tender areas should be identified. Rebound tenderness, which is a sudden sharp pain occurring when the pressure over a tender area is suddenly released, should be sought. Referred tenderness, pain in one portion of the abdomen elicited by pressure in another area (caused by the intestines shifting away

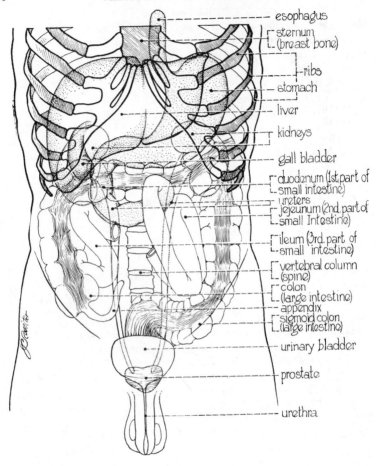

Figure 49. Organs of the abdominal cavity.

from the site being depressed and irritating the diseased organ), must be recognized.

Generally speaking, pain associated with diarrhea or pain that is not associated with nausea and vomiting is not a sign of disease requiring operation. Severe pain that lasts for more than six hours or that prevents the patient from sleeping is usually indicative of a condition requiring surgery. Abdominal distension and paralytic ileus, rebound pain, exactly localized tenderness, and rigidity of the abdominal muscles are indicative of a serious intraabdominal condition that is best treated by surgery. Jaundice is evidence of gallbladder or liver disease that is of such severity that the patient should be evacuated regardless of whether surgery is needed, since full recovery requires at least several weeks.

REPORTING HISTORY AND PHYSICAL FINDINGS

Because decisions about a climber with abdominal pain must almost always include consideration of a major disruption of the outing and the expense of evacuating the casualty, consultation by radio or telephone should be obtained if possible. An appropriate decision can be made only if the report of the history and physical examination is given to the consultant physician in a systematic manner. The outline for the history should be followed; all data must be written down prior to the discussion. In addition, answers to the following questions should be

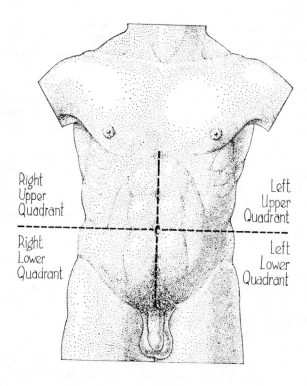

Figure 50. The four quadrants of the abdomen.

available in written form for the discussion:

1. What is the temperature, pulse, and respiratory rate?
2. Does the patient look sick?
3. Does the patient appear to be complaining for an ulterior or perhaps sub-conscious motive? Does he appear to overreact to pain?
4. Is the abdomen rigid due to involuntary muscle spasm?
5. Where is the pain most severe (a) as the patient lies unexamined? (b) with gentle probing? and (c) after sudden release of the probing fingers (rebound pain)?
6. Is a hernia or intraabdominal mass present?

CONDITIONS THAT DO *NOT* REQUIRE EVACUATION

Gastroenteritis

The most common cause of abdominal pain is acute gastroenteritis, which is discussed more thoroughly in Chapter Eighteen, "Gastrointestinal Diseases."

Gradually increasing, diffuse abdominal pain that culminates in waves of ab-dominal cramps and diarrhea is typical of acute gastroenteritis. During spasms of pain the patient frequently draws his knees up on his abdomen for relief, but the periods between spasms are relatively free from pain. Generalized abdominal tenderness is often present and may be slightly greater in the lower abdomen. Bowel sounds are louder than normal. Nausea and vomiting may be the most prominent symptoms; chills and fever may also be present.

Gastroenteritis must be distinguished principally from appendicitis. In appen-dicitis: (1) no evidence of food contamination or of other suffering from the same disease is found; (2) pain is not diffuse and usually is not cramping; and (3) diar-rhea is not prominent. The onset of appendicitis is usually gradual and the pain is relatively constant. Tenderness, if present, is localized in the right lower quadrant of the abdomen.

Mittelschmerz

Mittelschmerz, which is German for "middle pain," occurs in women midway between menstrual periods and is produced by minor bleeding accompanying ovulation. Women with this disorder usually have had previous episodes of such pain and can frequently identify the condition.

The pain comes on gradually, may be severe, and usually is localized in either the right or left lower abdominal quadrants, depending upon which ovary is in-volved. Vomiting or diarrhea usually does not occur. The abdomen is usually soft, but tenderness may be elicited by deep palpation in one of the lower quadrants.

Mittelschmerz may be difficult to differentiate from appendicitis if the right ovary is involved. The gynecologic condition should be suspected if the pain occurs halfway between menstrual periods.

No specific treatment is necessary. The pain can usually be controlled with aspirin and codeine and usually disappears within thirty-six to forty-eight hours. Symptoms persisting for a longer time should prompt reconsideration of the diagnosis.

Acute Salpingitis

Acute salpingitis is an infection of the fallopian tubes, the structures that conduct ova (eggs) from the ovaries to the uterus and sometimes referred to as oviducts. The infection is commonly gonorrheal in origin, but many other organisms can also cause such infections. The incidence of such infections is slightly increased in women using intrauterine contraceptive devices (IUDs).

The pain usually develops gradually, but can become quite severe. Both fallopian tubes are usually involved to some extent, causing pain in both the right and left lower quadrants of the abdomen. However, the pain commonly is much more severe on one side than the other. The pain may be accompanied by nausea and vomiting. Typically a high fever, 103° F (39.5° C) or higher, is present. Tenderness, muscle spasm, and rebound pain may be present in either or both of the lower abdominal quadrants.

Acute salpingitis may be impossible to differentiate from appendicitis if the right tube is involved. The presence of a high fever is suggestive of salpingitis but can also occur with appendicitis, particularly if the appendix has ruptured. A history of sexual exposure followed by a vaginal discharge is suggestive of gonorrhea, but patients with that infection can also develop appendicitis. Pain or tenderness in both sides of the abdomen is rather strong evidence of salpingitis.

If distinction from appendicitis is not possible, the patient should be treated as if she had appendicitis. If the disorder appears highly likely to be salpingitis, the patient does not have to be evacuated. Surgery is not required for acute salpingitis. However, treatment for gonorrhea should be instituted. (See Chapter Twenty, "Genitourinary Disorders.")

CONDITIONS THAT REQUIRE EVACUATION

Appendicitis

Appendicitis is the most common disorder producing acute abdominal pain that requires surgical treatment. Individuals who are frequently in remote areas for prolonged periods should discuss with their physician the advisability of having a prophylactic appendectomy.

The onset of appendicitis is characterized by vague abdominal discomfort that becomes progressively worse. Cramps are usually absent. The earliest symptoms are frequently located in the midabdomen. One to three hours later the pain shifts to the right lower quadrant. During this time the patient usually becomes nauseated and vomits several times. One or two bowel movements may occur, but diarrhea is uncommon. Rarely has the patient had any previous similar attacks.

The area of maximum tenderness is in the right lower quadrant of the abdomen. Later, referred tenderness, rebound tenderness, and muscle spasm appear in the same area. Usually a low fever of about 101 ° F (38.5 ° C) is present, but chills are rare.

If the appendix ruptures, pain may abruptly disappear. A few hours later the pain usually returns but is more diffuse and is associated with signs of peritonitis. However, the infection can remain localized to the area around the appendix, forming an abscess. With this complication a low fever usually persists and the patient does not feel well. However, he may have no other symptoms. Such patients still must be evacuated promptly. The abscess often ruptures a week or more later, and can produce an overwhelming, rapidly fatal peritonitis.

Antibiotic therapy should be started at once. If the patient is not vomiting, chloramphenicol should be given orally every six hours. If oral therapy is not possible, chloramphenicol can be given intravenously, or ampicillin and gentamycin can be given intramuscularly every six hours. If the patient is in severe pain, morphine can be given intramuscularly every four hours. However, morphine masks the physical findings characteristic of appendicitis and should not be administered within four hours of the time the patient is to be examined by a physician.

Appendicitis is best treated by immediate surgery. Therefore, the patient should be evacuated as fast as possible. Intravenous fluids may be required to avoid dehydration if the patient is vomiting and evacuation requires more than thirty-six hours. If gastric distension and paralytic ileus appear, nasogastric suction should be instituted. (See Appendix B, "Therapeutic Procedures.")

Some cases of appendicitis have been cured with antibiotics alone. In a truly remote area such therapy can be tried. If the patient's fever and all abdominal pain and tenderness completely disappear, a good, healthy appetite returns, and he feels completely well, he can probably resume climbing safely. However, only a physician with access to clinical laboratory services can determine whether the disease has actually been cured or is merely quiescent. Therefore, the patient should be evacuated in less remote circumstances or if there is any question about his condition.

Intestinal Obstruction

Intestinal obstruction is produced by a number of conditions that block the passage of food through the intestines. The symptoms are similar regardless of the cause of the obstruction but do vary somewhat according to the location of the obstruction in the gastrointestinal tract. Bands of fibrous tissue from previous abdominal operations are a frequent cause of this disorder. Some patients have a history of repeated episodes of obstruction.

The onset of symptoms is gradual and is characterized by cramping pain that occurs in waves and increases rapidly in severity. The patient is frequently free of pain between spasms. Nausea and vomiting, which are almost invariably present, occur early in obstructions located in the upper portion of the intestine. If the obstruction is lower in the small intestine or in the large intestine, vomiting may not occur for several hours or even longer after the onset of pain.

The patient appears quite ill and usually has a rapid pulse. Sometimes other signs of shock are present. The abdomen is distended, particularly with obstructions in the lower part of the intestinal tract. Scars from previous abdominal operations are frequently present. Bowel sounds are much louder than normal, occasionally being audible a considerable distance from the patient. However, twelve to twenty-four hours after onset of the obstruction, the intestines become so distended by fluid and air that contractions cease and the bowel sounds disappear. Signs of peritonitis — diffuse abdominal pain and tenderness and spasm of the abdominal muscles — are usually present at this stage.

The early stages of intestinal obstruction may simulate acute gastroenteritis. However, although one or two bowel movements occur, diarrhea is rarely present with obstruction.

Immediate evacuation is imperative since surgery is almost always necessary. Nasogastric suction should be instituted if possible. Intravenous fluid therapy (and the replacement, with balanced salt solution, of all fluids lost through vomiting or gastric suction) is necessary if evacuation requires more than thirty-six hours. Antibiotic treatment for peritonitis also should be instituted. No fluids or medications should be given orally.

Perforated Peptic Ulcer

Perforation is one of the complications that can occur with a peptic ulcer. (See Chapter Eighteen, "Gastrointestinal Diseases.") The same processes that have digested the lining of the stomach or intestine to form the ulcer crater continue their action until the ulcer extends through the entire wall of the organ. The resulting perforation permits stomach acids and other intestinal contents to enter the abdominal cavity. These substances cause an intense chemical irritation of the peritoneum and may initiate a severe infection.

The patient usually has a history of a peptic ulcer (upper abdominal pain coming on two to six hours after eating and relieved by food, milk, and antacids.) However, approximately twenty percent of the patients with a perforated ulcer do not have such prior symptoms.

(Parasitic infestation can also cause intestinal perforation but such events are limited almost entirely to porters or other residents of underdeveloped countries who usually carry numerous intestinal parasites at all times. The signs and symptoms are similar to a perforated peptic ulcer, and the treatment is essentially the same. The victim would not have a previous history suggestive of peptic ulcer, and most have lived with their parasites for so long they are not aware that symptoms produced by the infestation are abnormal.)

At the time of perforation the patient suffers the abrupt, almost instantaneous onset of severe upper abdominal pain that is sharp and continuous and may spread over the entire abdomen. The pain is followed shortly by the vomiting of recently ingested food or of bile. The patient appears quite sick and gets progressively worse for the next twelve to twenty-four hours.

The abdomen is diffusely tender, but pain is more marked in the upper quadrants. Spasm of the abdominal muscles is prominent, particularly in the upper abdomen. Bowel sounds disappear shortly after the perforation, and distention of the abdomen soon follows due to intestinal paralysis.

A perforated ulcer is a severe emergency requiring immediate evacuation. Treatment for peritonitis should be administered during evacuation. Occasionally the perforation seals, and the patient begins to get better, but he still must be evacuated to a medical facility where definitive treatment for his ulcer can be instituted and the complications following his perforation attended.

Incarcerated Hernia

A hernia (or "rupture") is a protrusion of the intestine from its proper location within the abdominal cavity. The most common hernia is an inguinal hernia that presents in the groin and may extend into the scrotum. Usually such hernias are easily reduced (pushed back into the abdomen) and have existed for months or even years. The hernia itself does not constitute an emergency, but the intestine may be trapped in the abnormal position, resulting in intestinal obstruction.

The surgical repair of a hernia is a relatively minor operation and should be carried out whenever one is detected, particularly before a mountaineering outing. Little justification exists for interruption of a significant mountaineering outing by this abnormality with the possible exception of hernias in back country inhabitants of underdeveloped nations.

A patient with an incarcerated hernia usually has a history of an ordinary hernia that has always been easily reduced but has become unreducible and very painful. The resulting intestinal obstruction causes vomiting, abdominal distension, and cessation of bowel movements. An obvious mass that is swollen and tender is usually present in the groin or scrotum. The abdomen may be distended and the patient may be vomiting.

The initial treatment should consist of trying to reduce the hernia. The patient should be flat on his back, preferably with his head and chest lower than his ab-

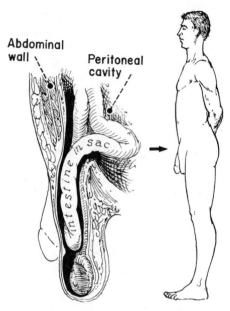

Figure 51. Anatomy of an inguinal hernia.

domen so gravity can help return the intestine into the abdominal cavity. If the patient is tense and straining, morphine should be given to produce relaxation and help reduce the hernia. Moderate, steady pressure on the hernia for ten minutes or longer may ultimately make the mass of intestine pop back into the abdominal cavity through the narrow neck of the sac and **temporarily** relieve the emergency.

If the hernia can not be reduced, the mass remains tender and inflamed, and the patient keeps vomiting and getting sicker. The bowel often becomes gangrenous. Immediate evacuation of the patient is mandatory. During evacuation the patient should be treated for intestinal obstruction. Intravenous fluids are required if evacuation takes more than thirty-six to forty-eight hours.

Occasionally the intestine is already gangrenous when the hernia is reduced. Therefore, anyone who has had an incarcerated hernia reduced must be closely watched for at least twenty-four hours for signs of peritonitis, intestinal obstruction, or both. If relief does not occur, gangrene of the intestine should be suspected and the victim urgently evacuated. On short outings the victim should be evacuated regardless of subsequent developments.

Acute Gallbladder Disease

The gallbladder is a saclike organ on the undersurface of the liver in which bile is stored until it is secreted into the small intestine. In some abnormal conditions, the bile salts may be precipitated, forming gallstones, a common disorder. Subsequent contractions of the gallbladder to expel bile are painful. This condition, known as chronic cholecystitis or chronic gallbladder disease, is characterized by recurrent episodes of colicky pain and tenderness in the right upper quadrant of the abdomen. Rarely, these attacks are associated with jaundice. Patients with gallstones poorly tolerate fried or fatty foods, which cause belching, indigestion, and abdominal pain.

A patient with acute gallbladder disease usually has a history of chronic cholecystitis. However, with acute cholecystitis he typically has much more severe pain, which may come on rather suddenly and is located immediately below the ribs on the right. The pain may be intermittent or continuous and may radiate to the back or to the shoulder blades. Vomiting is common; diarrhea is rare. The patient appears obviously ill and is frequently jaundiced. The urine is often dark and the stools may be light grey or clay colored, particularly two to three days after the onset.

Tenderness, rebound tenderness, and referred pain are all in the right upper quadrant. The temperature may be mildly elevated (99° to 101° F or 37.5° to 38.5° C).

Treatment consists of rest with nothing being taken by mouth until vomiting stops. Then only clear liquids should be ingested. All fried or fatty foods, including milk, must be avoided. Meperidine or morphine intramuscularly usually is required to control the pain. Meperidine is preferable. In an isolated area, ampicillin should be given intramuscularly every six hours as long as the pain continues.

The attack usually subsides spontaneously within one or two days. If the patient has had previous attacks, he may even be able to continue climbing after he has regained his strength. (If a climber has had previous attacks of acute cholecystitis, he should seriously consider having his gallbladder removed surgically (cholecystectomy) before a prolonged expedition.) The safest course is for the patient to be evacuated, particularly if jaundice is present. Although most patients with acute gallbladder disease do not require emergency surgery, such treatment is needed by some. Moving the patient to a hospital is by far the safest course. Occasionally gallbladder colic is difficult to differentiate from appendicitis, pancreatitis, or a perforated ulcer.

Acute Pancreatitis

Acute pancreatitis is a severe inflammatory disorder of unknown cause involving the pancreas, an organ located in the upper portion of the abdomen behind the lower border of the stomach. Some individuals suffer recurrent attacks of this disorder, which is reputed to be one of the most painful diseases that afflicts man.

Pancreatitis typically develops after a heavy meal or the ingestion of large amounts of alcohol. It also may follow severe hypothermia but can appear at any time. The pain is located in the upper part of the abdomen in the midline or on the left side, but frequently radiates to the back and to the shoulder blades. The onset is relatively rapid, building up to peak intensity over a few minutes to a few hours, but is not as abrupt as the onset of symptoms of a perforated ulcer. Loss of appetite is almost invariable; nausea and vomiting are usually present; diarrhea is rare.

In severe cases prostration and shock are obvious. The patient is frequently cyanotic and has a rapid pulse and a low blood pressure. Fever is usually present, particularly in severe cases, varies from 100° to 103°F (38° to 39°C), and persists as long as the disease is active.

Upper abdominal tenderness is almost always present. However, spasm of the abdominal muscles and rebound tenderness may be rather mild because the stomach is interposed between the pancreas and the abdominal wall.

Acute pancreatitis may be difficult to distinguish from acute inflammation of the gallbladder. In addition to a more rapid onset, the location of maximum pain and tenderness in the midline or on the left side of the upper abdomen rather than the right, and the presence of severe prostration and shock, pancreatitis is also characterized by the frequent failure of narcotics to completely relieve the pain. However, many patients with pancreatitis do have gallstones and a history of gallbladder disease, including intolerance for fried or fatty foods.

Therapy for pancreatitis consists of rapid evacuation, efforts to relieve pain, inactivation of the gastrointestinal system, and general care of the patient. Although the treatment of acute pancreatitis does not require surgery, it does require expert medical care. This disease causes an appreciable number of deaths, even with the best treatment currently available. Furthermore, complications that require a physician's attention are relatively common. Therefore, evacuation is essential.

Meperidine or morphine (preferably meperidine) should be administered intramuscularly every three to four hours for pain. Nitroglycerin tablets sublingually every two to three hours may provide some relief and should be given in conjunction with meperidine.

Nothing should be given by mouth and nasogastric suction should be instituted if possible. An antispasmodic given intramuscularly every four hours reduces stomach activity and diminishes the secretory activity of the pancreas. Intravenous fluids must be administered to provide the daily fluid requirements as well as to replace losses due to vomiting or gastric suction. Shock should be treated in the same manner as shock from other causes.

Peritonitis

A number of intraabdominal catastrophes produce gross infection of the abdominal cavity (peritonitis). The appearance of patients with peritonitis is similar regardless of the underlying cause. The patient lies very quietly, since motion is quite painful. He is pale, febrile with a temperature usually over 101 ° F (38.5 ° C), and is obviously very sick. The appetite is entirely gone, the patient is usually nauseated, and he may be vomiting. The abdomen may be somewhat distended and is diffusely tender and firm to palpation. No bowel sounds can be heard and the patient does not pass any flatus. Signs and symptoms of the disease causing the infection are also present.

The patient must be evacuated by stretcher as rapidly as possible. During evacuation he should be made comfortable with morphine or meperidine, given nothing by mouth, and kept supine, warm, and quiet. Gentamycin and clindamycin should be administered intramuscularly or intravenously every six to eight hours. Nasogastric suction should be instituted if gastric distension develops. Intravenous fluid administration is required if evacuation takes over thirty-six hours. All fluids lost by vomiting or nasogastric suction should be replaced with a balanced salt solution.

Kidney Stone

Occasionally minerals are precipitated from the urine and deposited in the kidney to form a stone. This stone may be swept into the bladder by the urinary stream, causing excruciating pain as it passes through the duct (ureter) that connects the kidney with the bladder.

The symptoms produced by a kidney stone usually appear suddenly and are characterized by sharp, stabbing pain, which may come and go in waves of increasing intensity. The pain usually begins in the back at the level of the lowest ribs but frequently radiates around the side to the lower abdomen and into the groin or scrotum. The patient typically writhes in pain and is unable to lie still.

Bright red blood is often found in the urine but may be present in only small amounts. (See Chapter Twenty, "Genitourinary Disorders.") Pain on urination and increased frequency of urination are common. Nausea, vomiting, and cold sweats are usually present; chills and fever may be present but are not typical.

A kidney stone rarely requires emergency surgical care and is not associated with any danger of severe blood loss. The pain may last for twenty-four hours or more but usually subsides spontaneously in a shorter period of time as the stone is passed into the bladder.

Morphine or meperidine can be given intramuscularly every four hours to afford relief from the pain. (Complete masking of the pain may not be achieved.) If the patient is not vomiting, he should drink as much water as possible to help flush out the stone.

Following subsidence of the pain, the likelihood of a subsequent attack is slight. The victim can resume his usual activities as soon as he feels capable. However, if the stone is not passed and pain continues for forty-eight hours or more, the patient should be evacuated. Serious renal damage can result if the stone remains in the ureter and obstructs the flow of urine.

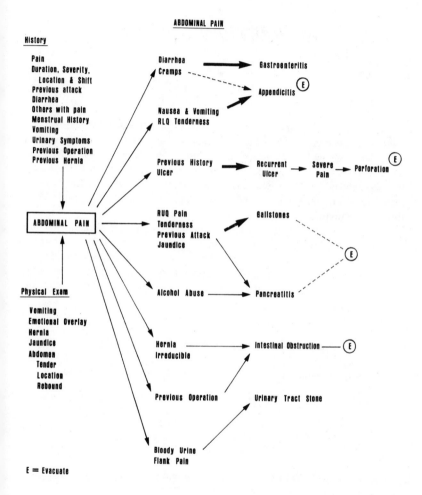

Figure 52. Algorithm for diagnosing acute abdominal pain.

CHAPTER TWENTY

Genitourinary Disorders

The urinary tract is made up of the kidneys, ureters, urinary bladder, and urethra. The genital system includes the ovaries, fallopian tubes, uterus, vagina, and external genitalia in females, and the testes, epididymides, vasa deferentia, seminal vesicles, prostate gland, and external genitalia in males. The kidneys filter the blood and excrete unneeded substances and water. The urine is transported by the ureters from the kidneys to the urinary bladder where it is held until voided through the urethra.

Normally hydrated adult males of average size with normal renal function form approximately 1 cc of urine per minute. At this rate about 60 cc are formed per hour; 1,500 cc are excreted per day. Persons with smaller or larger bodies produce somewhat smaller or larger urine volumes, although urinary output does not vary directly with size. Dehydration reduces urine volume; overhydration increases urinary output.

ACUTE URINARY TRACT DISORDERS

The most common symptoms or signs of acute urinary tract disease are:

1. Pain in the back or flank;
2. Burning with urination;
3. Blood in the urine;
4. Changes in urine volume.

Pain is usually indicative of kidney disease and is characteristically located to one side of the vertebral column at the point where it is joined by the lowest ribs. However, the pain frequently radiates to the sides just above the pelvis and around to the groin.

A burning sensation with voiding is unmistakable. Occasionally the patient complains of the sensation of passing gravel. Such symptoms are usually the result of inflammatory diseases of the urinary bladder, prostate, or urethra.

Bleeding can be obvious or may produce only cloudy or "smoky" urine. However, if the urine is allowed to stand so the cells can settle out, a red sludge

328

can be seen at the bottom of the container, confirming the presence of blood. Even small amounts of blood can be detected in this way.

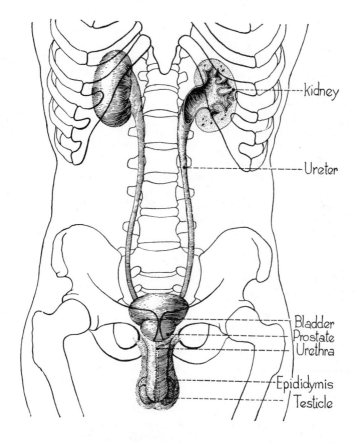

Figure 53. Anatomy of the urinary and male genital systems.

Changes in urinary volume, except for very large deviations, usually go unnoticed unless the urinary output is measured. In mountaineering circumstances dehydration is by far the most common cause for a change in urinary output. However, some renal diseases can result in almost total cessation of kidney function with almost no urine being formed. Uncommonly, a larger volume of very dilute urine is excreted.

Cystitis

Cystitis is an inflammation of the urinary bladder, which can occur with or without a concurrent infection. This disorder is rare in young males but is not uncommon in females. When cystitis is associated with pyelonephritis, symptoms of the latter disease predominate.

The principal symptom of cystitis is burning or pain during voiding. The pain may increase somewhat as the bladder is emptied but disappears gradually after urine flow has stopped. The frequency of voiding may also be increased because the irritated bladder feels full with a smaller urine volume. Fever, a feeling of being ill, or any other symptoms are rare. Slight bleeding sometimes occurs, and rarely bleeding may be severe enough to make the urine obviously bloody.

Usually no treatment is needed for cystitis and the symptoms disappear in two or three days. If symptoms are severe, persist for a longer time, or are associated with fever, ampicillin, trimethoprim-sulfamethoxazole, or a cephalosporin may be administered. These drugs are excreted by the kidneys and reach high concentrations in the urine. They should be given orally four times a day for at least one week or until the patient has been completely free of symptoms for two days, if that takes longer. The victim must also drink large quantities of fluids, considerably more than the usual requirements.

Pyelonephritis

Pyelonephritis is an infection of a kidney, or sometimes both kidneys, and is characterized by the sudden onset of high fever, often associated with chills. The patient feels and appears quite ill. Back pain of moderate severity is usually present. Pressing or gentle pounding with the fist just below the lower rib on either side of the vertebral column reveals tenderness. Symptoms of cystitis are often present, and slight to moderate bleeding may occur.

The patient should rest and drink large quantities of fluids, at least twice the usual daily requirement. Fluid intake and urinary output should be measured and recorded. Evacuation from very high altitudes is desirable.

Antibacterial therapy is important. Ampicillin, trimethoprim-sulfamethoxazole, or a cephalosporin should be given orally every six hours and should be continued for five days after all signs of disease have disappeared or for a minimum of ten days. Individuals with repeated episodes of pyelonephritis should consult a physician; irreversible kidney disease can result and some underlying disorder, such as renal stones, may be present.

Acute Renal Failure

Renal failure, a drastic reduction or total cessation of kidney function, occasionally follows a severe injury, particularly if the victim is in shock for several hours or longer. (Certain poisons, drug reactions, and other disorders can also cause acute renal failure.) If the patient can be kept alive through the period of reduced renal function, which may last from a few days to several months, complete recovery is usually possible.

The principal manifestation of renal failure is reduced urinary output. Dehydration may also cause a low urinary output. However, if a dehydrated subject is given fluid, the urinary volume increases. The victim of acute renal failure can not increase his urinary output, no matter how much fluid he is given. Additionally, with dehydration the urine is concentrated and has a deep yellow or orange color; with acute renal failure, the small amount of urine produced is typically dilute. Any adequately hydrated subject with a urinary output of less than 400 cc per day of dilute urine following a severe injury should be considered to be in renal failure.

Weakness, loss of appetite, nausea, vomiting, diarrhea, muscle twitching, confusion, convulsions, and eventually coma appear some time after the onset of renal failure. Usually the victim has almost no symptoms related to his diminished renal function for the first two or three days. However, weakness becomes apparent on about the third day, and the other symptoms soon follow.

Urinary retention due to spasm of the bladder muscles and rupture of the urinary bladder both simulate renal failure because urinary output ceases. However, urinary retention is usually accompanied by a strong urge to urinate as well as by pain in the bladder or lower abdomen. If urethral catheterization discloses the bladder to be empty, urinary retention can be ruled out. Following bladder rupture, evidence of an abdominal or pelvic injury as well as abdominal pain and tenderness are usually obvious. (See Chapter Eleven, "Abdominal Injuries.") However, acute renal failure can also be associated with an injury in which the bladder is ruptured.

Evacuation is urgent. Only a well equipped medical center would have the facilities to keep a victim of acute renal failure alive for more than a few days. Some form of dialysis (artificial kidney) is essential.

During evacuation, fluid intake must be carefully controlled to keep the patient from being overloaded with water. To establish the diagnosis of acute renal failure the patient's previous state of hydration must be determined. If he appears to have been dehydrated, enough fluids must be given to correct that situation. If renal output does not return, fluids subsequently must be administered very carefully. Each day's fluid intake should be limited to one quart plus a quantity roughly equal to the urine volume. However, fluid needs are increased by vomiting, sweating, and the increased pulmonary losses at high elevations with cold air temperatures. (See Dehydration at Altitude in Chapter Two, "Basic Medical Care and Evacuation.") Any unusual losses by these routes must also be replaced.

If the patient is not able to take fluids orally because he is nauseated or vomiting, which is the usual condition after about the third day, they must be given intravenously. The quart of water, the previous day's urinary output, and any unusual losses through the lungs should be replaced with a five or ten percent glucose solution. Fluids lost through vomiting and excessive sweating should be replaced with a balanced salt solution. To ensure that the volume replaced matches the amounts that have been lost, the urine volume, losses from other sources, and oral or intravenous intake must be measured as carefully as possible and recorded.

While he can, the patient should be encouraged to eat sweets such as hard candy or glucose tablets. However, citrus fruits and fruit juices must be avoided as they contain potassium, which is highly toxic for a subject with reduced renal function.

Medications should be avoided if possible because most drugs are excreted by the kidneys. In the absence of renal excretion, their concentration can rapidly build to toxic levels.

Acute Glomerulonephritis

Glomerulonephritis is a disease of the renal glomeruli, the portion of the kidneys in which the blood is filtered. Chronic glomerulonephritis is a relatively common disease. More patients require chronic dialysis or kidney transplants as the result of chronic glomerulonephritis than any other disorder. However, chronic glomerulonephritis would rarely have such a rapid onset that it could cause problems on even an extended mountaineering outing. Acute glomerulonephritis can appear much more rapidly.

Acute glomerulonephritis usually follows a "strep throat" or a streptococcal infection in some other location by a few days or a few weeks, but a number of patients do not have such preceding infections. (This disorder is usually caused by an immune reaction to a portion of the streptococcus organism. The products of that reaction are filtered from the blood by the glomeruli, where they incite a damaging inflammatory reaction.) Since the advent of antibiotics, the incidence of acute glomerulonephritis has been greatly reduced by treating the initial streptococcal infection with penicillin. This disorder is important because a small percentage of patients have potentially lethal renal disease.

If the disease is mild, which is much more common, swelling or puffiness of the face, blood in the urine, and headache are the most common observable abnormalities. More severe disease is characterized by edema and the signs of acute renal failure. A low fever and loss of appetite, nausea, and vomiting may be present with mild or severe disease.

Puffiness or swelling of the face, which is the most common symptom, may be noticed by someone other than the patient. The swelling is more striking early in the morning when the patient first awakens and is particularly prominent about the eyes. Swelling of the feet and ankles may also be present.

Many patients have an elevated blood pressure.

The urine may appear bloody, but more frequently blood can only be detected after the red blood cells have been permitted to settle to the bottom of a container. Protein is almost always present in the urine with acute glomerulonephritis. Boiling the urine causes the protein to precipitate as a thick, flocculent coagulum resembling egg albumen, which is a significant, reliable diagnostic finding.

Few patients with acute glomerulonephritis manifest all of these signs and symptoms. The presence of one or two should prompt a search for others, particularly protein in the urine. (In the absence of this abnormality, a diagnosis of acute glomerulonephritis must be seriously questioned.)

The patient should rest as much as possible. Salt, which tends to promote the formation of edema fluid, should be restricted. Penicillin, four times a day, should be given for ten days in case a lingering streptococcal infection is present elsewhere in the body. Evacuation is desirable, but in a truly remote area may not be mandatory if the patient can maintain a urinary output of more than 500 cc per day. If his urine volume falls below 400 cc per twenty-four hours, the patient should be considered to have acute renal failure, his fluid intake and output must be appropriately monitored, and he should be evacuated to a hospital.

OTHER URINARY TRACT DISORDERS

Renal Stones

Since the characteristic symptom of renal stones is severe pain, this disorder is discussed in Chapter Nineteen, "Acute Abdominal Pain." Bloody urine and burning with voiding can also accompany the passage of a stone.

Hematuria

Hematuria, which means bloody urine, may be associated with traumatic injuries, tuberculosis, or tumors of the urinary tract, as well as the disorders discussed above. Traumatic urinary disorders are discussed in Chapter Eleven, "Abdominal Injuries." Adequate treatment for tuberculosis or tumors is impossible in the field. Therefore, the appearance of obviously bloody urine, particularly in the absence of any evidence of another disorder, should prompt immediate medical consultation in order to determine the cause and institute appropriate therapy.

Obvious hematuria is frequently a sign of a serious disorder. (The loss of blood itself is almost never of sufficient volume to be disabling.)

Hemoglobinuria

Severe injuries, burns, severe infections, and other disorders cause the destruction of red blood cells. As these cells are broken down, their hemoglobin is released into the blood and is excreted by the kidneys. Urine containing large amounts of the pigment is faint pink to deep red in color and resembles bloody urine.

Hemoglobinuria must be distinguished from hematuria, which is caused by entirely different conditions. If urine that contains hemoglobin is permitted to stand, no blood settles to the bottom of the container. Acute renal failure sometimes follows disorders producing hemoglobinuria if the individual becomes dehydrated or goes into shock. A fluid intake high enough to significantly increase urinary output helps prevent this complication.

Occasionally, strenuous exercise alone results in hemoglobinuria or myoglobinuria. Myoglobin is a protein similar to hemoglobin that originates in muscle and can also be released by crushing injuries. Such disorders can also cause acute renal failure, but the conditions usually are benign and disappear with rest. The subjects must maintain a generous fluid intake to reduce the chances of renal failure.

The pigment from some foods or dyes, particularly beets, occasionally imparts a reddish color to the urine. However, the patient can usually remember the ingestion of these substances, and the pigment disappears from the urine within a few hours or days.

FEMALE GENITAL PROBLEMS

Although gynecologic problems are common and widely variable, few appear so rapidly they could create problems on a mountaineering outing. An examination by a physician beforehand should disclose any potential disorders and permit their correction before the outing is underway.

Two problems that could occur are dysmenorrhea and abnormal bleeding.

Dysmenorrhea

Dysmenorrhea means painful menstruation. The pain can be caused by many different abnormalities, including a wrongly positioned uterus and the passage of blood clots. Most women with dysmenorrhea have had it most of their postpubertal lives. Such pain encountered for the first time on a mountaineering outing must be most unusual. In fact, exercise is one of the remedies sometimes effective for dysmenorrhea.

The pain, which typically is cramping, may be disabling but usually is less severe. Pain may be worse the first day or two of the menstrual period. Treatment with aspirin and codeine every four hours is usually sufficient. Treatment with prostaglandin antagonists such as ibuprofen may be effective also.

Diminished physical activity may also be of some benefit. Women bothered with this problem — and they are numerous — have usually learned to deal with it long before it could create problems in a mountaineering situation.

Abnormal Bleeding

Abnormal uterine bleeding can take the form of excessive bleeding with menstrual periods, bleeding between periods, or both. Numerous disorders can produce such abnormal bleeding, but commonly no cause can be identified. No specific treatment can be given under mountaineering situations. The bleeding is rarely severe enough to create blood loss problems. If a hemorrhage of massive proportions does occur, packing the vagina with tampons, gauze, or anything available may help slow the bleeding during evacuation, although complete control of bleeding by such means probably can not be obtained. Such problems must be exceedingly rare; exercise seems to help control abnormal bleeding for many women.

PREGNANCY

Pregnancy, at least in its early stages, does not necessarily require curtailment of a woman's customary activities, but a more propitious time can be found to initially take up climbing. Prudence does dictate some precautions that should be observed when considering mountaineering activities. Fifteen to twenty percent of all pregnancies terminate in spontaneous abortions; most occur during the first three months of pregnancy. Occasionally such abortions are associated with severe bleeding, which can not be stopped without hospital facilities. Therefore, a woman in this stage of pregnancy should probably not enter an area so remote that evacuation within twelve to twenty-four hours by stretcher could not be readily accomplished.

During the last three months of pregnancy, the enlarged uterus and the baby it contains often cause problems with balance. Climbing that requires delicate balance may be unusually difficult. A fall, particularly if held by a rope tied with a conventional waist loop, could injure the mother, baby, or both, even though such falls would not injure a woman who was not pregnant. Premature labor, whether caused by a fall or occurring spontaneously, could result in delivery in less than optimal circumstances or the birth of a small immature baby who could not survive without the facilities available in a hospital.

Occasionally pregnancy creates or aggravates other medical problems, such as diabetes, hypertension, or cardiac disease. The mother should consult her physician for any special care such problems would require on a mountaineering outing.

Contraceptives

One aspect of pregnancy, its prevention, does have direct implications for high altitude mountaineering. Oral contraceptives appear to cause an increased incidence of venous thromboses and the resulting complication, pulmonary embolism. High altitude mountaineering also predisposes climbers to the development of these frequently lethal disorders. (See Chapter Sixteen, "Diseases of the Respiratory System.") Women taking part in a mountaineering outing requiring a significant stay at altitudes above 12,000 to 14,000 feet (3,700 to 4,300 m) should discontinue oral contraceptives at least several weeks in advance. If some other form of contraception is needed and an intrauterine contraceptive device (IUD) is selected, it should be inserted long enough in advance of the outing to be sure it is well tolerated. Rarely these devices cause perforation, bleeding, or infection that could be difficult or impossible to control in mountaineering circumstances, but most of these problems show up during the first few months the devices are used.

MALE GENITAL PROBLEMS

Few male genital problems appear with sufficient speed or at a young enough age to cause problems in mountaineering situations. Two exceptions are acute epididymitis and torsion of the testes, two entirely different disorders that are discussed together because their features are similar and differentiation may be quite difficult, even for a physician.

Epididymitis and Testicular Torsion

Epididymitis is an inflammatory condition of the epididymis, a part of the testicle in which sperm are collected before passing on through the vas deferens to the seminal vesicle where they are stored prior to ejaculation. Epididymitis sometimes is the result of gonorrheal infection, the organisms presumably passing backward from the urethra through the vas deferens. Rarely are cultures taken from the inflamed tissues, and it appears likely that most cases of epididymitis have no relation to a venereal infection. Many cases may not result from infection at all.

Torsion of the testis refers to twisting of the testis within the scrotum. The twisting movement involves the spermatic cord, which contains the vas deferens and the arteries and veins supplying the testis. As the spermatic cord is twisted, the blood vessels, particularly the veins, are occluded. If the occlusion is not relieved, which usually requires surgery, the testis that has been deprived of its blood supply dies within a few hours.

The presence of either of these disorders is unmistakable as they are both quite painful. The scrotum is often distended and may also be red and inflamed, particularly with epididymitis. The testis is usually swollen and quite tender. The pain of testicular torsion may appear rather rapidly, while that of epididymitis usually develops more slowly. An enlarged, firm, nodular epididymis may be felt in the presence of epididymitis. Elevation of the scrotum and the application of cold packs are frequently helpful with epididymitis, but elevation of the scrotum usually does not help relieve the pain of testicular torsion, a point of difference between the two disorders that may be helpful in diagnosis. With testicular torsion, the testis may be higher in the scrotum than the opposite testis because twisting the cord causes it to shorten.

The patient should rest as much as possible. In urban surroundings many physicians keep their patients with epididymitis confined to bed. (Such confinement is usually not difficult to impose because the disorder is too painful for the patient to be up and moving around.)

Tetracycline should be administered to patients with either disorder. If the patient has a history of gonorrhea or exposure to gonorrhea within the previous two months and he is not allergic to penicillin, that drug should be given instead of tetracycline. The dose should be the same as that used to treat gonorrhea. Patients with testicular torsion who can not be evacuated right away should receive antibiotics to prevent the establishment of an infection in the dead tissue of the testis.

Almost all patients with either of these disorders must be evacuated. Patients with testicular torsion require surgery, even if it can not be carried out quickly enough to save the testis. Patients with epididymitis require rest and antibiotics. Two to three weeks may be required for complete healing. Resumption of activity before all symptoms have completely cleared frequently reactivates the disease. However, epididymitis has little tendency to spread to other areas. Patients with this disorder could probably be adequately treated in base camp in truly remote circumstances.

VENEREAL DISEASES

The venereal diseases are a group of infectious diseases spread by sexual contact, both homosexual and heterosexual, and caused by a variety of organisms. Syphilis and gonorrhea are the most common bacterial infections. Herpes viral infections have achieved recent notoriety, although they have been around for many years. Hepatitis B is also spread by sexual contact to a large extent within developed nations, but is not considered a venereal disease and is discussed in Chapter Eighteen, "Gastrointestinal Diseases." The predominance of the acquired immune deficiency syndrome (AIDS) among male homosexuals suggests a sexually transmitted infection, but too little is known about that disorder at the present time for further discussion to have significant value.

All venereal diseases are spread by intimate personal contact. Infection from "toilet seats" or similar sources essentially does not occur because the organisms can not survive well enough outside of the body to produce infection by such means.

At the present time the only dependable way to prevent such infections is to avoid sexual contact with infected individuals. Condoms are of only limited value in preventing infection. Prophylactic antibiotic therapy has many disadvantages as well as the significant hazard of allergic reactions to the drugs.

Syphilis

Syphilis is produced by infection with the spirochete *Treponema pallidum*. This disease has an interesting history. It apparently originated in the western hemisphere, was transported to Europe by members of Columbus's crew, and in an amazingly short time was spread all over the world. The great variation in its clinical features, its long duration, and its potential for involving any of the body's organs and mimicking almost any other disease have long held a great fascination for medical investigators.

The discovery of penicillin therapy for this infection was a dramatic triumph. Some students of this disease feel that the treatment used before penicillin probably never cured a single case of syphilis. In contrast, no examples of syphilis resistant to penicillin have been documented.

Syphilitic infections have three stages. The primary stage is that of the chancre, a one-quarter to one-half inch (6 to 13 mm) ulcer that usually appears at the site of infectious contact. A characteristic and striking feature of this ulcer is that it is usually painless. Most chancres appear on the genitalia, but they are occasionally found on the mouth or lips or the skin of other parts of the body. In women, chancres may be located within the vagina or on the uterine cervix and may not be visible to external examination. Sometimes primary chancres never appear or go unnoticed, particularly when hidden in a location such as the vagina.

The secondary stage of syphilis is characterized by the appearance of a skin rash about six weeks after the primary lesion. Many patients do not manifest this stage of the disease. The appearance of this rash is highly variable, although it does not produce blisters, and it usually has a wide distribution, including the palms and soles of the feet and the mucous membranes of the mouth. The rash does not itch and generally is symptomless. It usually lasts from a few days to a few weeks.

In its third or tertiary stage, syphilis can affect any organ or tissue and can produce fatal cardiac disease or disabling brain disease. However, tertiary syphilis takes years to develop and can be prevented by appropriate therapy.

A precise diagnosis of syphilis requires laboratory facilities not available in most hospitals. Treatment in mountaineering circumstances should be based on a history of sexual contact and the presence of skin changes suggestive of a primary chancre or the secondary skin rash. The infection is most contagious during the primary and secondary stages.

The treatment of choice for a primary infection is penicillin. Benzathine penicillin G, an intramuscular injection of 2.4 million units (1.5 gm) in each buttock, is preferred in most urban settings because it ensures that adequate treatment has been given regardless of whether the patient returns for further injections. Alternatively, single daily intramuscular injections of 600,000 units (375 mg) of aqueous procaine penicillin G may be given for a period of eight days. Individuals allergic to penicillin can be treated with erythromycin or tetracycline, 0.5 gm four times a day for fifteen days. Follow-up care should be obtained from a physician after a mountaineering outing to be sure the infection has been totally eradicated.

Gonorrhea

Gonorrhea is an epidemic disease with an estimated 3 million cases in the United States and 150 million throughout the world in 1974. The infection in males is usually limited to the lower genital tract, principally the urethra. The urethral infection is associated with a purulent urethral discharge, but the characteristic symptom is pain, often severe, with voiding. The infection usually clears after seven to ten days, but treatment should be administered anyway. Residual infection may persist, particularly in the prostate, or the infection may spread to other parts of the body.

In females, gonorrhea is a much more insidious infection. Seventy-five percent of infected women have no initial symptoms at all. The infection usually must be diagnosed by bacterial cultures or smears from the vagina or uterine cervix. Treatment must be based on a history of sexual contact with a possibly infected individual in the absence of laboratory facilities for a definitive diagnosis.

Gonorrhea is also a much more threatening disorder in females. Spread of the infection to other organs is much more common. Extension to the fallopian tubes produces painful infections with symptoms similar to those of appendicitis. (See Acute Salpingitis in Chapter Nineteen, "Acute Abdominal Pain.") Permanent sterility is the usual result. Spread to one or more joints can produce a destructive arthritis; involvement of the heart can cause disabling cardiac disease. Infections also occur in other tissues.

The treatment of choice is penicillin. Procaine penicillin G, 4.8 million units (3.0 gm), should be injected intramuscularly, ideally together with 1.0 gm of probenecid orally. Subsequently, tetracycline (500 mg four times a day) should be given orally for seven days. For individuals allergic to penicillin, tetracycline (0.5 gm four times a day for at least seven days) can be substituted. A physician should be consulted after the mountaineering outing to ensure no residual infection persists.

Strains of gonorrhea resistant to penicillin have emerged in recent years, particularly in Southeast Asia. Persons suspected of having contracted an infection by such organisms should be treated with spectinomycin, but this antibiotic is less useful than other drugs for treating more common infections and would rarely be included in the medical supplies for a serious mountaineering outing.

Genital Herpes

In spite of the attention it has recently attracted, genital herpes infection is little different from herpes occurring on the lips and known as "fever blisters" except for its location. Recent studies have indicated that the same viral organisms are involved. Although the genital infection is transmitted by sexual contact, it has the same tendency to recur periodically in the same location that oral herpes does. Because the tissues are somewhat more sensitive, infections on the genitalia may be more uncomfortable than those around the mouth. No curative treatment has yet been developed.

Other Considerations

All patients with suspected or known venereal disease should consult a physician and be treated. The results of an untreated infection can be disastrous. The ease with which syphilis and gonorrhea can be treated has caused a lack of concern about all venereal disease. To encourage individuals to obtain treatment they need, many states have laws that permit physicians to treat minors with such infections without reporting the disease to the patient's parents or guardians.

CHAPTER TWENTY-ONE

Diseases of the Nervous System

The nervous system is made up of the brain and spinal cord, which comprise the central nervous system (CNS) and the peripheral nerves. Almost everything that happens in the body — voluntary and involuntary movement, respiration, blood circulation, even endocrine function — is controlled or regulated by the nervous system.

The diseases of this complex system are numerous and often disabling. However, most of these diseases are of a chronic nature and come on too slowly to create problems in mountaineering circumstances, even on expeditions lasting several months.

SIGNS AND SYMPTOMS

The signs and symptoms produced by diseases of the nervous system can consist of altered intellectual function, impaired control of movements (motor disturbances), sensory disorders, loss of function of specific nerves, and a group of unrelated, less specific signs.

Altered Intellect

Alterations of intellectual function produce personality changes, most commonly increased irritability or silliness, and impairment in the patient's contact with his surroundings, which shows up first as forgetfulness and confusion but can progress to hallucinations, delirium, or complete loss of consciousness (coma).

Motor Disturbances

Motor disturbances, when early or mild, result in loss of coordination, which causes the patient to stumble or fall repeatedly, or to be unable to perform delicate or repetitive movements with his hands. More severe dysfunction can cause weakness, convulsions, or total paralysis.

Sensory Disturbances

Sensory disturbances most commonly consist of tingling or prickly sensations, such as those felt when a limb "goes to sleep," and are not necessarily indicative of nervous system disease. Acetazolamide commonly produces similar symptoms that go away when the drug is stopped. Total anesthesia can occur but is rare. Anesthesia involving an entire limb or portion of a limb in a "stocking" fashion, with a sharp margin of demarcation circling the limb, is due to "hysteria" rather than organic disease. The distribution of the nerves is such that this pattern of anesthesia can be produced only by emotional disorders.

Individual Nerve Loss

Loss of function of individual nerves originating in the brain can cause many varied symptoms. Disorders involving the nerves to the eyes may cause double vision, blurred vision, or blindness, occasionally limited to only a portion of the field of vision. Impairment of the nerves to the eye muscles causes paralysis of eye movements. The pupils may fail to contract when exposed to light or may differ greatly in size.

Disorders involving nerves to the muscles of the face cause weakness or paralysis of facial movements and drooling on the affected side. Swallowing is impaired when the nerves to the muscles of the throat are affected, and fluids may be regurgitated through the nose or aspirated into the lungs. Disturbances of the nerves to the ear can cause ringing or buzzing in the ears, vertigo, or hearing loss. Damage to other nerves may cause loss of smell, loss of taste, severe facial pain, weakness of the muscles of the neck, or impairment of respiration.

Damage to the nerves originating in the spinal cord causes paralysis or sensory disturbances, commonly anesthesia, in the portion of the body supplied by the injured nerves. Reflexes such as the knee jerk may be lost.

Other Symptoms

Other symptoms associated with nervous system diseases include nausea and vomiting, the latter often occurring without warning. Headache, which is discussed further below, may accompany diseases of any organ; when associated with nervous system disease it is usually severe. Fever with central nervous system infections is often high; in other nervous system disorders the temperature is normal or only slightly elevated. Blood clots within the skull often cause a slower pulse rate and a wider than normal separation of diastolic and systolic blood pressures.

COMMON NERVOUS SYSTEM DISORDERS

The common nervous system disorders are usually not very serious and are frequently brief in duration.

Headache

Headache is a very common ailment suffered by all but a few fortunate individuals. Rarely can any specific cause for a headache be identified. Therefore, this disorder is frequently thought of as a disease in itself, although it is often only a symptom of another illness.

Headache after a rapid ascent to high altitude is quite common. Although many individuals have no symptoms other than headache, this is probably a mild form of acute mountain sickness.

The pain of a headache may be located in the back of the neck, behind the eyes, or all areas in between. Little significance can be attached to the location of the pain except when it is limited to one side of the head. One sided headaches are frequently caused by vascular disorders such as migraine.

A severe, persistent headache in an individual who usually does not suffer from headaches may be a sign of serious disease. Headache associated with confusion, forgetfulness, dizziness, nausea and vomiting, and occasionally convulsions or loss of consciousness may be the result of an acute increase in blood pressure (hypertensive encephalopathy). This disorder usually occurs in persons with preexisting hypertension but requires prompt treatment to avoid brain damage that can be disastrous. (See Chapter Seventeen, "Diseases of the Heart and Blood Vessels.") Headache associated with fever and a stiff neck are characteristic of meningitis. Following a head injury, increasing severity of a headache may be indicative of the development of a blood clot within the skull. (See Chapter Nine, "Injuries of the Head and Neck.")

Aspirin every three to four hours relieves the pain of most headaches; aspirin and codeine taken with the same frequency is adequate for most of the remainder. Any underlying disease causing the headache must obviously receive appropriate treatment.

Individuals with frequent headaches should consult a physician. Headaches resulting from vascular disorders can often be treated successfully. Some other causes of recurrent headaches, such as brain tumors or high blood pressure, are quite serious but usually come on so slowly they would cause problems only on a protracted expedition.

Fainting

Fainting is a common disorder that usually is not a sign of serious disease. It can follow strong emotion or pain but sometimes appears to occur almost spontaneously. Even when fainting is the result of disease, it is rarely a sign of a disease involving the nervous system. Fainting occurs following the dilatation of numerous peripheral blood vessels, particularly those in muscles. As the blood fills these vessels, the blood pressure falls, the blood supply to the brain is reduced, and unconsciousness results.

The episode of unconsciousness is usually preceded by a period of a few seconds to several minutes in which the person feels weak. This weakness is often accompanied by restlessness and occasionally by nausea. The victim frequently breaks out in a "cold sweat." He appears pale and his pulse is rapid.

These signs and symptoms are similar to those of shock. However, in fainting the physiological derangements are not as severe as they are in shock, and there is rarely any underlying illness that could be expected to produce shock.

If a person notices the onset of the symptoms that precede fainting he can usually avoid the period of unconsciousness. He must get off his feet, either by sitting or lying down, to avoid injury from falling. His head should be lower than the rest of his body so that gravity can help increase the flow of blood to the brain. The head can be placed between the knees or, preferably, the victim can lie down with the feet elevated. Help should be obtained if possible.

In taking care of someone who has fainted or is about to faint, the same measures should be carried out. Maintaining an open airway is rarely a problem because unconsciousness is almost never very deep. No medications are necessary. Aromatic spirits of ammonia are of no real benefit and probably should not be used to avoid injuring the nasal mucosa. Any injuries resulting from falling should receive attention.

Unconsciousness rarely lasts more than a few minutes. More persistent coma is a sign of a more serious disorder. As soon as the victim feels well he can be on his way again, although he must sit up for a few minutes first and then stand up slowly and carefully. If the victim has not eaten for some time, he should try to obtain food or a sugar-containing beverage such as orange juice.

A single episode of fainting is rarely significant. Repeated episodes can be indicative of a serious disease.

Convulsions

Convulsions often are a sign of disease of the nervous system and commonly occur during infections involving the brain or following brain injuries. However, convulsions also occur during the course of diseases that affect the brain only indirectly. (Convulsions associated with renal failure are not at all uncommon.) Occasionally a person suffers a single convulsion for which no cause can be determined and which never recurs.

Epilepsy is a condition in which a person suffers repeated convulsions over a long period of time. Sometimes a cause for these episodes can be found, but commonly the etiology remains undetermined. However, epilepsy can usually be controlled with medications even if the cause is unknown. Convulsions rarely recur as long as the person follows his prescribed treatment diligently.

A person with epilepsy need not refrain from mountaineering or similar activities provided his disorder is controlled and he is conscientious about taking his medications. In fairness to his companions, and in the interest of his own well being, his climbing partners should be informed of his condition so they can learn in advance what measures to take should a convulsion occur. The stigma formerly attached to convulsions and particularly epilepsy is now generally recognized to be completely unwarranted.

The onset of a convulsion is usually sudden and may be marked by an outcry of some kind. The victim characteristically loses consciousness and falls to the ground, his body twisting and writhing, and all four limbs twitching and jerking. The jaw may be involved also, and the victim can badly injure his tongue by biting. He may salivate profusely, resulting in drooling and frothing; he may defecate or void uncontrollably.

In any single convulsive episode all or none of these features may be present. Sometimes the victim exhibits only slight twitching of the extremities. A person who is unconscious from a head injury may exhibit only a series of jerking movements that gradually increase in intensity and then subside. If one or more limbs has been paralyzed as a result of the injury, it is not involved in the movements.

The convulsion usually lasts only one or two minutes but can persist for five minutes or even longer. Subsequently the patient is usually unconscious from a few minutes to several hours; he may be in a deep coma in which he is almost completely unresponsive, even to painful stimuli.

Essentially nothing can be done to shorten or terminate the convulsive episode. The most helpful measure is to prevent the victim's injuring himself. A folded handkerchief or similar padded object should be placed between his teeth to protect his tongue from being bitten. Clothing around his neck should be loosened to prevent strangulation. The arms and legs should be restrained only enough to prevent the victim from striking nearby objects and injuring himself as he flails about. No attempts should be made to hold the extremities still, as muscular or tendinous injuries may result.

During the postconvulsive stage, the victim requires the same care as any comatose person. If possible, he should be permitted to awaken from his coma without any stimulation and allowed to rest until he feels that his strength has returned and he has fully recovered. Thereafter, he must be closely attended for a period of at least twelve hours in case he should have a recurrence.

An individual suffering repeated convulsions can be treated with barbiturates such as phenobarbital or secobarbital if control of the convulsions is necessary for evacuation. Drugs should be administered orally only if the person is fully awake and able to swallow; otherwise, they should be injected intramuscularly. Administration of phenobarbital should be repeated at six to eight hour intervals (four to six hour intervals for secobarbital) until the person can be placed in the care of a physician. A person who has received this amount of a barbiturate is usually drowsy and must not be left alone, particularly where he could fall and get hurt.

Any underlying disorders and any injuries received during the convulsion should receive care. Anyone suffering an unexplained convulsion should be thoroughly examined by a physician as soon as possible so that any underlying disease can be diagnosed and treated.

INFECTIONS

Meningitis and Encephalitis

Meningitis is an infection of the membranes surrounding the brain and spinal cord, which is usually caused by bacteria. Encephalitis is an infection of the brain itself and is usually of viral origin. However, the facilities required for distinguishing between these infections and identifying the organisms that have caused them can be found only in a medical center. Since these diseases produce similar signs and symptoms and, in mountaineering circumstances, would be treated essentially the same, they are discussed as a single category. (Rabies, a form of encephalitis, is discussed in Chapter Fifteen, "Animal Bites and Stings.")

These diseases are usually spread by human contact. Some of the encephalitides are spread by insects, particularly mosquitoes. Meningitis can result from the direct spread by bacteria from another chronically infected area such as sinuses, ears, or mastoids, or from an open fracture of the skull.

A number of organisms can cause meningitis or encephalitis, and each organism varies in the effects it produces. As a result, this entire group of infections can present a considerable spectrum of signs, symptoms, and severity.

Severe headache is usually the initial symptom but is followed in a few hours by high fever and severe prostration. Confusion, delirium, or coma may ensue and are fairly common with encephalitis. Nausea, vomiting, and convulsions sometimes occur. Paralysis is not usually produced by most of these infections. When paralysis occurs it usually involves only one or two nerves, usually those originating in the brain, and most commonly causes impairment of eye movements and double vision, ringing or buzzing in the ears, dizziness or vertigo, or difficulty in swallowing. (Polio, a striking exception, is discussed below.)

The most specific diagnostic signs in central nervous system infections are those that result from involvement of the fibrous membranes that cover the brain. These membranes are severely inflamed with meningitis and to some extent with encephalitis. Any movement of these membranes such as bending the neck or back causes pain. In order to prevent such movement, the muscles surrounding the vertebral column go into spasm. When a patient with one of these disorders is asked to touch his chin to his chest he is unable to do so, although normally that maneuver is very easy. If the patient is placed on his back and his leg lifted with the knees bent, straightening the leg causes pain in the back. This maneuver pulls nerves in the leg which in turn produces movement of the spinal cord and its coverings, resulting in pain.

The treatment for meningitis and encephalitis consists of control of the infection and alleviation of some of its effects. To treat the infection, large amounts of antibiotics are needed. These should be given intravenously if preparations suitable for administration by that route are available, because high blood concentrations of the antibiotic are required in order for therapeutic quantities to get out of the blood and into the brain and cerebrospinal fluid where the infection is located. Penicillin or ampicillin is the drug of choice for individuals who are not allergic to penicillin. Eight to twelve grams per day, depending on the patient's size, should be given in six equally divided doses. If the patient is allergic to penicillin, chloramphenicol should be substituted. Four to six grams per day of this drug should be administered in four equal doses.

Fever in these infections can be very high; it should be lowered if it goes above 104°F (40°C) orally. Aspirin every four hours and cooling the arms and legs with wet cloths may be required.

The headache that accompanies these disorders is frequently very severe but can usually be controlled with aspirin and codeine every four hours. Should convulsions occur, they must be controlled to avoid injuring the victim further. However, in the absence of convulsions, medications for sleep or medications for pain stronger than codeine should not be given because they act synergistically with the infection to further depress the function of the brain.

Fluid balance must be maintained; intravenous fluids may be necessary. Coma requires the same care as unconsciousness from any cause. Evacuation to low altitudes or oxygen administration is desirable. The victim should be isolated with only one or two attendants to prevent spread of the disease. Evacuation to a hospital is always desirable and may be essential.

Poliomyelitis

Poliomyelitis is a type of encephalitis that can be recognized by the presence of paralysis. The paralysis may come on rapidly or gradually and is usually accompanied or preceded by pain in the involved muscles. Rarely swallowing and respiration are impaired, requiring careful maintenance of an open airway.

Treatment is the same as for other diseases in this group except that particular care must be taken to avoid any exertion by the patient. Exercise of any type appears to definitely increase the severity of the paralysis and the ultimate disability resulting from the disease. Such precautions are definitely worthwhile. Some individuals who are almost totally paralyzed during the acute stage of poliomyelitis can recover completely.

Poliomyelitis is essentially completely preventable by prior immunization;

failure to take this preventive measure by residents of developed countries is inexcusable. In underdeveloped countries such as Nepal polio immunization can not be afforded by most of the population and the infection is widespread.

STROKE

"Stroke" is a term applied to a group of disorders in which the blood supply to a portion of the brain is permanently disturbed. The most common of these disorders are hemorrhage, which may destroy much of the brain, and clotting within an artery, which causes the death of tissue supplied by that blood vessel.

Typically strokes result from arteriosclerosis (hardening of the arteries), are usually associated with high blood pressure, and occur predominately in older people. However, strokes can occur in younger adults with severe, untreated hypertension. The dehydration and increased numbers of red blood cells that occur at high altitudes tend to increase the risk of stroke. The most likely victims of strokes in expeditionary mountaineering are members of the support team such as porters. (The climbers should have been thoroughly examined prior to the expedition.) Many of these individuals have never had an opportunity for any type of medical care, not even a routine physical examination. High blood pressure in such individuals would not have been detected. If possible, porters should be screened for hypertension (as well as other diseases, particularly infectious diseases such as tuberculosis) and affected individuals excluded from the expedition. However, the political situation in some areas may not permit such discrimination.

Although many persons survive strokes, frequently with surprisingly little or no disability, the prognosis is still serious, particularly at high altitudes with the added stress resulting from cold and reduced atmospheric oxygen.

The onset is quite variable. With milder strokes, headache is commonly present. Other symptoms, which may be transient, include weakness of an arm or leg or one-half of the body; vague, unusual sensations such as tingling, "pins and needles" sensations, or numbness; visual disturbances such as blurred vision or partial blindness (which may not be noticed by the patient); and difficulties with speech, both speaking and understanding the speech of others. Personality changes such as combativeness, indecisiveness, or irritability may occur.

With more severe strokes headache is typically present. Unconsciousness may follow fairly quickly and rapidly progress to a deep coma in which the victim does not respond to any stimuli. (These events may take place almost instantaneously.) Breathing is noisy and may be very irregular (Cheyne-Stokes respirations). Paralysis is usually present, most commonly affects one side of the body, and may include the face as well as the extremities. However, the paralysis can involve the entire body and is often difficult to evaluate in the presence of coma.

Regardless of the severity of symptoms, a patient with evidence of a stroke should be evacuated to lower altitude without delay. Oxygen should be administered at altitudes above 8,000 feet (2,400 m). An open airway must be maintained. If the patient has an elevated blood pressure, he should be given sedatives unless they interfere with his evacuation. After a lower elevation is reached, a conscious patient with hypertension may benefit from several days rest before continuing. However, a physician's care is essential. If the patient has only transient symptoms, further, more disabling damage can often be prevented. For the patient with more severe disease, such recovery as will occur requires months.

CHAPTER TWENTY-TWO

Disorders of the Eye, Ear, Nose, and Throat

Diseases of the eye, ear, nose, and throat, which are the most common of all disorders if the common cold is included, are rarely disabling, usually cause only a moderate inconvenience, and are of relatively short duration. However, all diseases of these organs, even colds, carry some threat of severe complications. Therefore, these disorders must be respected and treated in a careful manner, particularly under expedition circumstances. Because loss of vision is such a devastating event, the eyes must be protected and their disorders must receive particularly careful attention.

DISORDERS OF THE EYE

Conjunctivitis

Conjunctivitis is an inflammatory disorder of the delicate membrane that covers the visible white portion of the surface of the eye (the sclera) and the undersurface of the eyelids. Inflammation is most frequently caused by irritation from a foreign body, smog, or smoke but is sometimes the result of a bacterial or viral infection. "Pink eye," a common type of conjunctivitis that can reach epidemic proportions among school children, is produced by pneumococci, the bacteria that were the most common cause of pneumonia in preantibiotic days. Trachoma, a much more severe form of viral conjunctivitis, is the most frequent cause of blindness in those areas of the world where it is commonly found, particularly Southeast Asia.

The patient with conjunctivitis characteristically feels as if he has something in his eye, even after the foreign body has been removed. Movement of the eye aggravates the irritation. The eye appears red and the blood vessels on its surface are engorged. The flow of tears is increased. Exudate may be crusted on the margins of the eyelids and the eyelashes and may seal the lids together at night during sleep.

If the conjunctivitis appears to result from irritation by smog, campfire smoke, or a similar source, steroid-free eye drops containing an antihistamine and a decongestant (such as Vasocon-A, Optihist, or Vernacel) can provide symptomatic relief, including the relief of swelling of the eyelids and excessive tearing.

350

If the presence of exudate indicates an infection is present, Neosporin Ophthalmic Ointment or Neosporin Ophthalmic Solution (eye drops) should be placed beneath the lower lid every four hours until symptoms have disappeared. Neosporin preparations should not be used except when clearly indicated. Allergy to Neosporin is fairly common, and the allergic reaction can be worse than the original condition.

If symptoms persist for more than three days and the conjunctivitis appears to be severe, tetracycline should be administered orally every six hours. Dark glasses or blinders with only a pinhole to see through help reduce the discomfort. Since many forms of conjunctivitis are infective, contact between the patient and other members of the party should be limited.

Subconjunctival Hemorrhage

Occasionally, following exertion or coughing (sometimes without any predisposing event) hemorrhages, which range in size from a few millimeters to almost the entire visible part of the eye, occur in the sclera. Although alarming, these hemorrhages are of no real significance, are not related to high altitude retinal hemorrhages, and require no treatment. They disappear in ten to fifteen days, depending upon the size of the hemorrhage. Hot compresses applied to the eye at frequent intervals may speed resolution a little but are not at all necessary.

Eyeglasses and Contact Lens

All eyeglasses to be worn for mountaineering, whether they are needed to correct visual defects or for protection from bright sunlight, should be made of shatter resistant (tempered) glass. A second pair should be carried in a secure place where they can not be broken or lost. In an emergency, "glasses" can be constructed of cardboard with a central pinhole for the person to see through. Such devices provide fairly good vision for individuals with refractive errors as well as providing effective sunlight protection.

Wearers of contact lenses frequently have greater problems with the lenses at higher altitudes, particularly at the elevations encountered in Himalayan mountaineering. Five members of the 1975 British Everest Expedition tried using contact lenses during an attempt on the southwest face. Two had little trouble with eyeglasses and reverted to them early in the expedition. The other three had problems with glasses misting up and were eager to try contact lenses. However, above 26,000 feet (7,900 m), all three had reverted to glasses due to a variety of problems, which included slipping of the lenses and their loss. The minimum surface oxygen tension for normal corneal function is estimated to be about 15 mm Hg. At extreme altitudes the oxygen level falls to nearly this level, particularly during sleep. Contact lenses may further decrease the surface oxygen tension, which may be the reason they are not as well tolerated at such elevations.

DISORDERS OF THE NOSE

The Common Cold

A large number of viruses cause upper respiratory infections (colds). However, secondary bacterial infections and allergy to the virus or bacteria cause many of the symptoms. Some generalized viral infections, particularly measles, often mimic a cold during their initial stages. The viruses are spread by personal contact. Chilling may play a role in contracting the disease by increasing susceptibility to infection, but in the absence of the causative viruses, cold exposure alone does not produce the disorder.

The symptoms of a cold are familiar. A sense of dryness, scratchiness, or tickling in the throat or back of the nose usually appears first and is followed in a few hours by nasal stuffiness, sneezing, and a thin, watery nasal discharge. After forty-eight hours, when the disease is fully developed, the eyes are often red and watery, the voice husky, and the nose obstructed. A fairly abundant nasal discharge is present, and taste and smell are diminished. A cough is commonly present and typically is dry at first. Later a moderate amount of mucoid material may be coughed up. The patient characteristically is uncomfortable but not seriously ill. Fever is usually absent but may be as high as 102° F (39° C). The throat may be sore but exudates are not present (see Streptococcal Pharyngitis) and the lymph nodes around the neck and jaw usually are not enlarged.

No effective treatment for a cold has been developed, although some measures to alleviate the symptoms are available. The disease usually lasts seven to ten days. Strenuous activity during the first few days when symptoms are most severe should probably be avoided, particularly at higher altitudes, in order to reduce the probability of complications such as sinusitis or bronchopneumonia. Low altitude climbs of moderate severity and limited work at high altitudes for the additional three to six days required for complete recovery are usually well tolerated.

A decongestant nasal spray such as Neo-Synephrine may be used every three to four hours to reduce nasal congestion and obstruction. However, symptoms may be worse after the decongestant wears off than they were beforehand (rebound phenomenon). Therefore, decongestant sprays should probably be reserved for the times when they are needed most, such as at night to permit restful sleep. When first administered, a decongestant usually relieves obstruction by reducing the swelling of the mucous membrane over the more prominent portions of the nasal passages. However, a second spraying ten minutes later is necessary to reach into the various recesses of the nasal cavity. The swelling in these areas should be relieved to promote drainage and lower the danger of sinusitis or a severe bacterial infection. A systemic decongestant or a combined decongestant and antihistamine may be beneficial when taken orally every four to six hours.

Antibiotics have no significant effect on the viruses that cause colds and for most individuals should not be administered. The rare serious complications of colds may require antibiotic therapy, but such therapy should not be given until the conditions actually develop. Prophylactic antibiotic therapy should be avoided, even at high altitudes, because the bacteria producing any subsequent infection would be resistant to the antibiotics.

Sinusitis

Sinusitis is an infection of one of the sinuses of the skull. These sinuses are open, air-filled spaces within the bone, which are lined by a thin mucous membrane similar to that of the nose and are connected with the nose by narrow canals. The sinuses serve to make the skull lighter in weight than it would be if these areas were occupied by solid bone.

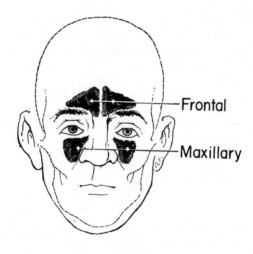

Figure 54. Location of the frontal and maxillary sinuses.

Sinusitis is most commonly caused by obstruction of the canals that drain the sinuses, usually as a result of swelling of the mucous membrane around the opening due to a cold or allergy. Mucous collects within the sinus, becomes infected, and the infection spreads to the surrounding tissues.

Sinusitis, although sometimes producing a painful headache, is rarely disabling by itself. However, complications do occur, and spread of the infection to the bones of the skull or to the brain itself can result in chronic osteomyelitis, meningitis, or a brain abscess. All of these disorders are lethal for a high percentage of the patients who develop them. However, such complications usually follow prolonged chronic sinusitis, which should be eradicated by a physician before a climber leaves on an extended outing.

Acute sinusitis usually accompanies or follows a cold or hay fever. The most prominent symptom is headache, which may be located in the front of the head, "behind the eyes," or occasionally in the back of the head. A purulent discharge frequently drains into the nose and back into the throat where it may be swallowed — the so-called "postnasal drip."

Fever rarely gets higher than 102° F (39° C) and may be entirely absent. Tenderness may be present over the involved sinus. Infection in the maxillary sinuses may produce pain or tenderness in the teeth of the upper jaw. If a small flashlight or penlight is placed in the victim's mouth with his lips closed over it, fluid in the maxillary sinuses can be detected by the failure of the sinus to be illuminated. (This examination must be carried out in total darkness, and a normal individual should be examined at the same time for comparison. If both sinuses are involved, as often happens, an inexperienced examiner would be unable to recognize any abnormality.) The frontal sinuses can be illuminated by pressing the flashlight into the upper inner corners of the eye sockets, just below the eyebrows.

The treatment of sinusitis consists of drainage and antibiotic therapy. A decongestant nasal spray should be administered every three to four hours to reduce the swelling of the nasal mucosa and permit drainage through the canals that enter the sinuses. Spraying should be repeated ten minutes after the first application to make sure the spray reaches the recesses where the openings of these canals are located. A systemic decongestant should also be administered. In a remote area, penicillin should be given orally every six hours. Treatment should be continued until all signs of sinusitis have been absent for two days.

Acute sinusitis usually clears up within a few days. Symptoms persisting for more than seven to ten days may be indicative of a complication and should prompt serious consideration of evacuation of the patient. Swelling around the eyes or nose is a definite sign of spread of the infection. If the swelling is prominent, the patient should be evacuated immediately.

Nose Bleed

Nose bleed is commonly a result of trauma, but most nose bleeds are spontaneous with no preceding injury. Regardless of the cause, the treatment is similar. Care for this problem is discussed in Chapter Nine, "Injuries of the Head and Neck."

SORE THROAT

Sore throat is a common symptom that is produced by a number of different conditions.

Drying

Prolonged breathing through the mouth, particularly in hot, dry climates or at high altitudes where the air is relatively low in moisture, causes drying of the mouth and throat resulting in a sore throat. An irritating, dry, hacking cough is also usually present. This condition can be diagnosed by recognizing the existence of conditions causing drying of the throat and excluding the presence of other diseases characterized by sore throat. Drying of the throat is not accompanied by chills or fever or enlargement of the lymph nodes of the neck or under the jaw. The throat may be a little red and inflamed but exudates are not present.

Treatment of any kind is usually disappointing. Lozenges containing anesthetics or antibiotics are available. However, hard candy or rock sugar melted in the mouth (not chewed) is probably just as effective, is much less expensive and easier to obtain, and does not carry the dangers associated with the indiscriminate use of antibiotics. Lozenges should be taken only about every four hours, but candy can be consumed freely. Finally, the candy has nutritional value, which is important at high altitudes where loss of appetite makes the ingestion of any food a problem.

Viral Pharyngitis

In conditions other than those that produce drying of the throat, viral infections are the most common cause of sore throats. Viral pharyngitis (viral sore throat) most commonly accompanies a cold but frequently is not associated with any other disorder. The victim usually does not feel or appear seriously ill, although a few individuals do feel much worse than most others. Fever may be present but is rarely higher than 101° F (38.5°C). The throat is inflamed, but exudates are not present and enlargement of lymph nodes is rare.

Before accepting a diagnosis of viral pharyngitis, the presence of streptococcal pharyngitis must be ruled out.

Viral sore throat usually clears up in three to six days without therapy. Lozenges may provide some relief, but hard candies melted in the mouth are probably equally effective. Antibiotics are of no benefit and should be avoided unless streptococcal infection is seriously suspected. However, it may be impossible to distinguish between these two infections without laboratory facilities.

Streptococcal Pharyngitis

Streptococcal pharyngitis, or "strep throat," is encountered less frequently than other causes of sore throat but can be treated much more satisfactorily. This infection, which is caused by streptococcal bacteria, is potentially dangerous because it can lead to rheumatic fever, which may damage the heart valves, or glomerulonephritis, a serious kidney disease.

The victim of streptococcal pharyngitis typically feels and appears ill. Fever is usually present and may reach 103° F (39.5° C) or higher. Chills often occur. The throat is beefy red and exudates, which are similar to the pus found in boils or infected wounds, appear as white or pale yellow points or patches scattered over the throat, particularly on the tonsils. The lymph nodes in the neck and under the jaw usually are enlarged and tender.

Fever, exudates, enlarged lymph nodes, and general malaise serve to differentiate "strep throat" from other forms of pharyngitis. However, malaise may not be marked, lymph node enlargement may not be prominent, and fever may not be very high. Therefore, any sore throat should be regarded with suspicion. In a remote area, if a significant possibility of streptococcal infection appears to be present, antibiotic therapy should be instituted.

The therapy for streptococcal pharyngitis consists of the oral administration of penicillin every six hours for ten days. Symptoms and signs of the disease usually disappear completely within twenty-four to forty-eight hours. Nonetheless, **therapy must be continued for ten days** to ensure complete eradication of the infection and the prevention of complications, particularly rheumatic fever. Patients allergic to penicillin should be treated with erythromycin.

DISORDERS OF THE MOUTH

Toothache

Toothache is almost invariably due to an infection. The infection initially produces a cavity in a tooth, but later it can spread to the surrounding bone and soft tissue to produce an abscess. Adequate dental care should almost completely prevent abscesses. However, such infections may occur among porters or similar members of an expedition for whom dental care is not available.

The diagnosis is based on the presence of pain around the involved tooth, which may be exquisitely sensitive. Frequently a cavity is obvious. The presence of swelling in the gum and jaw indicates that the tooth has become abscessed. Often fever and occasionally chills accompany an abscess, but they rarely occur with an uncomplicated cavity.

For a simple toothache, a small wad of cotton soaked in oil of cloves and inserted in the cavity usually reduces the pain. Aspirin or aspirin and codeine every four hours also help to relieve discomfort.

The presence of an abscess is an indication that the tooth should be pulled. However, extraction by anyone other than a dentist should be attempted only in remote situations and only when dental forceps are available. The patient should be given an antibiotic such as penicillin or ampicillin intramuscularly thirty minutes prior to the extraction to help destroy the bacteria invariably released into the bloodstream during the extraction. Chills and fever are common in the twenty-four hours after the tooth is pulled. If the victim is to be evacuated to a dentist for the extraction, he should be given penicillin or ampicillin every six hours until evacuation is completed.

An analgesic may or may not be needed. Sometimes extraction of an abscessed tooth is surprisingly painless.

Canker Sores

Canker sores are small painful ulcers that appear in the mouth without apparent cause. They first appear as small blisters which soon rupture, leaving small, white ulcers surrounded by an area of inflammation. Such sores may be caused by *Herpes simplex* infection.

No therapy is effective for curing these ulcers, but they disappear in a few days without treatment. A mouthwash consisting of a teaspoon (4 cc) of sodium bicarbonate (baking soda) in a glass of water is somewhat soothing; a mouthwash of half water and half three percent hydrogen peroxide solution helps prevent secondary infection.

Herpes

Oral herpes (also known as "cold sores" or "fever blisters") is a viral infection *(Herpes simplex)* that produces small, painful blisters on the lips and skin of the face and occasionally inside the mouth. The viruses persist in the tissues, and the blisters tend to recur in the same location time after time. Herpes sores commonly result from sunburn of the lips or face but frequently can not be associated with any other disorder. Additionally, herpes sores may accompany other severe infections such as pneumonia or meningitis.

An initial small, painful swelling rapidly develops into one or more small blisters containing a clear fluid and surrounded by a thin margin of inflamed skin. The blisters may rupture, particularly if they are traumatized, resulting in bleeding and crusting. Fever or other symptoms are rarely experienced.

The application of a local anesthetic ointment (Nupercainal) may provide some symptomatic relief, but no specific treatment is available. The blisters usually heal in five to ten days, and although uncomfortable and perhaps unsightly, they usually cause no significant disability. Preventing sunburn of the lips probably helps prevent the appearance of these sores.

EAR INFECTIONS

Ear infections frequently occur in infants and young children but are uncommon in older persons. The eustachian tube which drains the middle ear is easily blocked by swelling of the mucous membrane in the throat or enlargement of the adenoids in young people. However, this tube is much larger in adults and these disorders rarely produce obstruction. In the absence of eustachian obstruction, ear infections are uncommon.

A cold, sinusitis, or hay fever usually precedes the ear infection. The principal symptom is pain in the ear. Fever or malaise may be present. Infrequently a purulent discharge from the ear can be found.

Therapy consists of the oral administration of penicillin every six hours until all signs of infection have been absent for two days. A systemic decongestant should also be given to help reduce swelling around the opening of the eustachian tube. A hot water bottle applied to the ear and aspirin or aspirin and codeine every three to four hours help reduce the pain. A warm (not hot), bland oil such as olive oil inserted into the ear also helps relieve the pain.

CHAPTER TWENTY-THREE

Infections

Infections occur whenever microorganisms invade tissues of the body and multiply or develop within them. Humans normally have living organisms in many parts of their bodies such as the skin, throat, or intestines. Most of these organisms are harmless and usually do not cause disease. However, when the body's defenses against infection are deficient, when organisms that are not harmless are present, or when an injury allows organisms to enter tissues in which they are not normally present, an infection may result.

Most common infections, such as influenza or traveller's diarrhea, are directly or indirectly transmitted from one person to another and are labelled "contagious." Others, such as urinary tract infections or appendicitis, are not contagious. Many of the contagious infections of concern to outdoorsmen are transmitted by vectors such as the mosquitoes that transmit malaria and yellow fever or the ticks that transmit Rocky Mountain spotted fever. Few infections likely to occur in the wilderness are so contagious that special isolation precautions need to be taken for individuals who have them.

A boil or abscess in the skin typifies the pain, swelling, redness, and heat produced by the inflammation accompanying localized infections. If infections remain localized within a small area such as the superficial layers of the skin, fever and other symptoms are usually not present. However, an infection may be localized but extend deeply, it may involve a major organ such as a lung, or it may disseminate throughout the body if the organisms gain access to the bloodstream. Such infections typically produce chills, fever, and malaise, which may be accompanied by headache, nausea, vomiting, or back pain.

When fever is accompanied by signs of localized infection, identification of its cause is not difficult. For example, if someone has burning pain on urination, passes small amounts of urine frequently, and has discomfort over the bladder or kidneys, a urinary infection is probably the cause of any associated chills and fever. Similarly, if pleuritic chest pain is accompanied by a cough productive of thick yellow sputum, the diagnosis is pneumonia. The infections discussed in this chapter are those that involve the skin and selected generalized infections. Infections of specific organs are discussed in the chapters dealing with those organs or systems.

ANTIBIOTICS

Although a large number of antibiotics have been developed for the treatment of infectious diseases, organisms vary greatly in their sensitivity to individual antibiotics. An antibiotic that is effective against the specific causative organism must be used for each infection. Boils and similar skin infections, for example, are commonly caused by staphylococci that may be sensitive to the penicillin group of antibiotics. Typhoid fever and bacillary dysentery are caused by bacteria that may not be sensitive to penicillin but are susceptible to sulfa drugs and chloramphenicol. Identifying the organism causing an infection so that the most appropriate antibiotic can be administered is highly desirable but is rarely possible in wilderness situations or even in mountain towns and villages of underdeveloped countries.

In order to eradicate an infection, antibiotics must be given in quantities large enough to produce concentrations in the blood and tissues that kill or inhibit the growth of infectious organisms. Hence, dose recommendations must be carefully followed. If nausea or vomiting are present, or the antibiotic being given is not effective orally, it must be administered by intramuscular injection. Intravenous administration under field conditions can be hazardous but may be necessary if very high blood concentrations of antibiotics are required, as in meningitis or to prevent osteomyelitis, for example. Once therapy with an antibiotic has been started, it should be continued long enough to kill all the organisms and until all signs and symptoms of the infection have been absent for several days. The usual period of treatment varies from five to twenty days, depending on the type of infection. Shorter courses of therapy may result in relapse of the infection.

Antibiotics should not be given prophylactically to prevent infections except under special circumstances. For example, most individuals with colds or minor wounds should not be given penicillin to prevent pneumonia or a wound infection. Available evidence indicates that the administration of antibiotics in this manner does not prevent later infection. In addition, such treatment may allow organisms not sensitive to the antibiotic to multiply and produce an infection that may be very difficult to treat.

The most frequently used antibiotics are the penicillins. The potassium salt of penicillin (Pen Vee K and others) is well absorbed from the intestines and is the usual form given orally for a wide variety of infections. If intramuscular injection of penicillin is necessary, procaine penicillin G is the preparation most commonly employed. Cloxacillin is given for staphylococcal infections that are likely to be resistant to ordinary penicillin. Ampicillin is usually effective against organisms that produce typhoid fever, other types of severe infectious diarrhea (except cholera), and urinary tract infections. Trimethoprim-sulfamethoxazole (Bactrim, Septra), a combination of two sulfonamides, is useful in treating a wide variety of infections, particularly ampicillin resistant typhoid fever and bacillary dysentery.

Some individuals are allergic to the penicillins and may have severe, even fatal, reactions to either oral or intramuscular penicillin. Before anyone receives any of the penicillins, they must be carefully questioned about previous allergic reactions. If a patient has a history even suggestive of penicillin allergy, another totally different antibiotic effective against the infecting organism must be substituted. Allergies to other antibiotics and to sulfa drugs also occur.

BACTERIAL INFECTIONS

Infections of the respiratory tract and skin are the most common of all bacterial infections. Most of these disorders are relatively innocuous if treated properly. If mistreated, a disastrous, widespread infection can result.

Abscesses

Abscesses, boils, carbuncles, and pimples are localized skin infections that differ only in size. They are almost all caused by staphylococci, which frequently are resistant to penicillin. These organisms release enzymes that cause clotting and obstruction of the blood vessels and lymphatics surrounding the site of the infection. The vascular obstruction blocks the spread of the bacteria and the infections usually remain localized, but the vascular obstruction also shuts out white blood cells, antibiotics, antibodies, and other protective substances in the blood. Other enzymes released by these bacteria destroy the tissues in the area of infection, producing a cavity that is filled with the mixture of bacteria, white blood cells, and liquefied, dead tissue commonly known as "pus."

The treatment for such disorders consists primarily of drainage and is similar to the treatment for infected wounds. However, pimples and small abscesses do not need to be surgically opened. They should be covered with a Band-Aid or similar small dressing until they rupture and drain spontaneously. Squeezing pimples forces the bacteria into the surrounding tissues, tends to spread the infection, and is a common practice from which everyone should abstain. A particularly dangerous area for such infections is the face around the nose and below the eyes. Squeezing a pimple in this region may force bacteria into veins and lymphatics, which carry them directly to the brain.

Larger abscesses may have to be incised in order to drain. The abscess should be covered with hot, wet, sterile compresses until a white or pale area appears in the center, indicating the pus has extended beneath the skin, or "pointed." After the surrounding and overlying skin has been cleaned with a preparation such as povidone-iodine (Betadine), alcohol, or clean water and soap, a small incision should be made through this area with a sterile scalpel or razor blade. (A local anesthetic may be necessary.) When the abscess has drained, it should be gently probed with sterile forceps to make certain no pockets of infection remain. Then the skin should be cleansed again, and a small piece of vaseline impregnated gauze should be inserted into the opening so it can not seal off. Finally, the entire area should be covered with sterile dressings.

Antibiotics are not only unnecessary but are undesirable and usually ineffective for treating a small, uncomplicated abscess. However, if the abscess is larger than one inch (2.5 cm) in diameter, or if fever, chills, or other symptoms indicate the bacteria have invaded the blood stream or have produced a secondary infection at another location, cloxacillin should be given every six hours until all evidence of infection has been absent for two days. Cloxacillin is preferable to penicillin to which many staphylococci (which cause most skin infections) are resistant. If prompt improvement does not take place, the patient must be evacuated immediately.

Similar antibiotic therapy should be instituted, even if signs of bloodstream or secondary infection are not present, if the patient has multiple abscesses or if the person is a diabetic, since such persons are prone to develop severe infections.

Cellulitis

Cellulitis is a bacterial infection of the skin and underlying tissues that is produced by organisms that do not cause obstruction of blood vessels. Such infections do not tend to remain localized and the bacteria can spread to other areas more easily. The site of the infection is usually red, swollen, hot, and tender and is usually not sharply demarcated from the surrounding tissues. Fever is usually present.

Since the blood vessels remain open, these infections can be successfully treated with antibiotics. Cloxacillin should be administered every six hours until all signs of infection have been absent for two days. For periods of thirty minutes every three or four hours, the infected area should be covered with a hot, wet cloth or compress, which should be replaced when it cools. The heat causes the blood vessels in the area to dilate, which increases the quantity of antibiotics and similar substances to which the bacteria are exposed. Incision and drainage are of no benefit because the infection is not localized. The patient should rest quietly until the infection has cleared. Due to its propensity to spread, cellulitis is a more dangerous infection than an abscess and its potential for complications must be respected.

Bacteremia and Septicemia

Bacteremia and septicemia are similar conditions characterized by the presence of bacteria in the blood stream. The organisms may multiply in the blood and produce infections throughout the body. Bacteremia is usually preceded by a localized infection such as an infected wound, a urinary tract infection, or an abscess.

Bacterial blood stream invasion produces chills, high fever, sweating, and prostration. Signs may suggest spread of the infection to other parts of the body.

Severe headache, a stiff neck, and nausea and vomiting may indicate involvement of the brain or its covering (meningitis). Cough, shortness of breath, and pain with breathing are suggestive of pneumonia.

Prompt administration of antibiotics may be lifesaving. Nafcillin every six hours and gentamicin every eight hours is a good, broad coverage antibiotic combination. Patients allergic to penicillin should receive cefazolin (Kefzol), 500 mg intramuscularly every six hours, instead of nafcillin. If only penicillin G is available, 20 million units a day should be given intravenously. Patients who do not respond to treatment within three to four days should be evacuated, since complications may occur in spite of antibiotic therapy.

Patients with bacteremia or septicemia should be provided with rest, warmth, a soft or liquid diet, and adequate fluids. Medications for pain and sleep are often helpful; aspirin or acetaminophen may be given to reduce fever. A temperature record must be kept and should include the times any drugs are administered.

OTHER INFECTIONS

Influenza

Influenza, a viral infection caused by influenza viruses A or B, is an acute, self-limited disease of five to six days duration. Although the infection is limited to the respiratory tract, the symptoms may suggest a generalized disease. Spread occurs by sneezing, coughing, or close contact with an infected person. Epidemics are common, particularly in winter months.

The incubation period is one or two days. The onset is heralded by chilliness, fever, weakness, lassitude, headache, loss of appetite, and characteristic aching muscle pains. A dry, hacking cough is prominent and may be severe. Other respiratory tract symptoms are sometimes present but are usually not prominent. Fever usually lasts two to three days and occasionally reaches 104° F (40° C). The pulse rate may be quite rapid.

The signs and symptoms of upper respiratory tract involvement usually differentiate influenza from other systemic infections; the fever, muscle aches, and cough distinguish it from a common cold. A history of contact with other persons with influenza is helpful in making a diagnosis. Gastrointestinal symptoms are usually absent, but diarrhea may occur.

No specific treatment is available. Symptoms are partially relieved by rest, warmth, a light diet with abundant juices and other liquids, and medications such as aspirin every four hours to relieve discomfort. Medication to promote sleep may be helpful.

Antibiotics are not part of the treatment of influenza. However, if fever returns after several days and a cough productive of purulent sputum appears, a pneumococcal or secondary staphylococcal pneumonia may have developed and should be treated with nafcillin every six hours by intramuscular injection.

Infectious Mononucleosis

Infectious mononucleosis is a common viral infection of young adults which appears to be contracted through close personal contact. This disease is rarely severe, although sometimes it is incapacitating, and complications that can be fatal do occur.

The most common symptom of infectious mononucleosis is a persistent sore throat, which is present in eighty-five percent of all patients. Other complaints are not specific: most common are a feeling of tiredness, loss of energy, or easy fatigability. Lymph nodes in various portions of the body are usually enlarged. The nodes in the sides and back of the neck are most often involved. Fever is also present but varies widely from person to person.

The triad of sore throat, lymph node enlargement, and fever is characteristic of infectious mononucleosis, but this disease is notorious for its great variability. A skin rash, headache, weakness, loss of appetite, and generalized aching may also be present. Jaundice sometimes occurs (six percent of patients) and indicates the liver is involved.

No specific treatment is available; antibiotics are of no avail. Rest is important, and the patient's activity should be limited while any symptoms of disease persist. **Climbing must be avoided.** Minor abdominal trauma could easily rupture the spleen, which is enlarged and unusually susceptible to trauma in infectious mononucleosis. Recovery in most cases takes two to four weeks. If jaundice is present the patient should be evacuated.

Rocky Mountain Spotted Fever

Rocky Mountain spotted fever is caused by a bacterium, *Rickettsia rickettsii*, which is transmitted to man by the bite of a wood or dog tick. Three to fourteen days after the bite, mild chilliness, loss of appetite, and a general run-down feeling usually appear. These mild symptoms are followed by chills, fever, headache, pain in the bones and muscles, sensitivity of the eyes to light, and confusion. Between two and six days after the onset of symptoms, a red rash appears on the wrists and ankles and spreads over the entire body. The rash may be present on the palms of the hands and the soles of the feet and consists of small red spots. These spots are actually hemorrhages into the skin and in severe cases large blotchy red areas may appear all over the body. The fever lasts about two weeks. The patient appears seriously ill without an obvious cause. Untreated, the mortality rate is twenty to thirty percent; treatment reduces the rate to three to ten percent.

Diagnosis is aided by a history of a tick bite in an endemic area. The most important endemic area is the middle Atlantic coastal states; fewer cases are seen west of the Mississippi, but the disease can occur in any of the forty-eight contiguous states.

Tetracycline or chloramphenicol should be given every six hours until the temperature has been normal for two to three days. General measures such as bed rest, fluid replacement, aspirin every four hours if needed for high fever, and medication for sleep are also important.

Rocky Mountain spotted fever can be prevented by careful daily inspection for ticks when in an endemic area. The ticks should be touched with a gasoline or kerosene soaked cotton pledget to make them detach, and carefully extracted with tweezers so they are not crushed. The wound should be cleansed carefully. Individuals moving about in brush in an endemic area should keep their shirt sleeves rolled down with the cuffs buttoned. Shirt collars should also be buttoned, heads should be covered, and long trousers should be closed by gaiters or tucked into boot tops. No reliable vaccine is available for prevention of the disease.

Colorado Tick Fever

Colorado tick fever is a viral disease transmitted by the wood tick. It occurs in all western states and is far more common than Rocky Mountain spotted fever. Infections usually occur in spring and early summer when ticks are active. Four to six days after exposure, chills and fever appear, along with headache and generalized aching. The eyes may be unusually sensitive to light. The initial attack lasts about two days, at which time the fever and other symptoms disappear, only to recur two to five days later. The outlook for complete recovery is good, even though no specific treatment is available. Bed rest, fluids, and aspirin are helpful. A physician should evaluate the patient to be sure that Rocky Mountain spotted fever is not present, since that is a more serious disorder, but one that can be effectively treated with antibiotics. Precautions against tick bites help prevent infection.

Relapsing Fever (Tick Fever)

Tick fever occurs in western and west central states. It is a blood stream infection by a spiral bacterium transmitted to man by a tick bite or, in some areas, by a louse. The ticks live on rodents and small animals such as chipmunks, squirrels, and rabbits. About two to fifteen days after the bite, chills, fever, headache, muscle aches and pains, joint pains, a cough, and often nausea and vomiting appear. A red rash may appear on the body and limbs. Bleeding from the nose, lungs, or gastrointestinal tract may occur but usually is not severe. The initial attack lasts two to eight days and may be followed by a remission lasting three to ten days. During the remission, fever is absent and the patient may feel well. A relapse in which the fever and all previous symptoms return usually occurs seven to ten days later in untreated patients. Hospitalization for identification of the organism in the blood is desirable. Tetracycline or chloramphenicol should be given every six hours for five to ten days.

Yellow Fever

Yellow fever is an infection of man and monkeys caused by a virus transmitted by the *Aedes* mosquito. It is chiefly found in South America and in Africa below the Sahara. Following an incubation period of three to six days, the illness begins with chills, fever, headache, and backache. The heart rate may be slow in relation to the severity of the fever. After three days the fever often falls temporarily, at which time the patient is flushed, nauseated, often vomiting, and may appear seriously ill. The eyes may be bloodshot and the tongue appears red. Bleeding from the gums and under the skin may occur; vomiting "coffee ground" material or black stools may indicate bleeding in the stomach or intestines. Slight jaundice may be present. Mild cases may resemble influenza or malaria. Jaundice, however, does not occur in influenza and only rarely in malaria. When present, it is an important sign of yellow fever and is responsible for this infection's name.

The treatment of yellow fever consists of bed rest and a liquid or soft diet high in carbohydrates. Fluid and salt replacement may be necessary for vomiting, diarrhea, or high fever. Aspirin every four hours for discomfort and bedtime medications for sleep are helpful. No specific treatment is available. If travel into a yellow fever area is planned, vaccination must be obtained (See Chapter Five, "Preventive Measures.")

Malaria

Malaria is caused by protozoa of the genus *Plasmodium* and is transmitted by the bite of infected mosquitoes. When considered on a worldwide basis, malaria is one of the most common of all diseases.

Malarial parasites are ingested along with the blood of an infected person or animal at the time of biting by female *Anopheles* mosquitoes. The parasites undergo fertilization and produce sporozoites in the gut of the mosquito. The sporozoites are transmitted to humans as the mosquito injects saliva into the skin during a subsequent bite. Sporozoites invade red blood cells and multiply, producing daughter parasites. These daughter parasites are released, destroying the red blood cells in the process, and invade other red blood cells where the process is repeated. The periodic release of parasites produces fever; the destruction of red blood cells can, over a period of time, result in anemia.

The initial symptoms of malaria are muscular soreness and a low fever (without chills), which appear about six to ten days after the bite of an infected mosquito. Four to eight days later, the typical chills and fever appear. The chills are characterized by shivering, chattering teeth, blue and cold skin, and a feeling of chilliness which is not relieved by heating pads or blankets. An hour later the febrile stage begins with a flushed face, a feeling of intense heat, headache, often delirium, and temperature as high as 107° F (41.5° C). This stage lasts about two hours and is followed by intense sweating and a fall in temperature. Headache, backache, and muscular aches may be unusually severe.

The repeated occurrence of febrile episodes at regular intervals such as every day, every other day, every three days, or occasionally at irregular intervals, is characteristic of malaria. In severe cases vomiting, diarrhea, severe anemia, dark urine containing elements of destroyed red blood cells, shock, and coma may occur. Enlargement of the liver or spleen may be present.

Treatment should consist of general supportive measures and specific drug therapy. Rest in bed and maintenance of body warmth during the chill is highly desirable. Since water loss due to sweating may be severe, a large fluid intake should be encouraged. Fluids and salt lost by vomiting or diarrhea also must be replaced. A careful record of temperature and pulse should be kept. If possible, blood smears should be made a few hours after the chill for later identification of the parasites.

During an acute episode of malaria, the subsequent period of therapy, and for two weeks following recovery, strenuous exercise should be avoided to prevent rupture of the spleen.

Specific treatment for malaria should be given by a physician. The most effective general regimen consists of chloroquine and primaquine. One-half gram of chloroquine should be given initially and should be followed by a second one-half gram in six hours and one-half gram on the second and third days. Fifteen milligrams of primaquine should be given each day for fourteen days.

Plasmodium falciparum malaria is the most dangerous form, and several strains have been found in South America, southeast Asia, and eastern Africa that are resistant to most antimalarial drugs. (Future discovery of similar strains in additional areas appears highly likely.) Expeditions into such areas should carry quinine, pyrimethamine, and sulfonamides to treat chloroquine resistant falciparum malaria. However, a physician's advice should be obtained before using these drugs.

Chloroquine prophylaxis is an effective means for preventing malaria caused by strains that are not resistant to this drug. One-half gram of chloroquine should be taken on the same day of each week, beginning two weeks before entering the endemic area and continuing for five weeks after leaving. In addition, any illness occurring within five weeks after leaving a malarial area should be reported to a physician because malaria may first appear long after exposure.

If travel is anticipated into areas where chloroquine resistant malaria is present, Fansidar, a combination of sulfadoxine and pyrimethamine, should be taken on the same schedule.

Advance information regarding the presence of malaria in areas that are to be visited should be obtained. In cities and towns that are frequently visited by tourists malaria is uncommon, and malaria carrying mosquitoes are rarely found at elevations above 3,000 feet (900 m). In malarial areas, contact with mosquitoes should be minimized with screens or mosquito netting, protective clothing, and insect repellents. The best available repellent at present is N,N-diethyltoluamide, which remains effective for up to eighteen hours, a considerable advantage over the odor repellents, which are effective for only two to four hours. It may be easier to avoid malarial areas than to take chloroquine for five weeks, as this drug does occasionally cause itching and gastrointestinal complaints.

Trichinosis

Trichinosis is a parasitic disease caused by eating raw, improperly cooked, or improperly treated pork containing larvae of the roundworm *Trichinella spiralis*. After the larvae are ingested they attach themselves to the wall of the small bowel, mature, and produce eggs. The larvae released when these eggs hatch are spread throughout the body by the circulation and localize in the muscles.

The severity of symptoms depends upon the number of organisms in the ingested pork. If infestation is heavy, penetration of the intestinal wall by the larvae one to four days after ingestion produces nausea, vomiting, abdominal cramps, and diarrhea that resembles food poisoning. The migration of the larvae to the muscles seven days after ingestion produces fever, chills, muscular weakness, a skin rash, and swelling of the face and tissues around the eyes. Headache may be severe.

The diagnosis is based upon the onset of symptoms following the ingestion of raw or uncooked pork or improperly prepared pork products such as salami. Muscle soreness and swelling of the face are also important diagnostic findings. A differential white blood count may reveal the presence of a large number of eosinophils. A skin test is also available. No specific treatment for trichinosis has been of proven value except thiabendazole, which should be given by a physician. Symptomatic treatment consists of rest, aspirin and codeine, and sedatives to promote restful sleep. Prednisone may be beneficial in the early stages of the disease. Since trichinae are present in essentially all pork products, prevention of infection is imperative. All pork must be thoroughly cooked. In addition, freezing at 0° F (-18° C) for twenty-four hours or 5° F (-15° C) for twenty days usually kills all trichinae.

CHAPTER TWENTY-FOUR

Allergies

When foreign substances enter the body, the immune system responds by forming "antibodies," which combine with the foreign materials to facilitate their elimination by the body's defense mechanisms. When the foreign substances (antigens) are bacteria or viruses, antibodies play a large role in preventing or eradicating infection. Other foreign antigens also elicit an antibody response.

Once a person has contacted an antigen, antibodies persist in his blood for years or even his lifetime. These persistent antibodies provide permanent immunity following infections such as measles or mumps. Vaccines are composed of dead or weakened organisms which elicit an antibody response without producing a full blown infection, resulting in immunity. However, many vaccines do not elicit the full antibody response an actual infection does and must be repeated every few years.

Antibodies are proteins known as immunoglobulins. Various types of immunoglobulins are classified as G, M, A, E, and D and are usually abbreviated IgG, IgM, and so on. Occasionally a person reacts to an antigen by forming an excessive amount of antibody, particularly IgE, the principal antibody responsible for allergic reactions. Further contact with that antigen — or allergen, as antigens that produce allergic reactions are called — results in a strong IgE response, which causes the release of histamine and related substances that produce the allergic reaction.

The periodic injection of gradually increasing amounts of an allergen can sometimes overwhelm the antibody response. This process, known as desensitization, eliminates or greatly reduces the allergic reaction. If desensitization is stopped, the original allergic condition usually returns. Nonetheless, desensitization can be quite useful in helping to control allergic reactions such as hypersensitivity to insect stings.

The substances to which an individual may become allergic are unlimited. Foods, pollens, animal dander, and dust are the most frequent offenders. Reactions to therapeutic agents are also common. Insect stings and penicillin are notorious for causing anaphylactic reactions, an uncommon type of allergic reaction which is explosive in onset and often lethal.

HAY FEVER

Hay fever, or acute nasal allergy, is usually caused by pollens, dust, or other allergens in the air. Hay fever is rare in an ice and snow world but is a common problem — occasionally a severe problem — at lower altitudes. The nasal membranes are red and swollen, causing nasal stuffiness and nasal discharge. The eyes are often red; watering of the eyes is common.

An individual with recurrent hay fever that is so severe it handicaps his activities should consider desensitization. He should work out with his physician or allergist the medications that are most effective for him personally. Effective treatment for hay fever usually combines an antihistamine with a decongestant. However, some drugs and drug combinations are more effective for certain individuals than others. Actifed is a combination of an antihistamine with a decongestant that is widely used to help control nasal allergies and the stuffiness of colds. This preparation has recently become available without a physician's prescription. A four percent solution of cromalyn sodium sprayed into the nose has been found effective for preventing the nasal symptoms of hay fever but has little effect on eye symptoms.

HIVES

Hives are often caused by food allergies — chocolate, seafood, and fresh fruit being the most common offenders — but can occur as an allergic reaction to almost any substance, including dusts and pollen, insect bites and stings, or drugs, occasionally even to drugs as commonly used as aspirin. Hives appear quickly following contact with the allergen, are often widely scattered, and consist of red or white raised wheals (or "bumps") which itch intensely. Hives may rapidly appear and disappear several times from a single allergen exposure. Repeated exposures to the same allergen usually reproduce the attacks indefinitely. However, the condition is more miserable than serious.

The treatment for recurrent episodes of hives consists of antihistamines. Those used for motion sickness are usually effective. Cornstarch packs or baths, or bland lotions may help reduce itching. Spontaneous recovery occurs without treatment if further exposure to the allergen is avoided.

CONTACT DERMATITIS

A rash occasionally develops following contact with jewelry, the case of a wrist watch, or a similar material. Often the cause can not be determined, and the rash may not be located at the point of contact. The rash is usually more annoying than disabling, typically is composed of multiple small blisters on a red background, and may itch or burn. Severe cases should be treated like poison ivy dermatitis.

POISON IVY

Poison ivy, poison oak, and poison sumac produce an acute contact dermatitis due to allergy to urushiol, a component of the sap of these three plants. The rash typically develops at the point of contact with the plants but may appear at sites that are far removed. After only a few days the rash usually appears on the skin of the hands and face, but as long as a week may be required for it to appear at other locations. The rash usually disappears in the same order it appeared after four to seven days.

Red streaks or patches that itch appear first. Later, blisters develop and then break down, resulting in oozing and crusting from the surface. Usually swelling of the underlying tissues, burning, and itching are present. Scratching should be avoided because it can introduce infection or cause scarring, but scratching does not spread the rash. The blisters are filled with serum, not the urushiol that causes the dermatitis.

Treatment depends upon the extent of the rash. If the area covered is small, no therapy at all may be needed. Calamine lotion may relieve itching. For more extensive eruptions, itching may be relieved by cool salt water compresses (two teaspoons [8 cc or 8 gm] of salt per quart of water) applied for ten minutes four times a day. A steroid ointment such as 0.25 percent hydrocortisone (now available over the counter) can be applied in limited amounts after the compresses.

Patients with extensive, disabling poison ivy dermatitis require systemic steroid therapy. In urban surroundings such patients have been defined as those sick enough to seek a physician's care. The physician should prescribe the medication.

Desensitization for poison ivy with an injectable preparation is available, and efforts to develop an oral desensitizing agent are continuing. At the present time, however, the side effects from both preparations are just about as bad or worse than the disease.

Many over-the-counter preparations for the treatment of poison ivy dermatitis contain antihistamines, analgesics, or even antibiotics, which can produce a secondary allergic reaction that may be worse than the original problem.

ANAPHYLACTIC SHOCK

Anaphylactic shock is an acute, massive allergic reaction that involves essentially the entire body. Fortunately, such reactions are uncommon, for death can occur within five to ten minutes if treatment is not administered immediately. (Deaths due to anaphylactic reactions undoubtedly still go unrecognized, being attributed to heart attacks or some similar disorder, and may be significantly more common than appreciated.)

Insect stings are one of the more common causes of anaphylactic shock. In the United States, deaths due to allergic reactions to insect stings far outnumber those caused by all other venomous animals, including poisonous snakes, spiders, and scorpions. (See Chapter Fifteen, "Animal Bites and Stings.")

Drugs are another prominent cause of anaphylactic shock. The most common offenders are penicillin and foreign serum such as horse serum. The danger of anaphylactic shock demands that these medications be given to patients who may be allergic to them only if absolutely essential (such as a severely envenomated snake bite victim), and even then only in a hospital where allergic reactions can be controlled. Anaphylactic reactions are most common after drugs have been injected but have been caused by orally administered medications. Very rarely, anaphylactic reactions have been caused by food to which the individual was allergic.

Diagnosis

The symptoms of anaphylactic shock usually appear five to fifteen minutes after exposure to the allergen. Occasionally an hour may pass before symptoms appear, and very rarely twenty-four hours can elapse, particularly after oral ingestion of the offending substance.

Organ systems involved by the reaction include:

1. Respiratory:	Laryngeal edema;
	Bronchospasm;
	Rhinitis.
2. Skin:	Hives;
	Angioedema.
3. Gastrointestinal:	Nausea;
	Vomiting;
	Cramps;
	Diarrhea.
4. Eyes:	Conjunctivitis.
5. Cardiovascular:	Arrhythmia;
	Shock.

The most prominent feature of anaphylactic shock is respiratory distress, which usually is unmistakable. Laryngeal edema is characterized by swelling of the tissues of the upper air passages, particularly the larynx, where the airway is already narrowed by the vocal chords. The swelling further narrows the air passages and can produce lethal respiratory obstruction. Bronchospasm produces symptoms that are similar to the respiratory difficulty that occurs with asthma but that often are much more severe. The cause, spasm of the muscles in the smaller bronchi resulting in severe constriction of the air passages, is also similar. With anaphylaxis the onset is much more abrupt, usually developing within minutes. Sometimes a sense of pressure beneath the sternum is noted.

The skin is the next most common organ involved by anaphylaxis. Hives may be present and are widely distributed. Angioedema consists of a localized swelling, which may occur on an extremity or around the eyes or mouth.

Nausea, vomiting, abdominal pain, and diarrhea may reflect involvement of the gastrointestinal system. Involvement of the eyes and nose causes changes that resemble a sudden, severe attack of hay fever. The eyes are swollen and red and the flow of tears is greatly increased. The nose is plugged by a red, swollen mucosa and mucoid discharge. Rarely, involvement of the cardiovascular system can result in shock or a cardiac arrhythmia, which can be fatal.

Treatment

Anaphylactic shock is a true medical emergency in which minutes may make a difference between therapeutic success and failure. Treatment must be instituted without delay and consists of the injection of 0.3 cc of a 1:1,000 aqueous solution of epinephrine (adrenaline). The route of administration is determined by the patient's condition. If the reaction is caught early when it is rather mild and only moderate respiratory distress is present, the adrenaline should be injected subcutaneously. If the patient is in severe respiratory difficulty, the epinephrine should be injected intramuscularly where it is absorbed more rapidly.

Injections of epinephrine can be repeated every fifteen minutes if needed. In fact, patients must be closely watched because many individuals relapse in fifteen to twenty minutes as the epinephrine wears off.

Respiratory obstruction due to laryngeal edema usually responds to epinephrine but may require tracheostomy.

Other steps can help a patient with anaphylaxis, but none can substitute for epinephrine. If the allergen has been injected, placing tourniquets above the injection site and injecting epinephrine around the site helps slow absorption. Oxygen should be administered during the period of respiratory difficulty regardless of the altitude. Other forms of treatment for shock should be instituted; appropriate care should be given if the patient is unconscious. Antihistamines may help control the itching of hives or other symptoms, but should be administered only after anaphylaxis has been controlled.

Prevention of anaphylactic shock by avoiding the allergen or by desensitization is far safer than treatment. Desensitization for insect sting allergy with purified venoms is effective. However, even after desensitization, individuals subject to anaphylactic shock from insect stings or similar uncontrollable allergens should always carry an "insect sting kit" so that the necessary medications for treatment are available. Effective desensitization for allergies to drugs such as penicillin is not practical.

Section Five: Appendixes

APPENDIX A

Medications

The dosages for most of the medications recommended in this text are provided only in this appendix. By this means, anyone administering these agents can be informed of the precautions that must be observed without undue repetition in the text.

The doses that are listed are those that can be safely administered to a young or middle aged adult in good health. The doses for children or elderly individuals for some drugs are quite different. The doses for individuals with liver or kidney disease are also quite different. Administration of the stated doses of these drugs to such persons could have deleterious, possibly even lethal effects. For some medications a range of doses has been given, indicating the dose should be adjusted for the patient's weight or for the severity of his disease.

Most medications have been listed by their generic names, sometimes with proprietary or "trade" names in parentheses. Generic names may be relatively unfamiliar but should cause fewer problems than proprietary names. Generic names are known by most physicians through whom most of these drugs must be obtained. To a considerable extent the same or similar generic names are used in countries other than the United States, although some generic names are totally different, even in other English speaking nations.

MEDICATIONS FOR THE RELIEF OF PAIN

The major hazards of administering strong pain relieving drugs are side effects such as respiratory or cerebral depression. Addiction is not a major hazard, possibly not even a significant hazard, for individuals receiving narcotics for legitimate reasons. Almost everyone who undergoes major surgery — thousands of people every day — receives narcotics postoperatively to control pain. Subsequent addiction is vanishingly rare. Many of the drugs effective for the relief of severe pain also have a euphoric effect, which is clearly beneficial for the victim of a major accident or illness. Addiction results when these drugs are taken for euphoria alone.

These agents are legally classified as "controlled substances" in the United States, and their distribution is regulated by a nonmedical governmental agency. They are usually difficult to obtain for anyone who is not an appropriately licensed physician. Problems with the regulatory agency can be lessened by precise records which detail the total amount of narcotics on hand, the location where they are stored, their security in that location, persons authorized to remove the agents from storage, the time and reason for obtaining the drugs, the individuals treated, and the time, place, quantity, and reason for administering the drugs.

To minimize the risk of addiction, the following precautions should be observed:

1. Narcotics should never be administered except when clearly needed for the relief of pain (or the few other conditions for which some are effective, such as the treatment of the pulmonary edema of heart failure with morphine).
2. A less potent analgesic should be substituted for a stronger agent such as morphine or meperidine as soon as pain has diminished to a level at which the weaker drugs can provide relief.
3. If therapy with one of the stronger narcotics must be continued for more than seven days, a switch from one of the opiates (morphine and others) to meperidine or vice versa may help prevent addiction.
4. Narcotic administration should not be continued for more than twelve to fourteen days except under extraordinary circumstances.

If a potent analgesic is needed, one should be used, and should be given in adequate quantities to relieve pain. A person with severe pain desperately needs the rest and relief that these drugs alone can provide. Halfway measures such as inadequate doses or inadequate drugs do not suffice.

Aspirin

Aspirin is a minor analgesic which is as effective for the relief of minor pain as any available drug except those classified as narcotics. No other minor analgesics are as effective except acetaminophen and, for some purposes, ibuprofen. Aspirin is often not as highly regarded as it should be because it is so familiar.

All aspirin is the same, and all brands sold in the United States are identical in quality and effectiveness even though the prices differ as much as 1,000 percent. The addition of buffering agents or antacids does not increase analgesic potency but may reduce the gastric irritation that aspirin not uncommonly produces. Combination with other compounds offers no significant benefits.

An apparently unrelated action of aspirin is its ability to reduce fever, which is a major reason it can provide symptomatic relief for colds and respiratory infections. More significantly, aspirin is valuable for the reduction of high fevers which threaten brain damage.

PRECAUTIONS

Aspirin is poisonous when taken in large quantities. In the United States it is by far the most common cause of poisoning in children. Aspirin, particularly flavored "children's" aspirin, must be inaccessible to children, like all medications.

Aspirin does cause stomach irritation and should not be used by persons with peptic ulcers or related disorders. Probably it should not be used by individuals with severe indigestion.

Aspirin should not be used in circumstances in which it might mask a fever which could be the first indication of an infection. (Codeine is probably the best substitute in this situation.)

Rare individuals are allergic to aspirin, or react adversely in some other way, and should not receive this drug.

DOSE

Two tablets — 600 mg or 10 grains — orally every four hours.

Acetaminophen

Acetaminophen (Tylenol, Datril, and others) is a minor analgesic just as effective as aspirin for relieving minor pain and for reducing fever. However, acetaminophen has less tendency to cause stomach irritation. It is somewhat more expensive but is not a costly drug.

PRECAUTIONS

Acetaminophen in large quantities (10 to 15 gm) produces severe liver damage. (At one time this drug was the medication most commonly used for suicide in Great Britain. Unless treatment for an overdose is obtained within a few hours after the drug has been ingested, it is ineffective.) This medication should be used with caution for individuals known to have liver disease. Many over-the-counter preparations for treating colds or sinus problems include acetaminophen, but this information is contained only in the list of contents, which is usually in very small print.

DOSE

One or two tablets — 325 to 650 mg — three to four times a day.

Ibuprofen

Ibuprofen (Motrin, Rufen, and others) is a nonsteroidal antiinflammatory agent and prostaglandin antagonist which has recently been approved for over-the-counter sale as a minor analgesic. Its analgesic properties are no greater than aspirin or acetaminophen and ibuprofen is not usually used as a substitute for those drugs. Its greatest value has been for treating dysmenorrhea (painful menstrual cramps) because its antagonism to prostaglandins tends to make the uterine muscle relax. (The antiinflammatory effects make this drug useful for treating arthritis, but that is not an acute disorder that requires care in mountaineering circumstances.)

PRECAUTIONS

Ibuprofen is a gastric irritant just like aspirin, although some patients who can not tolerate aspirin have no problems with ibuprofen. It should not be taken by persons with a history of peptic ulcer or severe indigestion. Individuals receiving this drug must be aware of its potential to produce gastric and upper intestinal ulceration and bleeding and must be alert for signs or symptoms of those disorders.

Ibuprofen also has a tendency to cause fluid retention. Whether it would aggravate symptoms of acute mountain sickness or high altitude pulmonary edema has probably not been studied, but it should be used with caution in circumstances in which those disorders could appear.

DOSE

For dysmenorrhea — 400 to 600 mg every four hours. (Tablets may contain 200, 300, 400, or 600 mg each; most tablets sold over the counter are 200 mg.)

Codeine

Codeine is an opium derivative which can provide analgesia for pain that can not be relieved by aspirin alone but that does not require a stronger drug such as morphine or meperidine. Codeine is also a useful substitute for aspirin when masking a fever might delay recognition of an infection.

The analgesic effect of codeine alone is no stronger than aspirin. However, the analgesia produced by combining the two is almost twice that produced by either when given alone. Therefore, aspirin should be administered along with codeine except in those circumstances where codeine is being substituted for aspirin.

Codeine is legally classified as a narcotic in the United States, but not in many other countries. Codeine has very little of the euphoric effect of other narcotics, and true physical addiction is quite rare.

PRECAUTIONS

Symptoms of indigestion or heartburn occur fairly frequently in individuals who frequently have such symptoms with other drugs, alcohol, or spicy foods. Some individuals experience nausea and a small number may vomit. Constipation fairly commonly follows codeine administration.

Codeine, as do all of the opium derivatives, causes spasm of the muscles controlling outflow from the biliary system (sphincter of Oddi) and should be used sparingly for patients with liver disease, gallstones, acute cholecystitis, or acute or chronic pancreatitis.

DOSE

32 to 64 mg (1/2 to 1 grain) orally, usually in combination with 600 mg of aspirin.

Morphine

Morphine, an opium derivative, is a potent analgesic that has been so widely used for so long and is so effective for the relief of severe pain that it has been called "God's own medicine." It is one of the oldest and most valuable agents in the armamentarium of a physician.

In addition to its analgesic properties, morphine has a strong sedative effect that helps calm an injured patient and limit his thrashing about, which could aggravate his wounds or hinder evacuation. This sedation and morphine's euphoric effect also help relieve the anxiety many injured persons experience following an accident.

PRECAUTIONS

Morphine, like all sedatives, depresses brain function. Therefore, morphine must never be given to a patient with a central nervous system injury or disease, even a mild disorder. Morphine would usually act synergistically with the disorder to further impair cerebral function. Additionally, after the administration of morphine or a similar drug, determining whether subsequent changes in the patient's condition were the result of progression of his disorder or the effects of the drug would be quite difficult. A patient with a severe brain disorder would be unconscious and would not require analgesia.

Since the brain controls respiration, morphine also depresses respiratory function. It must be used quite cautiously for patients with chest injuries or pulmonary diseases, particularly at higher altitudes. However, relieving the pain of a severe chest injury may allow a patient to cough and breathe more deeply (in the absence of an accompanying brain disorder).

Morphine causes nausea and vomiting in some individuals; it is constipating for almost everyone and can contribute to the development of fecal impaction. This drug may cause spasm of the muscles controlling outflow from the urinary bladder, resulting in urinary retention requiring urethral catheterization, particularly following abdominal injuries. Like codeine, morphine causes spasm of the muscle controlling biliary outflow and should be used with caution for patients with liver, gallbladder, or pancreatic diseases. Meperidine produces such spasm much less frequently and should be used when these patients need a potent analgesic.

Morphine is addicting, should be used only when specifically needed for the relief of severe pain, and should be discontinued when less potent drugs can provide adequate analgesia.

DOSE

For individuals weighing 150 pounds (70 kg) or more, 16 mg (1/4 grain) intramuscularly, 12 to 16 mg intravenously, or 20 mg (1/3 grain) orally every four hours.

For individuals weighing less than 150 pounds (70 kg), 12 mg (3/16 grain) intramuscularly, 9 to 12 mg intravenously, or 15 mg (1/4 grain) orally every four hours.

Oral administration is as effective as intramuscular injection but absorption is slower and thirty to sixty minutes are required for the drug to take effect. Following intramuscular injection, analgesia can be expected after ten to fifteen minutes, and the onset following intravenous injection is almost immediate. The intravenous route of administration should be used for patients in shock, preferably by individuals with previous experience with intravenous drug administration. The drug must be injected slowly over a period of several minutes, and the injection should be stopped if pain relief is achieved before the full dose is administered.

Meperidine

Meperidine (Demerol) is a synthetic analgesic first introduced in 1938. It is not an opium derivative, as are codeine and morphine. The analgesia provided by meperidine is equal to that of morphine, but meperidine does not have as much sedative and euphoric effect and the overall relief from severe pain may not be as satisfactory as that obtainable with morphine. For individuals with less severe injuries, the absence of sedation and euphoria may be desirable.

PRECAUTIONS

Meperidine was developed as a potent analgesic because it was thought to have fewer side effects than morphine. However, meperidine definitely depresses cerebral function, must not be given to patients with central nervous system injuries or diseases, and must be used very carefully for patients with respiratory disorders.

Meperidine does cause fewer problems with biliary outflow than morphine; it appears to cause nausea and vomiting, constipation, or urinary retention less commonly, but such problems do occur.

Meperidine is definitely addicting, but addiction may take longer to develop and may occur less frequently because meperidine produces less euphoria. Precautions to avoid addiction must be observed. For patients who require a potent analgesic for longer than seven to ten days, switching from morphine to meperidine at that time may help avoid addiction.

DOSE

100 mg intramuscularly or orally, or 75 to 100 mg intravenously every three to four hours.

Dibucaine Ointment

Dibucaine (Nupercainal) is a local anesthetic that is neither a narcotic nor related to procaine or cocaine and can be used by individuals allergic to those agents. Although the ointment can provide temporary relief from the pain and discomfort of many minor disorders, it is probably used most commonly for hemorrhoids and related anal problems.

PRECAUTIONS

Few precautions are necessary, although no more than one ounce of the one percent ointment should be used in a single twenty-four hour period. Allergy to this agent may develop, usually produces a rash covering the area to which the ointment has been applied, and commonly causes more discomfort than the condition for which this medication was being used.

Lidocaine

Lidocaine (Xylocaine) is an injectable local anesthetic that is widely used for dental procedures and for minor surgery, including suturing lacerations. Epinephrine may be added to lidocaine solutions to constrict blood vessels at the site of injection, reduce the speed of absorption, and prolong local anesthesia. Lidocaine ointment is available and is used in the same manner as dibucaine ointment.

The concentrations of solutions for injection range from 0.5 to 2.0 percent; a 1.0 percent solution appears most useful for mountaineering circumstances, although the higher concentrations provide more of the agent in a smaller volume.

PRECAUTIONS

For the uncommon individuals who are allergic to lidocaine this drug must not be used. Adverse reactions include anaphylaxis (see Chapter Twenty-Four, "Allergies") and convulsions.

During injections of lidocaine, repeated aspirations should be made with the syringe to ensure the drug is not being injected into a blood vessel.

DOSE AND ADMINISTRATION

The usual injection consists of 5 to 10 cc of a one percent solution, although more is occasionally needed. The solution should be injected into and just beneath the skin first and into deeper tissues after the skin has been anesthetized. Before each injection the plunger of the syringe should be pulled back to ensure the needle is not in a blood vessel. Anesthesia is almost immediate in onset, usually persists for thirty to forty-five minutes, and can be tested by pricking the injected area with the tip of a sterile needle.

MEDICATIONS FOR SLEEP OR SEDATION

Conventional sleeping medications should not be taken at altitudes above 10,000 feet (3,000 m). Under the influence of these drugs, respirations can be slowed to such an extent that the blood oxygen level falls significantly, aggravating the symptoms of acute mountain sickness. Acetazolamide is the drug of choice for promoting sleep at higher elevations.

Barbiturates

Barbiturates are commonly used to induce sleep, for sedation, and for controlling convulsions. Pentobarbital (Nembutal) and secobarbital (Seconal) are short acting barbiturates which usually take effect fifteen to thirty minutes after oral administration. These preparations are useful for inducing sleep because their onset is so rapid, but their actions last only two to four hours. Amobarbital is an intermediate speed barbiturate, taking somewhat longer to take effect, but lasting for four to six hours. A combination of secobarbital and amobarbital (Tuinal) is used to obtain the fast onset of the short acting barbiturate and the longer duration of the other.

Phenobarbital is a long acting barbiturate. It takes effect in thirty to sixty minutes and persists for six to eight hours or occasionally considerably longer. Phenobarbital is used for controlling convulsions, but its slow onset and long duration make it less useful for inducing sleep.

All of the barbiturates are approximately equally effective for sedation. A choice should be based on the desired duration of the sedation. Currently, however, the benzodiazepines are more commonly used as sedatives and tranquilizers.

PRECAUTIONS

All of the barbiturates can cause a "drug hangover" consisting of lassitude and somnolence. Phenobarbital has the greatest tendency to cause hangovers and is so long acting its effects may last past the usual hours of sleep. For these reasons, phenobarbital is rarely used as a sleep medication. Individuals for whom the hangover is a handicap the following day should not use barbiturates.

Some persons are quite resistant to the sleep inducing action of barbiturates. Such individuals should use another medication (or none at all).

Barbiturates must not be given to individuals with head injuries or central nervous system disease because fatal depression of brain function, particularly respiration, can result. However, individuals with recurring convulsions can be given enough phenobarbital to control their convulsions.

Barbiturates and alcohol both have a depressive effect upon brain function. If the two are combined, the resulting depression is greater than would be expected from just the summation of their individual effects. A number of deaths have resulted from taking conventional doses of barbiturates to induce sleep after an evening of social drinking. Because the effects are unpredictable and hazardous, barbiturates should never be taken in combination with alcohol.

Individuals with hepatitis, heart failure, diabetes, or fever may be unusually sensitive to the effects of barbiturates. If such patients develop unusual lassitude or somnolence, the medication must be stopped or administered in smaller doses.

Barbiturates produce a hyperexcited state in some individuals, mostly elderly persons or individuals with uncontrolled pain from an injury.

Large doses of barbiturates can be lethal; these drugs are among those most commonly used for suicide. An overdose produces somnolence that progresses to coma with reduced respiratory function.

Barbiturates tend to be habit forming, although they are not physically addicting in the manner of narcotics. They should be used only when definitely needed.

DOSE

To induce sleep: 100 mg orally at bedtime; a second dose may be given one to two hours later if needed.

For sedation: 50 to 100 mg orally every four to eight hours.

For convulsions: 200 mg orally or intramuscularly for individuals weighing more than 150 pounds (70 kg); 150 mg for smaller adults. An additional 100 mg should be administered if convulsions recur.

Benzodiazepines

The benzodiazepines are a group of drugs with almost identical pharmacologic properties, but chlordiazepoxide (Librium) and diazepam (Valium) are most commonly used as tranquilizers, and flurazepam (Dalmane) is most commonly used for promoting sleep. These drugs are as effective as the barbiturates for inducing sleep.

The benzodiazepines are definitely safer than the barbiturates. A lethal overdose is quite rare unless some other drug, usually alcohol, is taken along with large quantities of the benzodiazepine.

PRECAUTIONS

The benzodiazepines can produce a hangover just like the barbiturates but do so much less commonly and not necessarily in the same persons. However, unusual drowsiness may persist the following day. Individuals who develop a hangover with barbiturates should try one of the benzodiazepines.

Like the barbiturates and narcotics, benzodiazepines depress brain function and should not be given to individuals with head injuries or central nervous system disease.

Benzodiazepines can potentiate the depressive effects of alcohol.

DOSE

To induce sleep: 15 to 30 mg at bedtime.

For sedation or as a tranquilizer: 5 to 10 mg two to four times per day.

Others

A number of additional medications are used for inducing sleep but would rarely be needed or available in mountaineering situations. Diphenhydramine (Benadryl) is an antihistamine that has occasionally been used as a sleeping medication for elderly individuals who become excited after taking barbiturates. Chloral hydrate is also widely used in hospitals, but is less convenient for wilderness use because it is a liquid. Glutethimide (Doriden) and methaqualone (Sopor and others) offer no advantages over barbiturates or benzodiazepines for legitimate uses and have been abused so extensively they have fallen into disrepute. Glutethimide has the singular disadvantage of not being removable by dialysis so that an overdose can not be effectively treated.

ANTIMICROBIAL AGENTS

The antimicrobial agents include drugs for treating established infections, primarily antibiotics and sulfonamides, and antiseptics such as povidone-iodine and benzalkonium chloride, which prevent infections by killing microorganisms on contact.

Bacteria are classified as positive or negative by their reaction with the gram stain, as cocci (spheres), bacilli (rods), or spirochetes (spirals), and as aerobic if they are able to grow in the presence of oxygen or anaerobic if they can not. This classification is used in the discussion that follows.

The Penicillins

Penicillin was the first antibiotic to be discovered and is still the most widely used and most effective of all antibiotics. Subsequently, similar drugs have been developed and the entire group is referred to as "the penicillins." The penicillins are bacteriocidal and actively destroy bacteria, whereas some antibiotics just keep them from multiplying (bacteriostatic). Organisms susceptible to the penicillins include most cocci, both gram positive and gram negative, such as streptococci ("strep" throat, cellulitis, impetigo); staphylococci (boils, abscesses, wound infections); pneumococci (conjunctivitis, pneumonia); and Neisseria (gonorrhea, meningitis). Also sensitive to the penicillins are the spirochete that causes syphilis, other related organisms, and many gram positive bacilli. Except for ampicillin, the penicillins have little effect against the gram negative bacilli likely to cause gastrointestinal infections such as traveller's diarrhea, dysentery, or typhoid fever.

Of the available penicillin preparations, phenoxymethyl penicillin is most suitable for oral administration because it is resistant to destruction by acid in the stomach. Procaine penicillin G is used for intramuscular administration because it is less painful and persists longer. Aqueous crystalline penicillin G is usually used for intravenous administration.

Ampicillin is a chemical variant of penicillin to which the gram negative bacilli that most commonly cause traveller's diarrhea are susceptible. Since the organisms susceptible to penicillin are also susceptible to ampicillin, that drug can always be used instead of penicillin, but it is more expensive.

Some of the staphylococci produce an enzyme called penicillinase that destroys penicillin and "protects" the organisms from that drug. Several semisynthetic penicillins that are penicillinase resistant have been developed and are effective against such organisms. Cloxacillin and dicloxacillin are penicillinase resistant penicillins that are effective when administered orally. Nafcillin and methicillin have similar properties but are usually administered intramuscularly and intravenously. Unless staphylococci have been proven to be sensitive to other antibiotics, infections caused by those organisms should always be treated with a penicillinase resistant agent.

PRECAUTIONS

The penicillins are essentially nontoxic but have been used so widely and indiscriminantly that allergic reactions occur in about ten percent of the patients receiving these drugs. Most of these reactions consist of skin rashes of varying kinds, a low fever, or other minor problems. However, a few individuals develop severe anaphylactic reactions that may be lethal within minutes.

Anyone who has suffered an anaphylactic reaction to any of the penicillins must never again be treated with that or any of the other penicillins. The danger of a potentially lethal reaction is significant. A history of previous minor allergic reactions is not predictive of such a life threatening event, but penicillins should be avoided in such individuals if possible.

If signs of allergy occur in a patient receiving a penicillin, the drug should be discontinued immediately. The patient should be warned of his allergy to penicillin and must transmit that information to his physician or anyone subsequently caring for him in an emergency. He should wear a bracelet or a tag warning of his allergy. A climber with an allergy to penicillin should inform other members of a major climbing party and must make preparations in advance to have other antibiotics available in case he needs them.

DOSE

Phenoxymethyl penicillin: 500 to 1,000 mg every six hours orally.

Procaine penicillin G: 375 to 3,000 mg (0.375 to 3.0 gm or 0.6 to 4.8 million units) per day in equally divided doses every six to twelve hours intramuscularly.

Aqueous crystalline penicillin G: 375 to 12,500 mg (0.375 to 12.5 gm or 0.6 to

20 million units) per day in equally divided doses every two to six hours intravenously.

Ampicillin: 500 to 1,000 mg every six hours orally.

Cloxacillin: 500 to 1,000 mg every six hours orally.

Dicloxacillin: 250 to 500 mg every six hours orally.

Nafcillin: 1.0 to 2.0 gm every two to six hours intravenously or intramuscularly.

The Cephalosporins

The cephalosporins are a group of antibiotics that are chemically similar and have antibacterial actions similar to the penicillins. Cefazolin (Kefzol and Ancef) and cephalothin (Keflin) are useful for treating serious staphylococcal and gram negative infections. Cefamandole (Mandole) is effective against many gram negative bacteria. Cefoxitin (Mefoxin) may prove a useful alternative to either clindamycin or chloramphenicol for treating anaerobic bacterial infections such as peritonitis.

PRECAUTIONS

Some patients allergic to penicillin are also allergic to the cephalosporins. Individuals who have had a severe reaction to penicillin, particularly an anaphylactic reaction, should not be treated with cephalosporins.

The cephalosporins enter the cerebrospinal fluid poorly and should not be used for treating meningitis.

DOSE

Cefamandole: 1,000 to 2,000 mg every six to eight hours intramuscularly or intravenously.

Cefoxitin: 1,000 to 2,000 mg every six to eight hours intramuscularly or intravenously.

Cephalothin: 1,000 to 2,000 mg every six to eight hours intramuscularly or intravenously.

Cefazolin: 500 to 1,000 mg every six hours intramuscularly or intravenously.

Erythromycin

Erythromycin is effective against pneumococci, streptococci, and most staphylococci. It is used primarily as a substitute for penicillin in individuals who are allergic to that drug. Erythromycin is a bacteriostatic agent and may not be as effective as penicillin. Even as a penicillin substitute it probably should not be used for severe staphylococcal infections.

PRECAUTIONS

Very few adverse reactions to erythromycin occur, and those that do appear are mild.

DOSE

500 to 1,000 mg every six hours orally.

Clindamycin

Clindamycin is another antibiotic with antibacterial effects similar to penicillin and is a suitable substitute for penicillin for individuals allergic to that drug. In addition, clindamycin is effective against a number of anaerobic organisms, particularly *Bacteroides fragilis,* one of the most common of the anaerobic organisms that cause peritonitis. Therefore, clindamycin is helpful in the treatment of peritonitis.

PRECAUTIONS

Approximately twenty to thirty percent of patients being treated with clindamycin develop diarrhea. Usually the diarrhea is mild and treatment with this antibiotic does not have to be suspended. However, rare individuals develop a life threatening colitis, which causes copious fluid and electrolyte loss and the passage of large amounts of blood and mucus in the stools. Clindamycin must be stopped at once if this type of diarrhea appears, and the lost fluids must be restored, intravenously if necessary.

DOSE

100 to 300 mg every six hours orally.

200 to 1,500 mg every eight hours intramuscularly or intravenously.

The Aminoglycosides

The aminoglycosides are a group of antibiotics that include streptomycin, neomycin, kanamycin, and gentamicin. Streptomycin is now used only for tuberculous infections because less toxic drugs are available. Neomycin is also highly toxic and its use is limited to preparations from which it can not be absorbed, such as ophthalmic ointments. Kanamycin and gentamicin are effective against a large number of gram negative bacilli and are used for severe infections caused by those organisms, such as peritonitis. Due to their toxicity these antibiotics should not be used for relatively minor infections. They are ineffective against anaerobic bacteria.

PRECAUTIONS

The aminoglycosides are excreted by the kidneys and can damage those organs. Patients with renal disease should not receive these drugs or should receive them in smaller doses.

The aminoglycosides can cause damage to the inner ear and the auditory and vestibular nerves, resulting in deafness, ringing or buzzing in the ears, loss of balance — particularly with the eyes closed — or vertigo.

The aminoglycosides should not be injected directly into a body cavity or be given rapidly by vein. Respiratory arrest due to a form of nerve block can result.

DOSE

Gentamicin: 1.7 mg per kg of body weight intramuscularly, followed by 1.0 mg per kg every eight hours.

Kanamycin: 5 mg per kg of body weight intramuscularly every eight hours.

Chloramphenicol

Chloramphenicol is a potent antibiotic with such a wide spectrum of antibacterial activity that it could be one of the most valuable antibacterial agents but for one flaw. In about one of every 25,000 to 50,000 patients receiving this drug, a lethal bone marrow suppression occurs. This reaction is idiosyncratic and can not be predicted before the drug is administered.

Some investigators have claimed that the death rate due to adverse reactions to chloramphenicol is no greater than the death rate caused by reactions to penicillin. Nonetheless, administration of chloramphenicol is usually limited to a few specific life threatening conditions, which include: (1) severe bacterial meningitis in patients allergic to penicillin, (2) severe anaerobic infections for which clindamycin is not effective, (3) infections by gram negative bacilli that do not respond to other antibiotics, and (4) severe rickettsial infections for which tetracycline is not effective.

PRECAUTIONS

In view of the severe bone marrow depression that can result from chloramphenicol therapy, this drug must only be used for those specific infections for which it is indicated.

DOSE

250 to 1,000 mg or 12.5 mg per kg of body weight, either orally or intravenously, every six hours.

Tetracycline

The tetracyclines have a very broad spectrum of activity, which includes rickettsia and some viruslike organisms as well as a large number of gram positive and gram negative bacteria. However, the tetracyclines are bacteriostatic drugs, and a number of more effective agents have replaced them for the treatment of many infections. Currently the disorders for which tetracycline is the antibiotic of choice are: (1) the treatment of certain viral and rickettsial infections, (2) treatment of gonorrhea, syphilis, and occasionally other infections in patients allergic to penicillin, and (3) the treatment of urinary tract infections caused by gram negative organisms. Tetracycline is also useful for treating cholera and is frequently effective for traveller's diarrhea, for which it can be administered to patients allergic to penicillin.

PRECAUTIONS

Tetracycline therapy may be associated with a mild diarrhea due to the suppression of the bacteria that normally predominate in the intestines and their replacement by other organisms. The diarrhea is rarely severe and usually stops after administration of the drug has been terminated.

Nausea and vomiting commonly occur in patients receiving tetracycline therapy.

Tetracycline can permanently stain the dental enamel in young children and should be avoided for such patients and pregnant women whenever other agents are available.

Tetracycline and penicillin tend to be antagonistic and the two drugs should not be administered together. Tetracycline also is inactivated in the stomach by food and should be given before meals.

DOSE

250 to 500 mg every six hours orally.

Polymyxin B, Bacitracin, and Neomycin Ophthalmic Mixture

This antibiotic mixture (Neosporin) is prepared as an ophthalmic ointment and as an ophthalmic solution (drops). It is used to treat conjunctivitis caused by a wide variety of organisms.

PRECAUTIONS

Some individuals are allergic to one or more of the components of this mixture and should not be treated with it.

A similar ointment produced for use on other tissues such as skin is called simply Neosporin Ointment. This preparation must not be confused with the ophthalmic ointment because it is not prepared to meet the same standards and may contain minor impurities that could be irritating or injurious to the eye even though they would not harm less sensitive tissues.

The antibiotics used in this preparation are valuable for treating infections in locations where they are not absorbed by the body. However, these antibiotics produce side effects that preclude their use for infections anywhere except on the body surface. They must never be taken internally.

DOSE

A small amount of the ointment or one or two drops of the solution should be installed behind the lower eyelid every three to four hours.

Trimethoprim-Sulfamethoxazole

Trimethoprim-sulfamethoxazole (Bactrim, Septra, or "trimethoprim-sulfa") is a combination of two agents, one of which is a sulfonamide. Sulfonamides are useful for treating many gastrointestinal or urinary tract infections because they can be administered in preparations that produce high concentrations of the drugs in these organs. Additionally, some infectious organisms resistant to antibiotics are readily destroyed by sulfonamides.

PRECAUTIONS

Sulfonamides in general are not very soluble in water and tend to precipitate in the urine, in effect forming small kidney stones which can cause significant damage. In order to prevent such damage, patients receiving these drugs must consume large quantities of fluids to maintain a high urinary volume (at least one to one and one-half liters per day) and to keep the drug in solution.

Some patients are allergic to sulfonamides and should not be treated with them. This preparation should not be taken by individuals with glucose-6-phosphatase deficiency. (This disorder, which must be diagnosed by a physician, usually causes mild anemia and is aggravated by certain drugs, particularly some sulfonamides.) These drugs block folic acid metabolism in bacteria and should not be taken by individuals being treated for folic acid deficiency (another type of anemia) since the drug might aggravate the deficiency.

Sulfonamides cross the placenta, are excreted in milk, and can have harmful effects on a fetus or newborn. They should be administered during the last months of pregnancy and to nursing mothers only by a physician.

DOSE

Two regular strength tablets (80 mg of trimethoprim and 400 mg of sulfamethoxazole) or one double strength tablet, orally every six to twelve hours.

Chloroquin

Chloroquin is used primarily for malaria and is highly effective for both prevention and treatment, except for chloroquin resistant *falciparum* malaria for which Fansidar is the prophylactic agent of choice. Chloroquin is also effective to some extent in the treatment of amebiasis.

PRECAUTIONS

In the dosages used for preventing or treating malaria, chloroquin has almost no serious side effects. Therapeutic doses may cause minor gastrointestinal disturbances. Skin rashes or itching occasionally occur. However, these symptoms often do not require interruption of therapy or prophylaxis and rapidly disappear when administration is ended.

DOSE

Prevention: 0.5 gm orally as a single dose once weekly on the same day of the week, starting two weeks before entering a malaria endemic area and continuing for five weeks after leaving.

Therapy: 1.0 gm orally followed in six to eight hours by 0.5 gm, with single doses of 0.5 gm being administered on each of the next three days. (Total dose: 3.0 gm over a period of four days.)

Sulfadoxine and Pyrimethamine

Sulfadoxine and pyrimethamine combined (Fansidar) provide effective prophylaxis for chloroquin resistant *falciparum* malaria.

PRECAUTIONS

Sulfadoxine is a sulfonamide and should not be taken by individuals allergic to sulfa drugs. Other precautions that should be observed during the administration of sulfonamides, particularly the maintenance of a high fluid intake, are discussed under trimethoprim-sulfamethoxazole.

The drugs contained in this combination can cross the placenta and are secreted in milk. They may be teratogenic and can cause disorders in newborn infants. Therefore, these drugs should not be taken during pregnancy or by nursing mothers.

Fansidar should not be given at the same time as other sulfonamides such as trimethoprim-sulfamethoxazole. Since all of these drugs are folic acid antagonists, taking them simultaneously could produce folic acid deficiency and anemia in the recipient.

DOSE

Prevention: One tablet (500 mg sulfadoxine and 25 mg pyrimethamine) orally on the same day each week starting two weeks before entering a malaria endemic area and continuing for five weeks after leaving.

Therapy for an established infestation should be administered by a physician familiar with the complexities of treating this disorder.

Benzalkonium Chloride

Benzalkonium chloride (Zephiran) is a cationic quaternary ammonium surface acting agent that is a highly effective antiseptic. Aqueous solutions of benzalkonium and povidone-iodine are the only agents currently readily available that are capable of killing bacteria in the depths of a wound without killing or seriously damaging the tissues.

When used as intended benzalkonium chloride has very little toxic effect. However, serious results, including collapse, coma, and death, can result if the solution is ingested.

Alcoholic solutions (tinctures) as well as aqueous solutions are available, but the aqueous are more suitable for wound antisepsis and do not burn or sting as do the tincture.

Solutions of benzalkonium must be kept in glass bottles.

DOSE

Benzalkonium chloride is usually supplied as a 1:750 solution. For disinfecting intact skin prior to needle puncture or for cleaning minor wounds, this solution can be used without dilution. For washing out deep or dirty wounds, the original solution should be diluted with disinfected water to about 1:3000. Copious quantities of the solution should be used to thoroughly rinse all wounds, particularly bites inflicted by a possibly rabid animal.

Povidone-Iodine

Povidone-iodine, an iodophor, is a loose complex of iodine with polyvinylpyrrolidone which was patented in 1956 and subsequently has become widely available as a ten percent solution under the trade names Betadine, Povidine, Pharmadine, and others. These preparations offer two significant advantages for wilderness use: (1) they can be kept in polyethylene containers instead of glass, and (2) they are effective disinfectants in dilute solutions so that less must be carried.

Povidone-iodine retains the strong bacteriocidal activity of iodine but eliminates many of the disadvantages, such as skin irritation, staining of the skin, and the odor of iodine. A 1:100 dilution of a ten percent solution has been found to have much greater bacteriocidal action than the original stock solution, and 1:1000 dilutions are almost equally effective.

PRECAUTIONS

Rare individuals are allergic to iodine; a chronic skin rash is the usual manifestation. Such individuals should not use povidone-iodine.

Povidone-iodine has been recommended for water disinfection, but no substantiating data has been provided. The 1:10,000 dilution that would result has been found to have no significant antimicrobial activity. At the present time these agents can not be considered reliable for water disinfection.

DOSE

For skin disinfection prior to injections a small quantity of an undiluted solution is suitable and convenient. For rinsing a larger wound, the original solution should be diluted several hundred times and the wound thoroughly rinsed with large quantities of the solution, particularly following the bite of a possibly rabid animal.

MEDICATIONS AFFECTING THE HEART, RESPIRATORY SYSTEM, AND BLOOD VESSELS

Acetazolamide

Acetazolamide (Diamox) inhibits the enzyme carbonic anhydrase, which catalyzes the reversible combination of carbon dioxide with water to form carbonic acid. This drug promotes renal bicarbonate excretion and tends to reduce the increase in blood pH (respiratory alkalosis) resulting from carbon dioxide loss produced by the faster and deeper breathing typical of high altitudes.

Acetazolamide reduces the severity of acute mountain sickness symptoms in individuals who must ascend from sea level to 12,000 to 14,000 feet (3,700 to 4,300 m) without adequate time for acclimatization. It does not eliminate such symptoms entirely. A significant effect on high altitude pulmonary edema has not been demonstrated. Perhaps the greatest benefit from acetazolamide is relief of sleep problems at high altitude. Elimination of episodes of severe hypoxia during sleep may be responsible for better tolerance of high altitude during waking hours.

PRECAUTIONS

Acetazolamide is a sulfonamide, although it does not have any antibacterial actions. Persons allergic to sulfonamides are allergic to this drug.

Persons with liver or kidney disease should not be treated with acetazolamide, and the drug should not be given during the last months of pregnancy or to nursing mothers.

Some individuals develop tingling sensations in the lips and finger tips, blurring of vision, and alterations of taste when taking this drug. These sensations disappear when the medication is stopped.

DOSE

250 mg every twelve hours starting one to two days before ascent and continuing for three to five days after arrival.

Furosemide

Furosemide (Lasix, or frusemide in the United Kingdom) is a potent diuretic which inhibits chloride and sodium reabsorption in the renal tubules. Its administration leads to the loss of large quantities of water and electrolytes through the kidneys.

PRECAUTIONS

The U.S. Food and Drug Administration requires the following warning in the manufacturer's information about this drug: "Warning — Lasix (furosemide) is a potent diuretic which if given in excessive amounts can lead to a profound diuresis with water and electrolyte depletion. Therefore, careful medical supervision is required, and dose schedules have to be adjusted to the individual patient's needs."

One climber who developed high altitude pulmonary edema was given furosemide and then walked unaided to a location several thousand feet lower. At that elevation his pulmonary edema disappeared, but he had to be evacuated by stretcher because he was so dehydrated and electrolyte depleted by the furosemide.

Excessive diuresis may cause dehydration and reduction in blood volume, resulting in circulatory collapse (shock) and increasing the possibility of venous thromboses and pulmonary embolism.

Patients with liver or renal disease should not receive this drug.

Persons allergic to sulfonamides may be allergic to furosemide.

Some cases of irreversible hearing loss have resulted from high doses of furosemide.

DOSE

20 to 40 mg orally; a second dose may be given twelve to twenty-four hours later.

Nitroglycerin

Nitroglycerin relaxes the walls of small blood vessels, permitting them to dilate and increase the flow of blood. This compound (which is the explosive) is most commonly used to treat angina pectoris (severe chest pain associated with inadequacy of the blood supply to the heart) but dilates all small arteries and can be used to increase the blood flow to other organs or tissues. As the result of dilatation of cerebral arteries, throbbing headaches frequently follow the use of nitroglycerin.

PRECAUTIONS

The most serious side effect of nitroglycerin therapy is a drop in blood pressure due to the dilatation of blood vessels. Fainting or — even worse — aggravation of the cardiac damage could result. Therefore, a patient receiving this drug must be closely attended. He should lie down with his head lowered if symptoms of faintness or dizziness appear.

The tablets should be kept in their original brown bottle and should not be kept longer than six months after purchase as they begin to lose their potency. Cotton wads should not be kept in the bottle, which must be kept tightly stoppered.

DOSE

One or two 0.4 mg (1/150 grain) tablets held under the tongue at the onset of an attack. If the pain persists, additional tablets may be taken at fifteen or thirty minute intervals for a total of four tablets during one hour. The tablets may be chewed but must not be swallowed. About three minutes is required for the medication to take effect.

Digoxin

Digoxin is one of the digitalis preparations, which are the oldest and most valuable drugs available for the treatment of a variety of heart disorders. Digitalis strengthens the contraction of the heart muscle, permitting more effective cardiac function for patients in heart failure. Digitalis preparations also help restore normal cardiac rhythm for patients with many types of abnormal rhythms. (These drugs are not beneficial and may be quite harmful for persons with normal hearts.)

PRECAUTIONS

Loss of appetite, nausea or vomiting, or slowing of the heart rate to less than sixty per minute are indications of digoxin toxicity. If such signs appear in a patient receiving this drug, the dose must be reduced.

Digoxin must be given with great care to anyone who has taken any digitalis preparation within the previous week. These drugs are excreted slowly over a period of several days or longer. An overdose could result if treatment was restarted (without an appropriate reduction in the quantity of the drug administered) shortly after it had been discontinued.

A number of digitalis preparations, such as digitoxin, have similar names. These preparations must not be confused because the therapeutic doses are significantly different.

DOSE

Initially: one 0.25 mg tablet orally every two hours for a total of six tablets (1.5 mg).

Maintenance: one 0.25 mg tablet at the same time once every twenty-four hours.

Epinephrine

Epinephrine (adrenalin) is a hormone secreted by the medulla of the adrenal gland. It is used to treat spasm of the bronchi due to anaphylactic shock or severe asthma, or to relieve the spasm and respiratory obstruction of laryngeal edema. Adrenalin is effective when injected or when applied directly to the involved tissues. It is destroyed by the acid and digestive enzymes in the stomach and is ineffective when administered orally.

PRECAUTIONS

Epinephrine must be administered very slowly and carefully to elderly individuals or to persons with heart disease of any kind, high blood pressure, thyroid disease, or diabetes. It also should not be given to persons in shock from blood loss. Epinephrine is a powerful cardiac stimulant; its effect on individuals with these disorders could be lethal.

Repeat injections of epinephrine should not be given until all effects of a previous injection have disappeared. An overdose of epinephrine could be lethal for persons with normal hearts.

The epinephrine preparation must be discarded without being used if it has turned brown or contains a precipitate.

The solutions of epinephrine for injection (1:1,000) and for inhalation (1:100) must be clearly and carefully marked. Confusion would probably prove fatal if the solution for inhalation were injected.

Following use of the nebulizer, the patient should rinse his mouth carefully to avoid swallowing the epinephrine, which can cause rather severe stomach distress.

DOSE

Subcutaneously: 0.3 to 0.5 cc (depending upon the patient's size) of a 1:1,000 solution every fifteen to thirty minutes.

Inhalation: Prepared aerosols have different dose schedules. The Medihaler-Epi dose is one inhalation every two minutes until relief is obtained. Such prepackaged aerosols are most convenient and reliable. If one is used, the directions accompanying the kit should be followed. If a prepared aerosol is not available, one can be made up by placing 0.5 cc of a one percent (1:100) solution of epinephrine in a nebulizer. Four to six inhalations should provide relief within one to three minutes. An overdose must be carefully avoided.

Aminophylline

Aminophylline is closely related to caffeine chemically and pharmacologically but does not have as much stimulating effect on the central nervous system. This drug is used to treat asthma because it relaxes the bronchial walls and permits the bronchi to dilate, relieving respiratory difficulty. At high altitudes aminophylline can prevent the interruption of sleep by Cheyne-Stokes respirations, but acetazolamide is probably preferable for that purpose.

PRECAUTIONS

Aminophylline in therapeutic doses has few toxic effects.

DOSE

One 500 mg suppository inserted well up into the rectum.

Isoproterenol

Isoproterenol (Isuprel) is chemically and pharmacologically similar to epinephrine and can provide relief for bronchial spasm and obstruction in asthma. It offers the advantage of being effective orally.

PRECAUTIONS

Isoproterenol must not be administered in combination with epinephrine. Their combined action on the heart could be disastrous. Only a physician should administer isoproterenol to a patient known to have serious cardiac disease.

Individuals allergic to iodine should not use this preparation.

DOSE

One or two tablespoons (15 to 30 cc) of the elixir (which also contains phenobarbital, ephedrine [a compound similar to epinephrine], theophylline [a compound almost identical to aminophylline], potassium iodide, and nineteen percent alcohol) three or four times daily. The dose should be adjusted to the severity of the asthma.

Phenylephrine

Phenylephrine hydrochloride, a decongestant well known in the United States as Neo-Synephrine, is present in many other preparations. This agent causes the blood vessels in the nasal mucosa to contract, reducing their volume, but also reducing the amount of fluid collected in the tissue (edema) around the vessels.

As a nasal spray, phenylephrine is used to shrink the swollen mucosa of the nose for patients with colds, hay fever, or sinusitis. This agent not only relieves obstruction to the passage of air, but also relieves obstruction and promotes drainage from the small canals opening into the sinuses.

The nasal spray can be used as an inhalant for treating asthma if epinephrine or isoproterenol are not available. Although not as effective as those agents, phenylephrine has a definite beneficial action in asthma and produces no significant side effects.

PRECAUTIONS

Administration of the nasal spray should be repeated ten minutes after the first application. Initially the spray only reaches the mucosa over the more prominent structures in the nasal cavity. Not until this portion of the mucosa has been shrunken can a subsequent application extend into the recesses where the small canals draining the sinuses open.

After the effects of the nasal spray have worn off, swelling of the nasal mucosa and airway obstruction recur. Such "rebound" symptoms may be worse than the initial symptoms. With each subsequent application, the duration of the spray's effects tends to become shorter. For this reason, use of the spray perhaps should be limited to the hours when decongestant action is needed to promote restful sleep. An oral decongestant should be used in conjunction with the spray to obtain more complete and longer lasting results.

DOSE

A 0.25 to 0.50 percent solution sprayed into each nostril and repeated after a ten minute interval. Administration may be repeated every three to four hours.

Pseudoephedrine

Pseudoephedrine (Sudafed and others) is a systemic decongestant. The drug acts through the nerves supplying the blood vessels in the mucosa of the upper respiratory tract, causing those vessels to contract. Excess fluid in the mucosa (edema) is reduced, the mucosa shrinks to normal thickness, and obstruction to the passage of air is relieved. This drug also shrinks the mucosa lining the small canals that drain the sinuses and the eustachian tubes that drain the middle ears, allowing air or fluid to move through these structures and helping to avoid aerotitis media, aerosinusitis, or infectious sinusitis.

PRECAUTIONS

Pseudoephedrine should be given to individuals with high blood pressure, heart disease, thyroid disease, or diabetes only by a physician.

Pseudoephedrine acts as a mild stimulant and makes some individuals restless or jumpy, which can inhibit restful sleep. Reducing the dose of the drug by only taking part of a tablet usually relieves these side effects.

DOSE

60 mg every six to eight hours.

Pseudoephedrine with Triprolidine

This combination of an antihistamine with a systemic decongestant (Actifed) is one of the most popular for controlling the symptoms of allergic reactions such as hay fever or for colds.

PRECAUTIONS

The precautions that must be observed are those for both the antihistamines and pseudoephedrine.

DOSE

One tablet every eight hours.

ANTIHISTAMINES

Antihistamines are a group of drugs that block the effects of histamine, a substance released during allergic and inflammatory reactions and considered responsible for many symptoms of allergy. In addition, some of these agents can prevent or reduce symptoms of motion sickness.

Chlorpheniramine and Triprolidine

Chlorpheniramine and triprolidine are two widely used antihistamines administered to relieve the symptoms of hay fever and similar allergies. They may also provide some relief with colds. Chlorpheniramine is present in Alka-Seltzer Plus Cold Tablets, Allerest, Chlor-Trimeton, Coricidin, Co-Tylenol, Novahistine, Sinarest, Teldrin, Tuss-Ornade, and many others. Some of these products are available in delayed release forms, which extend drug action after a single administration for as long as twelve hours. Triprolidine is present in Actidil, which is not as widely used as other antihistamines, but is combined with pseudoephedrine in Actifed, one of the most widely used combinations of an antihistamine with a decongestant.

Dimenhydrinate, Meclizine, and Cyclizine

Dimenhydrinate (Dramamine), meclizine (Bonine and Antivert), and cyclizine (Marezine) are antihistamines used primarily to control motion sickness. All should be taken about one hour before embarking on a trip. An advantage of meclizine is that a single dose is effective for twenty-four hours. All are fairly effective against allergies.

Diphenhydramine

Diphenhydramine (Benadryl) is an antihistamine that is highly effective for treating allergies. However, all antihistamines have some tendency to make recipients drowsy. This effect is so pronounced with diphenhydramine that it is effectively used as a sleep medication.

PRECAUTIONS

All antihistamines have a tendency to cause drowsiness, although individual susceptibility to this effect varies. Anyone who has taken an antihistamine must be very careful about engaging in activities for which drowsiness could be a hazard, particularly driving a car.

DOSE

Chlorpheniramine: dose depends upon the preparation being used.

Triprolidine: Actifed — one tablet every eight hours.

Dimenhydrinate: one 50 mg tablet every four hours.

Meclizine: one or two 25 mg tablets every twenty-four hours.

Cyclizine: one 50 mg tablet every four to six hours.

Diphenhydramine: one 50 mg tablet at bedtime (for sleep) or every six to eight hours (for allergies).

MEDICATIONS FOR GASTROINTESTINAL DISORDERS

Paregoric

Paregoric (camphorated tincture of opium) is a mixture of several compounds, the most important of which is morphine. This mixture is used to control diarrhea through the immobilizing action of opium derivatives on the lower gastrointestinal tract.

PRECAUTIONS

The problems related to using any drug to control diarrhea are discussed in Chapter Eighteen, "Gastrointestinal Diseases."

Paregoric is classified as a controlled substance due to its opium content. Addiction to paregoric does occur rarely, but not from reasonable use.

DOSE

One teaspoonful (5 cc) orally every two hours or after each bowel movement.

Diphenoxylate

Diphenoxylate (Lomotil) is a combination of two compounds that is used to control diarrhea through slowing of intestinal mobility.

PRECAUTIONS

The most important complications resulting from the administration of diphenoxylate are those from using any drug to control diarrhea.

This drug is chemically very similar to meperidine, although lacking its analgesic and euphoric properties. Addiction is at least theoretically possible and diphenoxylate is classified as a controlled substance.

DOSE

Two tablets four times a day is the maximum recommended dose. Smaller amounts should be used if they are effective.

Loperamide

Loperamide (Imodium) helps control diarrhea by reducing intestinal mobility.

PRECAUTIONS

The most important complications associated with the administration of loperamide are those resulting from using any drug to control diarrhea.

Loperamide is at least potentially addicting, although no addicted humans have been reported, and is classified as a controlled substance by U.S. federal law.

DOSE

Two 2 mg capsules followed by one 2 mg capsule after each unformed stool, not to exceed eight capsules in any twenty-four hour period.

Antacids

Antacids are preparations that contain various combinations of compounds, such as aluminum hydroxide, calcium carbonate, magnesium carbonate, magnesium hydroxide, and magnesium trisilicate. They are administered to neutralize acids in the stomach in the treatment of peptic ulcers and for relief of symptoms of indigestion. Some of the preparations are flavored. Among the better known antacids are Alka-Seltzer, Alka-2, Amphojel, Gaviscom, Gelusil, Maalox, and WinGel.

PRECAUTIONS

Magnesium-containing antacids sometimes produce a mild diarrhea, but this side effect rarely requires treatment or interruption of therapy. These drugs are absorbed from the gastrointestinal tract in minimal amounts, if at all, and have no effects on the rest of the body. They are of no value in preventing acute mountain sickness.

Antacids should not be taken indiscriminately over long periods of time. Prolonged consumption of antacids and calcium-containing foods such as milk can lead to calcium deposits in the kidneys and impaired renal function.

DOSE

The dose depends upon the preparation being used but usually consists of one or two tablets as often as required for the pain or distress of an ulcer or indigestion.

Antispasmodics

Antispasmodics reduce the amount of acid produced by the stomach as well as reducing peristaltic activity, both of which are desirable in the treatment of indigestion, peptic ulcer, or acute pancreatitis. Some of the better known antispasmodics are Donnatal, Pamine, Pro-Banthine, and tincture of belladonna. Many others of equal effectiveness are produced.

PRECAUTIONS

Antispasmodics produce blurring of vision and dryness of the mouth as their most common side effects. Following ingestion of one of these drugs, a patient might not be able to participate in activities requiring visual acuity, such as driving a car.

Individuals with a history of glaucoma should not be treated with these drugs. Blurring of vision by antispasmodics results from dilatation of the pupil and immobilization of the muscles that focus the eyes. Dilatation of the pupils in this manner can seriously aggravate glaucoma, a condition characterized by increased intraocular pressure.

Some antispasmodics have a significant constipating effect and should not be used alone. A generous fluid intake and the use of antacids that have a laxative action, as most do, counteracts this tendency.

These drugs also have a tendency to immobilize the urinary bladder, resulting in urinary retention that requires urethral catheterization. Although this complication would be rare in climbers, therapy may have to be discontinued for several days and then resumed at a lower dose if it occurs.

DOSE

The dose depends upon the preparation being used. The drugs are usually given one-half hour before meals and at bedtime. A double dose may be given at bedtime if the patient tends to be awakened at night by ulcer pain.

Preparations for intramuscular injection are available for treating patients with acute pancreatitis for whom oral therapy is undesirable.

APPENDIX B

Therapeutic Procedures

ADMINISTERING MEDICATIONS

Oral Medications

The oral route is the easiest, most convenient, and generally the safest method for administering drugs. This route has two major disadvantages: the time required for a drug to be absorbed, which delays the onset of its effects, and variations in the rate and completeness of absorption. The acid and digestive enzymes of the stomach and small intestine completely inactivate some therapeutic agents, and they must be given by another route.

Patients who are not fully conscious may aspirate medications given orally, resulting in pneumonia or even respiratory obstruction. Unconscious or stuporous patients must never be given any medications, food, or fluids orally.

Usually oral therapy is useless for patients who are vomiting. The drugs are most commonly expelled before they can be absorbed. Even if the patient is able to keep them down, emptying of the stomach is greatly retarded, resulting in a prolonged delay in the onset of action because orally administered drugs are usually absorbed only in the small intestine.

With the exception of drugs that are irritating to the stomach, such as aspirin or codeine, medications should be taken at least one-half hour before meals. The stomach empties more slowly and irregularly when it is filled with food, delaying the onset of the drug's effects. Additionally, the food may interfere with absorption of the drug.

Intramuscular Injections

The intramuscular route for administration of drugs is more reliable than the oral since the vagaries of intestinal absorption are avoided. However, intramuscular injections are associated with several hazards, of which the most serious is the risk of an overdose. An excessive dose of a drug or the wrong drug given orally can be partially recovered by making the patient vomit. No similar "safety valve" is available for medications that have been injected. In addition, with intramuscular injections there is a slight risk of injecting the drug directly into a blood vessel inside the muscle, producing much higher and more toxic concentrations of the agent in the blood than occur with the slower absorption from a true intramuscular site.

Intramuscular injections are usually not absorbed well by patients in shock. If several injections of a drug are given, the medication may not be absorbed until the patient recovers from shock. At that time, however, all of the injections are absorbed at once, leading to an overdose and possibly serious toxic effects.

The needle used for an intramuscular injection may injure nerves, blood vessels, or other structures if the site for the injection is not carefully chosen.

The most common complication of intramuscular injections is the production of an abscess by bacteria which are introduced with the needle. Although the needle may be free of bacteria, the skin through which it must pass can not be completely sterilized. Bacteria from this site are essentially always carried deeper into the tissues. However, thorough cleansing of the skin before the injection, and care to avoid contamination of the needle, usually reduce the quantity of bacteria that are introduced to a number that the body's defenses can destroy without such complications.

The following steps should be followed in administering any therapeutic agent intramuscularly:

1. The skin over the injection site should be cleaned with soap and water, swabbed with alcohol (or preferably a disinfectant such as Betadine or Zephiran), and permitted to dry.
2. The label on the drug container should be examined closely to ensure the proper medication in the correct dose is being administered.
3. A syringe of appropriate size should be fitted with a twenty-three gauge needle.
4. The top of the bottle through which the needle is to be inserted should be swabbed with alcohol or a disinfectant.
5. The drug should be extracted from the bottle by inserting the needle through the rubber top, injecting a volume of air equal to the volume of fluid to be removed, and then withdrawing the medication.
6. The needle should be pointed upward and any air bubbles or excess drug expressed from the syringe.
7. The label on the bottle must be examined again to make sure no mistakes have occurred. Such errors are far easier to prevent than they are to correct.
8. Without touching the injection site, a mound of skin and muscle should be pinched up so that the needle does not strike the underlying bone, and the needle should be inserted with a quick, jabbing motion.
9. Before injecting the medication, the plunger of the syringe must be pulled back to make certain the needle is not in a blood vessel. If blood is pulled back into the syringe, the needle must be removed and inserted in a different location.
10. The contents of the syringe should be injected fairly slowly to minimize discomfort, and the needle should be withdrawn quickly.

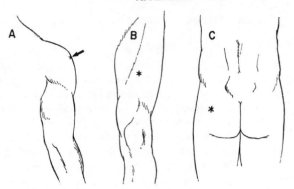

Figure 55. Sites for the administration of intramuscular injections.
(A-shoulder; B-thigh; C-buttock.)

Subcutaneous Injections

Subcutaneous injections are desirable for a few drugs, principally epinephrine, to provide somewhat slower absorption than intramuscular injections. The technique for subcutaneous injections is the same as for intramuscular injections, but the needle should be inserted at an angle so that it stays in the subcutaneous fatty tissue and does not enter the muscle. Injections can be made any place where there is a significant amount of fat beneath the skin.

Intravenous Medications

Intravenous drug administration is required in a few medical emergencies and for some infections in order to get medications into the blood faster or in higher concentrations than can be attained with other routes of administration. Additionally, intravenous injection can maintain a constant high blood concentration of a drug without the ups and downs associated with other methods of administration, which are by necessity intermittent. However, intravenous injections are more hazardous than intramuscular because the drugs can reach very high concentrations in the blood quite rapidly. If a medication is injected too quickly, the resulting high concentration can produce severe complications — even death.

Intravenous drug administration is associated with additional risks. Once the drug has been injected it can not be recovered. If the wrong drug or too much of a medication is injected, no "safety valve" is available. If the patient has an allergic reaction to the drug, little can be done to reverse the process. Such injections must be given only when necessary; specified rates of injection and other precautions must be closely observed.

The technique for administering intravenous medications over a long period of time is that for intravenous fluid administration. Intravenous antibiotics are administered by injecting the antibiotic directly into a bottle of intravenous fluids.

If the injections are intermittent, such as the injection of epinephrine for anaphylactic shock or the periodic injection of morphine to provide analgesia for a patient in shock, the large veins located in the fold of the arm at the elbow should be used. Preparation of the injection and the injection site should be the same as for intramuscular injections. After the needle has been inserted into a vein, a small amount of blood should be withdrawn to dilute the drug and make certain the needle is in the proper location. Subsequently, the drug should be injected very slowly but as continuously as possible over a period of no less than two to three minutes — preferably longer.

INTRAVENOUS FLUID THERAPY

Intravenous fluid therapy is required to replace normal and abnormal fluid losses for patients who are not able to take fluids orally, to administer blood or plasma following a severe hemorrhage, and for the intravenous administration of some medications. The technique for administering fluids intravenously is basically simple, although it may appear otherwise. Climbers planning outings to an area where intravenous fluids might be required should learn the technique under the guidance of a nurse or physician.

Although details in the way intravenous fluids are administered vary between individuals, the basic technique is as follows:

1. The patient should be placed in a supine position and a tourniquet that blocks venous but not arterial blood flow should be placed around the upper arm. (The pulse must be palpable at the wrist.)
2. The patient should open and close his fist several times to engorge the superficial veins with blood. Letting the arm hang down for a few minutes or covering it with a warm, moist towel helps make the veins more prominent if they are small or obscured by subcutaneous fat.
3. A large, prominent vein on the inner, flat surface of the arm should be selected and the overlying skin cleaned with soap and water followed by swabbing with alcohol and a disinfectant.
4. The protective cap should be removed from the bottle of fluids to be administered, and the dispensing apparatus inserted into the proper opening. The air intake for the bottle should be opened and the dispensing tubing filled with fluid. To avoid forcing air bubbles into the patient's vein, the drip chamber just below the bottle should be filled to an appropriate depth by lowering the bottle and letting the fluid in the tube run back into the chamber. The tube should be refilled, clamped, and an eighteen or nineteen gauge needle attached. The needle should be sharp, and a small amount of fluid should be allowed to run out to ensure it is not obstructed.

5. The patient's arm should be held in one hand with the thumb stretching the skin tight over the vein into which the needle is to be inserted.

6. The needle should be held parallel to the vein with the bevel upward. It should be inserted quickly through the skin and more slowly into the vein. A slight amount of "give" may be felt as the vein is entered. To prevent its being dislodged, the needle should be threaded upward inside the vein for a short distance. This step usually causes the most trouble because the needle can be thrust through the opposite side of the vein. If the tip of the needle is lifted slightly, pulling the bevel toward the upper vein wall and holding the point in the center of the lumen, the danger of penetrating the opposite wall is reduced.

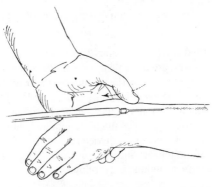

Figure 56. Technique for inserting a needle for intravenous fluid therapy.

7. If the needle has been properly inserted, blood may be seen in the tubing. Squeezing the tubing or lowering the bottle of fluids below the level of the patient and opening the clamp causes blood to flow back into the tubing if the needle is correctly located within the vein, and indicates that administration of fluids can be started.

8. The bottle of fluids should be suspended two to three feet above the patient's body, the clamp on the tubing released, and the tourniquet removed from the patient's arm.

9. Once the fluids are flowing satisfactorily, the needle should be anchored with tape. Gauze pads may be helpful in securing the hub of the needle. The last eight to ten inches of tubing should be formed into an "S" or "U" and taped to the patient's arm. Such loops should absorb any accidental pulls on the apparatus and prevent dislodging the needle. If the victim is not fully conscious or is thrashing about, his arm should be anchored in some manner while fluids are being given. During all manipulations with the needle or dispensing apparatus, caution must be exercised to prevent penetrating the wall of the vein with the needle.

10. Usually the clamp on the tubing should be partially closed so that the fluid is flowing at approximately 125 drops per minute (500 cc per hour). However, plasma administration following a severe hemorrhage or fluid replacement for disorders such as cholera may have to be made at much faster rates in order for the patient to receive adequate quantities in a limited time. Occasionally fluids must be given at more than one site in order to achieve the needed speed of administration.

11. Swelling at the site of the needle tip indicates the needle has punctured the vein and fluids are being infiltrated into the tissue. The needle must be withdrawn and inserted at another site. No effort should be made to reinsert the needle in the original vein until all swelling has disappeared, which usually requires several hours. The swelling usually produces little or no discomfort and requires no specific treatment.

12. If the fluid fails to flow when the tubing is unclamped, the needle may be obstructed. Changing its position slightly may move the bevel away from the wall of the vein and restart the flow. Squeezing the tubing may force out small clots or plugs of tissue blocking the needle. If the tourniquet on the upper arm is not removed the fluid can not flow. Occasionally such measures are not successful in starting or restarting flow and the needle must be withdrawn, a new needle attached to the tubing, and the fluids administered at another site.

13. When more than one bottle of fluids is to be given, as is usual, a dispensing apparatus often can be inserted into the second bottle, the tubing filled as described, and the tip of the tubing inserted into the air intake of the first bottle. This measure eliminates the need for clamping the tubing to the patient just as the last fluid runs out of the bottle but before the drip chamber empties and then trying to insert the dispenser into the second bottle before blood clots in the needle and obstructs it.

14. The veins used for intravenous fluid therapy frequently clot after the needle is withdrawn and are not suitable for subsequent use. In situations where intravenous fluid therapy for several days or more is anticipated, the first infusions should be placed near the patient's wrists and subsequent infusions placed higher up the arms as the veins become obstructed.

15. The veins on the back of the hands should not be used for intravenous therapy if other sites are available as this area is quite sensitive. Also, the veins in this location move about quite readily and needles inserted into them tend to be easily dislodged. The veins in the fold of the arm at the elbow, where blood for laboratory analysis is usually withdrawn, are also less suitable for fluid administration because very slight flexing of the arm can dislodge the needle.

16. Occasionally veins for intravenous therapy are impossible to find, particularly in fat people or patients who are in shock or severely dehydrated. In such circumstances, fluids can be administered by inserting the needle

beneath the skin of the back, abdomen, or upper thighs and letting the fluid infiltrate the subcutaneous space. Absorption from such sites is erratic, and administration may produce some discomfort, but when the fluids are needed, this route is better than not giving fluids at all. Medications should not be administered in this manner.

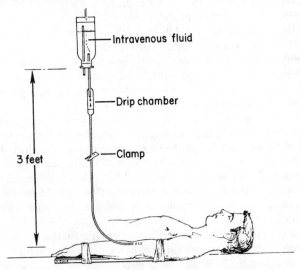

Figure 57. Apparatus for the administration of intravenous fluids.

NASOGASTRIC INTUBATION

Nasogastric intubation is highly desirable for the care of patients with paralytic ileus (intestinal paralysis). All of the serious diseases associated with severe, acute abdominal pain produce such paralysis, but the effects are most severe in disorders causing peritonitis or intestinal obstruction.

Everyone swallows large quantities of air when eating or drinking and at other times. This air is the source of most of the gas always present in the gastrointestinal tract. If the stomach is paralyzed and its contents can not be expelled into the intestine, it quickly becomes ballooned with air. The distended stomach impinges on the diaphragm, interfering with respiration; it also presses on the veins in the abdomen, impeding the return of blood from the lower half of the body to the heart. In addition, large quantities of digestive juices, partially digested food, and other fluids are pooled in the stomach. Fluid accumulation and distension eventually lead to vomiting, loss of the fluids and electrolytes, and the danger of pneumonia or respiratory obstruction if the vomitus is aspirated.

A tube inserted through the nose and esophagus into the stomach permits the air that is swallowed to escape and prevents most of these complications. The tube is uncomfortable because it causes a sore throat, but it usually does not cause gagging or similar symptoms.

The use of nasogastric suction is not without hazard since fluids are removed from the stomach as well as air. If these fluids are not replaced intravenously with a balanced salt solution or saline, serious salt and water depletion inevitably results. If fluids for intravenous therapy are not available, the nasogastric tube should be used only to remove air that has collected. After the air has escaped, the tube should be clamped and only reopened when significant quantities of air have reaccumulated.

The technique for nasogastric intubation is as follows:

1. The tube, at least a size eighteen French, should be chilled and the tip lubricated with a bland jelly, mineral oil, or at least water before it is inserted.
2. The patient should be sitting up and should have a container of cold water and a straw, a few pieces of crushed ice, or a handful of snow to swallow.
3. The tube should be inserted through one nostril, along the floor of the nasal cavity, to the back of the throat. Then the patient should be instructed to swallow. As he swallows the tube should be thrust further so the tongue and muscles of the throat can guide it into the esophagus. Several attempts are usually necessary, and when the tube does enter the esophagus the patient should be told to keep swallowing. With each swallow the tube should be rapidly thrust further down until a previously marked length equal to the distance from the patient's nose to his stomach has been inserted.
4. A small amount of air should be injected through the tube after it is in place. If the tube is in the stomach, bubbling sounds made by the injected air can be clearly heard. However, if the tube has coiled in the back of the patient's throat or turned on itself in his esophagus and did not enter the stomach, such sounds are not heard and the tube must be partially withdrawn and reinserted.
5. Rarely the tube may enter the patient's trachea, causing him to cough and sometimes to be unable to talk. If the tube is withdrawn promptly, no harm is done, but the patient may be understandably reluctant to undergo further attempts at intubation.
6. After the tube is in place it should be taped to the patient's nose or forehead to prevent its being expelled or swallowed entirely. Air and fluid in the stomach can be withdrawn with a syringe equipped with an attachment to fit the tubing. After the stomach is emptied, the tube should be attached to a suction apparatus constructed by suspending a jar filled with water several feet above the patient's body, as shown in the accompanying diagram.

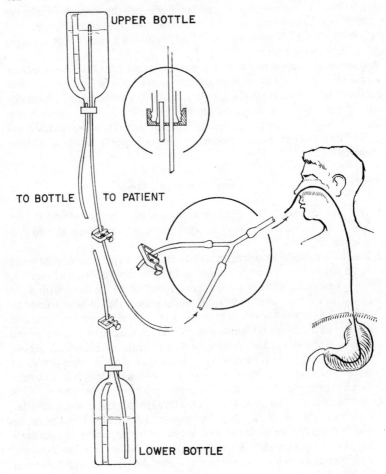

Figure 58. Apparatus for applying gentle suction to a nasogastric tube.

7. Nasogastric tubes have a tendency to become obstructed by mucus or particles of food. Therefore, the tube should be flushed with a small amount of a salt solution every two hours. (Water should not be used if a salt solution is available.) The fluid used to irrigate the tube must be subtracted from the total volume lost through the tube when calculating the patient's fluid requirements.

8. The total volume of fluid lost through the nasogastric tube must be carefully measured and recorded. All of the fluid lost in this manner should be replaced intravenously with a balanced salt solution or saline.

URETHRAL CATHETERIZATION

Following prolonged periods of unconsciousness or after severe injuries, particularly injuries in which the lower portion of the body is paralyzed, the urinary bladder may become severely distended. Due to stretching of the bladder muscles and pressure against the opening of the bladder, the patient may be unable to void. To relieve the distension a catheter must be inserted into the bladder through the urethra. The discomfort from this procedure is surprisingly small, usually much less than the pain from a distended bladder.

Urethral catheterization is rarely required for females, whose much shorter urethra offers far less resistance to voiding, particularly for young women who would be partaking in a mountaineering outing. If urethral catheterization is needed for a female, it must be carried out by someone with enough knowledge of female anatomy to correctly identify the urethral opening.

Rarely an individual with a distended bladder repeatedly voids a small amount but does not completely empty his bladder. For such individuals, distension requires longer to develop but can become much more severe because it is less obvious. Since the individual is voiding, the primary symptom is the severe discomfort from the distended bladder.

Usually about eight to ten hours are required for the bladder to become distended. Urethral catheterization can often be avoided if the patient can be induced to void before that much time has elapsed. Having him stand up and walk around for a few minutes or placing his hand in warm water is frequently helpful in achieving his goal.

The greatest hazard from urethral catheterization is the danger of introducing infection. Meticulous care to avoid contamination of the catheter greatly reduces the incidence of such complications.

The following procedure should be followed for urethral catheterization:

1. Everything needed must be assembled before the procedure is begun. Any break to obtain a forgotten item invites contamination and infection. The required supplies consist of a sterile urinary catheter, size sixteen or eighteen French, sterile rubber or plastic gloves or sterile instruments to handle the catheter, sterile lubricating ointment, and alcohol swabs. A sterile towel on which to place the items is a great convenience and helps avoid contamination. The sterile wrapper from the gloves may be an appropriate substitute. A receptacle to collect the urine should also be on hand, particularly if the volume of urine must be measured.

2. The glans penis must be cleaned with alcohol, a disinfectant, or just soap and water and the catheter must be removed from its container without being contaminated. The circumstances and assistance available should determine which is done first, but the glans should not touch any nonsterile objects after it has been cleaned.
3. A small amount of a sterile lubricant should be applied to the catheter tip.
4. With the patient in the supine position, the catheter should be inserted into the urethra and gently threaded upward until urine begins to flow from the open end. This maneuver is facilitated if the penis is pulled upward to straighten the urethra and eliminate any folds in the mucosa lining this passage.
5. After the urine has ceased to flow the catheter should be gently withdrawn.
6. Most patients require only a single catheterization and are subsequently able to void without difficulty. However, patients with paralysis of the lower portion of their bodies usually have to be catheterized every eight hours to prevent overdistention of the bladder and possible renal injury. In such patients, an indwelling (Foley) catheter should be inserted. This type of catheter has a small balloon just below the tip. After the catheter has been inserted this balloon can be inflated by injecting fluid with a syringe and needle into the nipple provided for this purpose on the external end of the catheter. The balloon must be deflated by clipping off the end of this nipple before the catheter is withdrawn. However, a catheter of this kind can usually be left in place for three to five days. To reduce the risk of infection, the patient may be treated with trimethoprim-sulfamethoxazole.

TUBE THORACOTOMY

Tube thoracotomy is a severely hazardous procedure. The possible complications include infection, puncture of the heart or a major blood vessel, laceration of the lung, or even penetration of the diaphragm and laceration of the liver or spleen, all of which would probably be disastrous in a wilderness situation. This procedure must only be attempted when all of the following conditions can be met:

1. The patient is dying as the result of impaired respiratory function due to air or fluid in the chest, which would almost always be the result of traumatic injury.
2. All of the required equipment is available: flutter valve, trochar or means for inserting the tube, and the necessary tubing. A local anesthetic and means for preventing infection are also desirable.
3. The person performing the procedure has received prior instruction from a physician.

In spite of the hazards it presents, this procedure may be lifesaving if performed properly for patients with a severe pneumothorax, particularly at high altitudes. Tube thoracotomy should be performed as follows:

1. If possible, the patient should be sitting up with his arms forward, propped in this position if necessary. If he can not sit up, he should have his head and chest higher than the rest of his body, and the side of the chest in which the tube is to be inserted should be uppermost.

2. If the patient's condition allows time, the attendant should scrub his hands and arms with soap, preferably one containing hexachlorophene, or Betadine and a brush for ten minutes by the clock.

3. A wide area of the patient's chest wall above the nipple on the injured side should be similarly scrubbed. Subsequently this area should be swabbed with iodine followed by alcohol, Zephiran, Betadine, or just alcohol if nothing else is available.

4. If sterile rubber gloves are available, they should be put on after the attendant's hands have been scrubbed and the patient's chest has been scrubbed and swabbed with an antiseptic.

5. The rib at the same level as the nipple or at its upper margin should be identified. A point just lateral to the nipple, or just beyond the edge of the breast for females, and at the upper margin of the rib should be selected for the thoracotomy.

6. The point selected should be anesthetized by infiltration with a local anesthetic (lidocaine). The infiltration should extend down to the rib and over its upper border.

7. A flutter valve (Heimlich valve) should be attached to one end of the chest tubing before the thoracotomy is begun. The valve must be checked to be certain it is not attached backwards.

8a. If a trochar is available, a small nick about one-quarter inch (6 mm) in length should be made in the skin with a sterile scalpel blade to facilitate its insertion. The trochar should be pushed firmly through the chest wall until it stops against the rib. Then the tip should be moved upward slightly until it passes over the top of the rib, thus avoiding the blood vessels that course along the bottom of every rib. The chest wall is one and one-half to two and one-half inches (4 to 6.5 cm) thick, depending upon the individual's muscularity and the amount of fat present.

8b. If a trochar is not available, a one inch (2.5 cm) incision should be made with a sterile scalpel and carried down to the rib. The bleeding that accompanies this incision can safely be ignored. The rib should be palpated with a sterile finger to ensure its upper margin is located.

9a. After the trochar passes over the top of the rib, it should be pushed into the chest cavity. A gush of air or fluid should be encountered as the pleura is entered. The tubing with flutter valve attached should be passed through the trochar so that two to three inches of tubing extends beyond the trochar into the chest. While holding the tubing to make sure it is not pulled out, the trochar should be withdrawn. (Leaking of air around the tubing is prevented by the muscles and other tissues of the chest wall.)

9b. With a pair of forceps or with a scalpel — carefully — the muscle above the rib and the underlying pleura should be punctured. A gush of air or blood should be encountered. Puncturing the pleura is usually painful in spite of the local anesthetic and the patient may require reassurance. A sterile finger can briefly palpate the inner surface of the pleura to ensure the chest has been entered. Then the tubing should be inserted, using the finger in the incision to guide it into position with about two inches extending into the pleural cavity.

10. Usually the patient experiences marked relief of his respiratory difficulties immediately or within a few minutes after the tube has been inserted.

11. The tube should be anchored to the chest wall with tape so that it can not be pulled out or forced farther into the chest. A sterile bandage should be placed around the opening in the chest wall.

12. After the tube is in place, air and perhaps a little blood can be seen to pass through the valve whenever the patient coughs. With severe lung injuries such emissions can be seen during quiet respiration. The valve should collapse during inspiration to prevent air being sucked into the chest.

13. If a large amount of fluid or blood is being lost through the tube, a sterile receptacle of some type should be attached to the end away from the patient, preferably with a second length of tubing, in order to measure the volume of the loss and prevent soiling the the patient's clothing, sleeping bag, or other items.

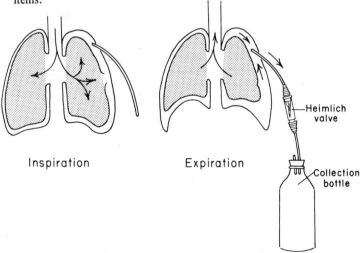

Inspiration   Expiration   —Heimlich valve

Collection bottle

Figure 59. Pulmonary function with a pneumothorax treated by tube thoracotomy. (Adapted from *Surgery of the Chest,* 3rd ed.)

STERILIZATION

Sterilization of instruments before they can be used is sometimes necessary. At sea level, boiling in water for fifteen minutes provides adequate sterilization, but equipment must be available for removing the items from the water without contaminating them. At altitudes above 3,000 to 4,000 feet (900 to 1,200 m), the boiling temperature of water is lower and boiling must be continued for an hour to obtain adequate sterilization. However, boiling in a pressure cooker for fifteen minutes under fifteen pounds pressure should be adequate at almost any altitude.

Scalpels, forceps, scissors, and similar metal instruments can be sterilized by washing them thoroughly, dipping them in alcohol, and lighting the alcohol. The instruments must be permitted to cool before they are used. However, blowing on the items to cool them causes contamination with bacteria from the nose and mouth.

Regardless of the manner they have been sterilized, needles and syringes used for one individual must never be used to administer injections to another. The methods of sterilization in the field are too uncertain and the risk of transmitting hepatitis too great to chance such a dangerous infection in this manner. Most needles and syringes currently available are disposable — designed to be used only once and then discarded. Supplies of this type should be secured for mountaineering outings. Other items such as forceps and scalpels are also being produced in sterile, disposable kits which are equally convenient and relatively inexpensive.

Dressings and instruments should be wrapped in paper and autoclaved. Items protected in this manner remain sterile for several months if they are undisturbed and stay dry. However, if the items are wet, sterility is lost.

Medical Supplies

No climbing party can be completely prepared for any and all accidents or illnesses. Only the materials needed for common medical problems can be carried. However, the additional materials needed for severe accidents or prolonged major illnesses should be available: at a base camp for expeditions, or at a central location in popular climbing areas. Obviously, larger parties can carry a larger quantity and a greater variety of medical supplies.

The following lists contain the materials most likely to be needed for treating acute medical disorders. Personal Medical Supplies suggests the items that probably should be carried by everyone on almost any outing. Outing Medical Supplies suggests supplies that should be available in major climbing areas and on smaller expeditions to remote areas. The Air Drop Medical Kit suggests supplies that should be available by air drop to victims of major accidents and possibly should be carried by major expeditions. Physicians should be consulted when determining the dosages and quantities of the items to be included.

Medications for preexisting disorders, such as diabetes or asthma, must be supplied by the individuals with such conditions.

Personal Medical Supplies

Aspirin, 300 mg tablets	20 or more
Meperidine, 50 mg tablets	10 or more
or	
Morphine, 16 mg tablets	10 or more
Band-Aids, large	10 or more
Sterile gauze pads, four-inch squares	6 or more
Porous adhesive tape, two-inch width	1 roll
Moleskin, four-inch squares	4 to 6
Elastic bandage, three-inch width	1 or 2
Triangular bandage	2 or 3
Tweezers	1 per party
Sunburn preventative containing para-aminobenzoic acid	
Antiseptic such as Betadine, Zepharin, or seventy percent ethyl or isopropyl alcohol	
Personal medications	

Outing Medical Kit

Medications (oral unless otherwise specified)
  Analgesics
    Aspirin and/or acetominophen
    Codeine
    Morphine (oral and injectable)
        or
    Meperidine (oral and injectable)
    Dibucaine ointment
  Antimicrobial preparations
    Penicillins
      Phenoxymethyl penicillin
      Ampicillin (oral and intramuscular)
      Cloxicillin
    Tetracycline
    Trimethaprim-sulfamethaoxazole
    Neosporin opthalmic drops
    Substitute antibiotics for members allergic to penicillin or sulfa drugs
    Antimalarials appropriate for area
    Wound antiseptic
  Gastrointestinal medications
    One or more antacids
    One or more motion sickness agents
    One or more antispasmodics
    One or more laxatives
    One or more antidiarrheal agents
  Cardiac and respiratory drugs
    A systemic decongestant
    A local decongestant spray
    Epinephrine
  Others
    One or more antihistamines
    Sunburn preventatives
    Antiinflammatory steroids

Bandages and dressings
  Sterile gauze pads
  Vaseline gauze
  Band-Aids
  Sterile absorbent cotton
  Eye pads
  Triangular bandages

    Adhesive tape
    Elastic bandages
    Moleskin

Equipment
    Surgical forceps and tweezers
    Scissors
    Scalpel with blades
    Syringes and needles
    Stethoscope
    Sphygmomanometer
    Plastic oral airway
    Tracheostomy device
    Tongue blades
    Inflatable splints
    Hot water bottle

Items in personal medical kit

Air Drop Medical Kit

Items in outing medical kit

Intravenous fluids (plastic containers)
    Balanced salt solution
    Five or ten percent glucose
    Plasma or plasma expander
    Tubing and needles for administration
    Intravenous antibiotics

Oxygen bottles, masks, valves, and tubing

Equipment for therapeutic procedures
    Sterile gloves, lidocaine, syringes and needles
    Trochar, tubing, and valves for thoracostomy
    Tubes, bottles, and syringes for nasogastric intubation
    Catheters and lubricant for urethral catheterization

Inflatable leg and arm splints

Additional medications for known medical problems

Rescue gear
    Ropes, carabiners, nuts or pitons, bolts, hammers, and pulleys
    Ice axes, ice screws
    Collapsible or wheel equipped stretchers

Camping gear
    Sleeping bags
    Tents
    Clothing

Food and potable water

Two way radio

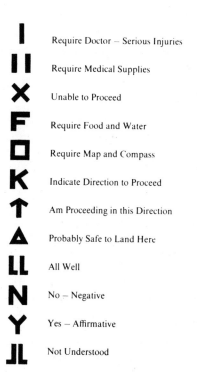

I	Require Doctor – Serious Injuries
II	Require Medical Supplies
X	Unable to Proceed
F	Require Food and Water
□	Require Map and Compass
K	Indicate Direction to Proceed
↑	Am Proceeding in this Direction
▲	Probably Safe to Land Here
LL	All Well
N	No – Negative
Y	Yes – Affirmative
JL	Not Understood

Figure 60. Standard symbols for ground-to-air communication.

APPENDIX D

Legal Considerations

Few climbers would question their obligation to provide medical care or assist in the evacuation of an ill or injured climber, whether a member of their party or another. None of the following should raise doubts about that responsibility. However, some discussion of the legal rights and obligations of persons rendering medical aid to others appears appropriate.

These comments are intended to provide only a general outline of the laws applicable in the United States and Canada. Each state, province, and nation makes its own rules concerning many problems, and the variation from place to place is often considerable. Anyone concerned about such problems must obtain specific information about the area with which he is involved.

PERSONAL LIABILITY

Almost no country has laws that require anyone to help a stranger in distress. A climber can decline to provide medical assistance to anyone with legal impunity. Any obligation that might exist in mountaineering circumstances is ethical or traditional, not legal. A legal obligation to provide medical care or other assistance does exist if the climber has negligently caused injury to another.

If medical assistance is provided, even though not required by law, it must be performed in a reasonable and careful manner. The diligence that would be exercised by an ordinarily prudent person under similar circumstances must be observed. Anyone providing medical care is legally liable for harm caused to the injured person if the harm could have been avoided by reasonable carefulness. Additionally, more severe injuries or diseases are recognized to require closer attention and more extensive and sophisticated medical assistance.

The circumstances in which assistance is rendered are also significant. **The care legally required is that which is reasonable under the circumstances.** The law takes into account such factors as the location of the victim, hazards for the person rendering aid, the equipment available, and the physical condition of the parties.

A physician is held to a higher standard. He must conduct himself as an ordinarily prudent doctor of medicine. Similarly, since the need for familiarity with basic first aid by climbers is well recognized, and many have such knowledge, a climber could be held liable for injuries resulting from his failure to be familiar with first aid techniques generally known to climbers if he had indicated in some manner beforehand that he did have such knowledge.

Although a legal basis for claims sometimes does exist, lawsuits arising from voluntary medical assistance are rare. For mountaineering accidents and illnesses only a few such claims have been filed.

ESTABLISHING DEATH

The problem of establishing that a person is dead is primarily medical — not legal. A doctor's death certificate is the customary method. If a doctor is not available, a statement by persons who have actually seen the body and checked it for life usually suffices. Following a fall or an avalanche in which the body can not be recovered or can not even be found, the statements of those who witnessed the accident is ordinarily adequate. If no one saw the accident, death may still be established satisfactorily by circumstantial evidence, such as abandoned equipment, a deserted automobile or campsite, or the last statements of the deceased.

However, if such evidence can not be found, and only the disappearance of the missing person into a mountainous area can be demonstrated, particularly if the mountainous area is one from which he would be expected to be able to walk out of without unusual difficulty — not the Himalayas — death might be impossible to establish, and enough time must pass to allow a legal "presumption" of death, usually seven years.

DISPOSAL OF THE BODY

The next of kin and the local law enforcement agencies both have a legal interest in the body. The next of kin usually have the right to determine whether the body shall be cremated or buried, where this shall be done, what religious ceremony shall be performed, and what other customs are to be followed. The law enforcement agencies must determine the cause of death, ensuring no crimes have been committed and no threat of an epidemic or similar public health hazard exists, and make certain the body is disposed of promptly without offending public sensibilities. Ordinarily, cremation or burial must be performed within a few days and the remains placed in a cemetery or similar appropriate site.

If the body is in a remote, inaccessible location, the next of kin and the law enforcement officials may decide to leave the body where it is. Following a mountaineering death, the members of a climbing party are not legally obligated to retrieve or even find the body.

APPENDIX D

ESTATE AND LIFE INSURANCE

Death occurring in the mountains, even if the body is not recoverable, does not pose insurmountable problems in the administration of an estate or in the settlement of life insurance claims. For administration of the estate, death must be proven, but the testimony of persons who actually saw the body is sufficient to establish the fact of death.

If the deceased had life insurance, proof of death is a necessary condition for the payment of benefits from such insurance. In general, proof of death that is adequate for administration of the estate is sufficient for life insurance.

A different problem is raised by insurance that had a double indemnity provision. Such clauses provide a payment that is double the face amount of insurance if death is accidental. Therefore, the exact cause of death must be ascertained so far as is possible. For example, after a fall the question of whether death resulted from a heart attack which precipitated the fall might be raised. If a heart attack caused a fall but injuries from the fall killed the victim, death would have been accidental and the double indemnity provision would apply. However, if the victim died before the fall as the result of a heart attack, death would not have been accidental and the double indemnity provision would not apply. Deciding which occurred is not easy and may be impossible. In single vehicle automobile accidents in which the victim has a heart attack and then wrecks his car, double indemnity is commonly paid because injuries from the wreck can not be proven not to have caused the victim's death. (Many individuals survive heart attacks.)

The best method for answering such questions is to carefully examine the accident site and the victims, thoroughly question all witnesses to the accident, and record all details of the findings as soon as possible after the accident has occurred. The body may need to be evacuated for an autopsy in order to establish the cause of death.

Glossary

ACUTE 1. Appearing after or persisting for a relatively brief period of time. (This term does not indicate a specific time period, but refers to a short interval of time relative to the condition for which it is used. An acute onset would mean minutes for some diseases, weeks for others.) 2. Requiring immediate or urgent attention.

AIRWAY The passages through which air enters and leaves the lungs.

ANALGESIA The relief of pain.

ANALGESIC A medication that relieves pain.

ANEMIA A condition in which the number of red blood cells in the circulating blood is smaller than normal.

ARRHYTHMIA An abnormal rhythm, usually referring to the heart.

ASPIRATE To breathe in (air is aspirated into the lungs); to draw in by suction (fluid is aspirated into a syringe).

AVULSION An injury in which tissue is torn away or forcibly separated.

BLEB A large blister.

CARRIER A person who is immune to an infection but transmits it to others as a result of carrying the organisms in his body.

CATHETER A slender, tubular instrument introduced through an anatomical passage into an internal organ. (A urethral or urinary catheter is passed into the urinary bladder through the urethra.)

CENTRAL NERVOUS SYSTEM The brain and spinal cord.

CERVICAL Pertaining to the neck.

CHRONIC Appearing after or persisting for a relatively long time; opposite of acute. (See Acute.)

COMA A state of total unconsciousness.

COMATOSE Totally unconscious.

CYANOSIS A purple or bluish discoloration observed in the lips and nails, and sometimes the skin, resulting from reduced amounts of oxygen in the blood.

DIAGNOSE To distinguish one disease or injury from another; to identify an illness or injury.

DIAGNOSIS The identification of an illness or injury.

DYSPNEA Abnormal shortness of breath; awareness of the need to breathe.

EDEMA An abnormal collection of fluid in some part of the body. (Pulmonary edema — an abnormal collection of fluid in the lungs.)

EMBOLISM Sudden obstruction of a blood vessel by an embolus.

EMBOLUS A clot or similar obstruction brought by the bloodstream from a distant blood vessel, such as a leg vein, through the more proximal larger vessels and heart and forced into a smaller artery, most commonly in the lung.

ENDEMIC Peculiar to or prevailing in or among some (specified) country or people.

EXUDATE Any substance, most commonly inflammatory cells and protein, that passes through blood vessel walls in living cellular tissue and is available for removal or extraction. Most frequently associated with inflammation.

FASCIA A sheet or membrane of fibrous tissue investing muscles or various other structures.

FLACCID Completely relaxed.

FLATUS Gas or air in the intestines.

GANGRENE The death of a part of the body, such as an arm or leg, usually as the result of an inadequate blood supply.

GENERALIZED Spread throughout the body as opposed to localized.

HALLUCINATION A sound, sight, or other sensation perceived by a person as a reality in the absence of an actually existing object or source.

HYDRATED Containing water. (Normally hydrated — containing a normal amount of water.)

INCUBATION PERIOD The period of time between infection by microorganisms and the onset of detectable signs or symptoms of the disease.

INTRAMUSCULAR Within muscle; commonly used to indicate the site for injection of a medication.

INTRAVENOUS Within a vein; commonly used to indicate the site for injection of a medication.

JAUNDICE An abnormal condition caused by the accumulation of bile pigments in the blood, usually resulting from liver disease, and characterized by yellow discoloration of the skin and eyes.

LUMEN The passageway within a tubular organ such as the intestines or a blood vessel.

MACERATE To reduce to a soft mass by soaking; to digest.

MALAISE A feeling of generalized discomfort or indisposition; feeling ill.

MENINGITIS Inflammation of the thin membranes that surround the brain and spinal cord, usually the result of infection.

METABOLISM In living organisms, the processes taking place that use energy to build substances from assimilated materials or break them down to release energy.

NEUROLOGIC Of or pertaining to the nervous system.

OSMOSIS The diffusion of a solution through a semipermeable membrane.

OSMOTIC PRESSURE The hydrostatic pressure created by diffusion through a semipermeable membrane.

PALPATE To feel or examine by touch.

PALPATION The process of examining the body by touch.

PALPITATION A rapid or irregular heartbeat of which the patient is aware.

PARALYTIC ILEUS Paralysis of the intestine producing functional obstruction, most often caused by peritonitis.

PATHOGENIC Producing disease.

PERITONITIS Inflammation of the thin membrane lining the abdominal cavity, usually resulting from infection or chemical irritation by intestinal contents or blood.

PROGNOSIS A prediction or conclusion regarding the course and termination of a disease or injury.

PRONE Lying flat in a face down position.

PROPHYLAXIS Preventive treatment for disease.

PULMONARY Of or pertaining to the lungs.

PURULENT Consisting of or containing pus; associated with the formation of or caused by pus.

RADIATION OF PAIN The sensation of pain experienced in an area other than the anatomical site of the injury or disease producing the pain.

RENAL Of or pertaining to the kidneys.

RESORB To reabsorb.

SOFT TISSUE The nonosseous tissues of the body. (The joint ligaments and internal organs are not included as this term is most commonly used.)

SOMNOLENCE Oppressive drowsiness or sleepiness.

SPASM An involuntary muscular contraction.

SPINAL CANAL The canal within the vertebral column which contains the spinal cord.

SPRAIN An injury characterized by incomplete rupture of the supporting ligaments around a joint.

STRAIN An injury characterized by stretching, with or without mild tearing, of a muscle or tendon.

SUBACUTE Appearing after or persisting for a period of time that is intermediate between acute and chronic and duration. (See Acute.)

SUBCUTANEOUS Beneath the skin.

SUPINE Lying flat in a face up position.

SUTURE To unite parts by stitching; to sew together the cut edges of injured tissues.

SYNDROME A group of signs and symptoms that occur together and comprise a disease entity.

TOXIC Having a poisonous or noxious effect.

TOXIN A noxious or poisonous substance.

TRAUMA A physical force that injures the body; an injury produced by physical force. Any external force that produces injury, such as emotional trauma.

TRAUMATIC Of or pertaining to trauma.

VASCULAR Of or pertaining to blood vessels.

INDEX

Abdominal injuries 164–70
  bleeding 167–68
  contusion 167
  nonpenetrating 167–69
  penetrating 169–70
  See also specific organ
Abdominal pain 314–40
  appendicitis 319–20
  gallbladder disease 324
  gastroenteritis 318
  hernia 322–23
  intestinal obstruction 320–21
  kidney stone 326–27, 333
  mittelschmerz 318–19
  pancreatitis 324–25
  peritonitis 326
  salpingitis 319
  ulcer 321–22
Abrasions 102
Abscesses 361–62
Acclimatization, altitude 178–81
Acetaminophen 378
Acetazolamide 394
Actifed 399
Adrenalin 396–97
Airway 46–51
Allergies 369–73
  anaphylactic shock 371–73
  contact dermatitis 370–71
  food 292

hay fever 370
hives 370
poison ivy dermatitis 371
Altitude 172–98
  acclimatization 178–81
  edema, cerebral 190–92
  edema, pulmonary 183–89
  edema, systemic 192–93
  mountain sickness, acute 182–83
  mountain sickness, persistent
    193–96
  nutrition 196
  physical performance 174–77
  retinal hemorrhage 192
  sleep hypoxia 177
  tolerance 181
Ambulation 30
Amebiasis 303–304
Aminoglycosides 388–89
Aminophylline 397
Amobarbital 383–84
Ampicillin 386–87
Anal fissure 306
Anaphylactic shock 371–73
Angina pectoris 279
Animal bites 230–50
  rabies 230–34
  scorpion stings 250–52
  snake bite 234–47
  spider bite 247–50

Ankle fractures 116
Antacids 402
Antibacterials 360-61, 385-92
  aminoglycosides 388-89
  ampicillin 386-87
  bacitracin 390
  Bactrim 391
  benzalkonium chloride 392-93
  cephalosporins 387
  chloramphenicol 389
  chloroquin 391-92
  clindamycin 388
  cloxacillin 386-87
  dicloxacillin 386-87
  erythromycin 387-88
  Fansidar 392
  gentamicin 388-89
  kanamycin 388-89
  methicillin 386-87
  Nafcillin 386-87
  neomycin 388-89, 390
  Neosporin 390
  penicillin 385-87
  polymyxin B 390
  pyrimethamine 392
  Septra 391
  streptomycin 388-89
  sulfadoxine 392
  tetracycline 389-90
  Trimethoprim-Sulfamethoxazole
    391
  Zephiran 392-93
Antihistamines 400-401
  Antivert 400
  Benadryl 400-401
  Bonine 400
  chlorpheniramine 400
  cyclizine 400
  dimenhydrinate 400
  diphenhydramine 400-401
  Dramamine 400
  Marezine 400
  meclizine 400
Antiseptics 96
  Betadine 92, 393-94
  Zephiran (benzalkonium chloride)
    392-93

Antispasmodics 402-403
Antivenom, snake 243
  spider 249
Antivert 400
Appendicitis 319-20
Artificial respiration 55-56
Aspirin 377-78
Asthma 266-68
Atrial fibrillation 282
Avalanches 36
Avulsions 102-103

Bacitracin 390
Back, fracture 120-21
  injuries 131-32
  ruptured disc 131-32
  strain 131
Bacteremia 362-63
Bactrim 391
Bandaging 100-101
Barbiturates 383-84
Barotrauma 152-53
Benadryl 385, 400
Benzalkonium chloride 392-93
Benzodiazepines 384-85
Betadine 92, 393-94
Black widow spider, bite 248-49
Bleeding, abdominal 167-68
  chest 160-61
  control 94-95
  gastrointestinal 310-11
  in fractures 111
  kidney 333
  lung 160-61
  uterine 335
Blisters 106-107
Blood pressure 276-77
  high 285-86
  stroke 348-49
Blood vessels 274, 285-87
  varicose veins 286-87
Bonine 400
Brain disorders 341-49
  convulsions 344-46
  headache 343
  infections 346-47
  stroke 348-49

Brain injuries 142–46
Breathing. *See* Respiratory disorders
Breathing abnormalities 260–62
　hyperventilation 261–62
　rhythm disorders 260–61
Bronchitis 263
Brown recluse spider, bite 249–50
Burns 133–41
　evacuation 134–35
　facial 140
　fluid balance 137–39
　pain 139–40
　shock 134
Bursitis 129–30

"Cafe coronary" 51–53
Calluses 131
Canker sores 357
Cardiac, resuscitation 56–58
　syncope 283
Cardiopulmonary resuscitation 53–59
Catheterization 413–14
Cellulitis 362
Cephalosporins 387
Cerebral edema 190–92
Chest injuries 154–63
　bleeding 160–61
　closed 155
　flail chest 156–57
　hemothorax 160–61
　perforating 161–63
　pneumothorax 158–60
　rib fractures 155
Chest pain 279
Chest tube 414–16
Chills 41–42
Chloral hydrate 385
Chloramphenicol 389
Chloroquin 391–92
Chlorpheniramine 400
Choking 51–53
Cholecystitis 324
Cholera 82, 300
Clavicle fractures 115
Clindamycin 388
Cloxacillin 386–87
Codeine 379

Cold injuries 199–216
Cold sores 357
Colds 352–53
Collar bone fractures 115
Colorado tick fever 365
Compartmental syndromes 128–29
Conjunctivitis 350–51
Constipation 304–308
Contact lens 351
Contraceptives 335–36
Contusions 103–104
　bone 126
Convulsions 344–46
Corns 131
"CPR" (cardiopulmonary
　resuscitation) 53–59
Cyclizine 400
Cystitis 330

Dalmane 384–85
Datril 378
Death 77–78, 423
Dehydration 32
Demerol 381
Dermatitis, contact 370–71
　poison ivy 371
Diamox 394
Diarrhea 290–304
Dibucaine 381–82
Dicloxacillin 386–87
Digitalis 283, 396
Digoxin 396
Dimenhydrinate 400
Diphenhydramine 400
Diphenoxylate 401
Disc 131–32
Dislocations 122–26
　elbow 123–24
　fingers 123
　jaw 125–26
　knee 125
　shoulder 124–25
Diuretics 394–95
Donnatal 403
Dramamine 400
Drugs. *See* Medications
Dysentery, bacillary 301–302

Dysmenorrhea 334

Ear, infections 357–58
  injuries 151–52
  middle 152–53
Earache 281
Edema, cerebral 190–92
  pulmonary 183–89
  systemic 192–93
Elbow fractures 114
Embolism 195, 269–73
Emergencies 34–35
  anaphylactic shock 371–73
Encephalitis 346–47
Epididymitis 336–37
Epinephrine 396–97
Erythromycin 387–88
Evacuation 37–39, 112–13, 121,
  142–43
  burns 134–35
Examination 20–21, 23–25
Extrasystoles 284–85
Eye disorders 350–51
  conjunctivitis 350–51
  hemorrhage 351
Eye injuries 149–51
  retinal hemorrhage 192
  snow blindness 222–23
Eyeglasses 351
Eyelid injuries 150–51

Facial injuries 148–49
  fractures 148–49
Fainting 343–44
Fansidar 392
Fecal impaction 305–306
Femur fractures 116–18
Fever 40–41. *See also specific disease
  or injury*
Fever blisters 357
Fibrillation, atrial 282
Fingers, dislocations 123
  fractures 113–14
First aid kits 418–21
Flail chest 156–57
Fluid balance 31–34
  burns 137–39

dehydration 32–33
Fluid therapy (intravenous) 407–10
Food, allergy 292
  aspiration 51–53
Foot, fractures 115–16
  injury 104
Forearm fractures 114
Fractures 108–126
  ankle 116
  arm, upper 114
  back 120–21
  clavicle 115
  collar bone 115
  elbow 114
  facial 148–49
  femur 116–18
  fingers 113–14
  foot 115–16
  forearm 114
  hand 113–14
  hip 118
  humerus 114
  jaw 115
  knee 116
  kneecap 116
  leg 116
  neck 120–21
  open 112
  pain of 112
  pelvis 119–20
  rib 155
  shoulder 114
  skull 146–47
  spine 120–21
  thigh 116–119
  toes 115
  vertebra 120–21
Frostbite 213–16
Frusemide 394–95
Furosemide 394–95

Gallbladder disease 324
Gastroenteritis 290–93, 318
Gastrointestinal diseases 288–313
  amebiasis 303–304
  bacillary dysentery 301–302
  cholera 300–301

constipation and rectal problems 304–305
diarrhea 290–304
food allergy 292
giardiasis 298–99
irritable colon syndrome 296
motion sickness 290
staphylococcal enteritis 291
typhoid fever 302–303
ulcer and related problems 308–11
viral enteritis 292
Gastrointestinal medications 401–403
antacids 402
antispasmodics 402–403
diphenoxylate 401
Donnatal 403
Imodium 402
Lomotil 401
Loperamide 402
Pamine 403
paregoric 401
Pro-Banthine 403
Genital herpes 340
Genital problems, female 334–36
male 336–37
Genitourinary disorders 328–40
cystitis 330
dysmenorrhea 334
epididymitis 336–37
glomerulonephritis 332–33
gonorrhea 339
kidney failure 330–32
kidney stones 326–27, 333
pylonephritis 330
syphilis 338–39
testicular pain 336–37
uterine bleeding 335
venereal diseases 337–40
Gentamicin 388–89
Giardiasis 298–99
Glomerulonephritis 332–33
Gonorrhea 339
Grief 60–62

Hand, fractures 113–14
injuries 104–105
Hay fever 370

Head injuries 142–53
brain 142–46
ear 151–52
eye 149–51
facial 148–49
scalp 147
skull fracture 146–47
Headache 343. See also specific disease or injury
Heart 207–218, 274–85
at altitude 278–79
blood pressure 276–77
diseases 279–85
medicines 394–96
pulse 275–77
Heart rhythm abnormalities 282–85
atrial fibrillation 282
cardiac syncope 283
extrasystoles 284–85
paroxysmal tachycardia 282
sinus tachycardia 284
"skipped beats" 284–85
Heartburn 310
Heat illness 223–29
heat exhaustion 226–27
heat stroke 227–28
heat syncope 226–27
muscle cramps 228–29
sunstroke 227–28
Heimlich maneuver 51–53
Helicopters 38–39
Hematoma, subdural 143–46
Hematuria 333
Hemoglobinuria 333–34
Hemorrhage. See Bleeding
Hemorrhoids 306–307
Hemothorax 160–61
Hepatitis 83–85, 311–13
Hernia 322–23
Herpes, genital 340
Herpes simplex 357
High altitude. See Altitude
High blood pressure 285–86
Hip fractures 118
Hives 370
Humerus fractures 114
Hyperventilation 261–62

Hypothermia 199–212
 mild 208–10
 prevention 204–207
 recognition 207–10
 severe 209–12
 treatment 210–12

Ibuprofen 378–79
Immersion foot 216
Immunizations 79–85
 cholera 82
 hepatitis 83–85
 measles 81
 poliomyelitis 81
 rubella 81
 smallpox 81
 tetanus 81–82
 typhoid fever 82
 yellow fever 82
Imodium 402
Indigestion 310
Infections 359–68
 abscesses 361–62
 antibiotics for 360–61
 bacteremia 362–63
 brain 346–47
 cellulitis 362
 Colorado tick fever 365
 ear 357–58
 influenza 363
 lungs 262–66
 malaria 366–68
 mononucleosis, infectious 364
 pulmonary 262–66
 relapsing fever 365
 Rocky Mountain spotted fever
  364–65
 septicemia 362–63
 tick fever 365
 trichinosis 368
 wound 95–100
 yellow fever 366
Influenza 363
Injections, intramuscular 404–405
Insect stings 252–53
Intestinal obstruction 320–21
Intravenous fluids 407–10

Intravenous medications 406–407
Iodine (treatment of water) 86–92
 Betadine 92
 iodine solutions, alcoholic 91
 iodine solution, saturated 89–90
 Kahn-Visscher 89–90, 91
 Lugol's solution 92
 povidone-iodine solutions 92
 resin bound iodine 89, 91
 tetraglycine hydroperiodide 88, 91
 tincture of iodine 89, 91
Irritable colon 296
Isoproterenol 398
Isuprel 398

Jaundice 311
Jaw, dislocation 125–26
 fractures 115
Joints 130

Kahn-Visscher 89–90
Kanamycin 388–89
Kidney disorders 328–34
 bleeding 333
 failure 330–32
 injuries 168
Kidney stone 326–27, 333
Knee, dislocations 125
 fractures 116

Lacerations 101
Lasix 394–95
Leg fractures 116
Legal considerations 422–24
 death, establishing 423
 disposal of body 423
 estate 424
 liability, personal 422–23
 life insurance 424
Librium 384–85
Lidocaine 382
Lightning 36–37
Liver, injuries 168–69
Liver disease 311–13
 hepatitis 311–13
 jaundice 311
Lomotil 401

Loperamide 402
Lugol's solution 92
Lung, bleeding 160–61
  flail chest 156–57
  hyperventilation 261–62
  infections 262–66
  perforating injuries 161–63
  pneumothorax 158–60, 268–69
Lung disorders 256–73
  asthma 266–68
  bronchitis 263
  chronic disease 260
  embolism 195, 269–73
  pleurisy 263–64
  pneumonia 264–66
  rhythm disorders 260–61
Lymph nodes 97–98

Malaria 366–68
Marezine 400
Measles 81
Meclizine 400
Medical history 21–23
Medical record 25–27
Medical supplies 418–21
  air drop 420–21
  outing 419–20
  personal 418
Medications 376–403
  antibiotics 385–94
  antihistamines 400–401
  gastrointestinal 401–403
  heart 394–96
  pain, relief of 376–82
  respiratory 396–401
  sleep or sedation 383–85
Medications, administering 404–407
  intramuscular 404–405
  intravenous 406–407
  oral 404
  subcutaneous 406
Meningitis 346–47
Menstrual, abnormal bleeding 335
  pain 334
Meperidine 381
Methicillin 386–87
Mittelschmerz 318–19

Monge's Syndrome 194–95
Mononucleosis, infectious 364
Morphine 380–81
Motion sickness 290
Motrin 378–79
Mountain sickness, acute 182–83
  chronic 194–95
  persistent 193–96
  subacute 193–94
Mouth disorders 356–57
  canker sores 357
  herpes simplex 357
  toothache 356–57
Muscle cramps 228–29
Muscle pulls 128
Muscle tears 128

Nafcillin 386–87
Nasogastric intubation 410–13
Neck, fractures 120–21
  injuries 106, 153
Nembutal 383–84
Neomycin 388–89, 390
Neosporin 390
Neo-Synephrine 398–99
Nervous system diseases 341–49
  convulsions 344–46
  headache 343
  infections 346–47
  poliomyelitis 347–48
  stroke 348–49
Nitroglycerin 395–96
Nose disorders 352–54
  nose bleeds 149
Nupercainal 381–82
Nursing care 28–31
Nutrition at altitude 196

Oral medications 404

Pain 44
  burns 139–40
Pain medications 376–82
  acetaminophen 378
  aspirin 377–78
  codeine 79
  Demerol 381

Dibucaine 381–82
ibuprofen 378–79
lidocaine 382
meperidine 381
morphine 380–81
Nupercainal 381–82
Xylocaine 382
Pamine 403
Pancreatitis 324–25
Paratyphoid fever 297–98
Paregoric 401
Paroxysmal tachycardia 282
Pelvic fractures 119–20
Penetrating injury, abdomen 169–70
  chest 161–63
Penicillin 385–87
Pentobarbital 383–84
Peptic ulcer 308–11
Peritonitis 326
Pharmadine 393–94
Pharyngitis 355–56
  streptococcal 355–56
  viral 355
Phenobarbital 383–84
Phenylephrine 398–99
Photophthalmia 222–23
Physical examination 20–21, 23–25
Pleurisy 263–64
Pneumonia 264–66
Pneumothorax 158–60, 268–69
Poison ivy dermatitis 371
Poisonous snake bite 234–47
Poliomyelitis 81, 347–48
Polymyxin B 390
Post traumatic stress disorder 74–76
Povidone-Iodine solutions 92, 393–94
Pregnancy 335
Pro-Banthine 403
Pseudoephedrine 399
Psychologic aid 68
Psychological responses 60–78
  by rescuers 70–76
  by victims 62–67
  grief 60–62
  to dead bodies 77–78
  to stress 72–76
Pulled muscles 128

Pulmonary edema, high altitude
  183–89
Pulmonary embolism 195, 269–73
Puncture wounds 101–102
Pyelonephritis 330
Pyrimethamine 392

Rabies 230–34
Rectal, abscess 307–308
  fissure 306
  hemorrhoids 306–307
Relapsing fever 365
Renal. See Kidney
Rescuers, selection 76–77
Resin bound iodine 89
Respiratory disorders 256–73
  anaphylactic shock 371–73
  See also Breathing abnormalities,
  Lung disorders
Respiratory system medicines
  396–401
  Actifed 399
  adrenalin 396–97
  aminophylline 397
  epinephrine 396–97
  isoproternol 398
  Isuprel 398
  Neo-Synephrine 398–99
  phenylephrine 398–99
  pseudoephedrine 399
  Sudafed 399
Resuscitation 53–59
Retinal hemorrhage 192
Rib fractures 155
Rocky Mountain spotted fever
  364–65
Rubella 81
Rufen 378–79

Salmonellosis 297–98
Salpingitis 319
Sanitation 85–86
Scalp injuries 147
Scorpion stings 250–52
Secobarbital 383–84
Seconal 383–84
Septicemia 362–63

Septra 391
Shigellosis 301-302
Shin splints 129-30
Shock 42-45
  burns 134
Shortness of breath, hyperventilation 261-62
Shoulder, dislocation 124-25
  fracture 114
Sinus tachycardia 284
Sinuses 152-53
Sinusitis 353-54
Skin cancer 221-22
Skin flaps 102-103
"Skipped heart beats" 284-85
Skull fracture 146-47
Sleep hypoxia 177
Sleep medications 383-85
  barbiturates 383-84
  Benadryl 385
  benzodiazepines 384-85
  chloral hydrate 385
  Dalmane 384-85
  Librium 384-85
  Nembutal 383-84
  Phenobarbital 383-84
  Seconal 383-84
  Tuinal 383-84
  Valium 384-85
Smallpox 81
Snake bite 234-47
  antivenom 243
  coral snake 244-45
  crotalid envenomation 239-40
  envenomation 238-39
Snow blindness 222-23
Soft tissue injuries 94-107
  bandaging 100-101
  bleeding 94-95
  infection 95-100
Solar injuries 217-23
Sore throat 354-56
Spider bites 247-50
  black widow spider 248-49
  brown recluse spider 249-50
  brown spider 249-50
Spine fractures 120-21

Spleen injuries 168-69
Sprains 126-28
Staphylococcal enteritis 291
Sterilization, instruments 417
  water 86-92
Stings 250-53
Stomach, bleeding 310-11
  ulcer 308-11, 321-22
Stomach tube 410-13
Stone, kidney 326-27, 333
Strains 126-28
  back 131
Strep throat 355-56
Streptomycin 388-89
Stress, psychological response to 72-76
Stroke 348-49
Subdural hematoma 143-46
Sudafed 399
Sulfadoxine 392
Sun protection factor 220
Sunburn 217-21
Sunstroke 227-28
Sutures 96-97
Syncope 283
Syphilis 338-39

Tendinitis 129-30
Tenosynovitis 130
Testicular pain 336-37
Tetanus 81-82
Tetracycline 389-90
Tetraglycine hydroperiodide 88
Thigh fractures 116-19
Thoracotomy 414-16
Throat disorders 354-56
Thrombophlebitis 195, 269-73
Tick fever 365
Tincture of iodine 89
Toenails, ingrown 131
Toothache 365-57
Tracheostomy 49-51
Transportation 37-39, 112-113
Traveller's diarrhea 292-93
Trench foot 216
Trichinosis 368
Trimethoprim-Sulfamethoxazole 391

Tuinal 383–84
"Turista" 292–93
Tylenol 378
Typhoid fever 82, 302–303

Ulcer, stomach 308–11, 321–22
Unconsciousness 46, 142–43
Urethral catheterization 413–14
Urinary disorders 328–34
  cystitis 330
  glomerulonephritis 332–33
  pyelonephritis 330
  renal failure 330–32

Valium 384–85
Varicose veins 286–87
Vascular disease 286–87
Veins, thrombophlebitis 195, 269–73
Venereal diseases 337–40
  gonorrhea 339
  syphilis 338–39
Vertebral column fractures 120–21
Viral enteritis 292
Vomiting 288–89

Water disinfection 86–92
  iodine in 86–92
Wind chill 202
Wounds 94–107
  abrasions 102
  antiseptics 96
  avulsions 102–103
  contusions 103–104
  infections 95–100
  lacerations 101
  puncture 101–102
  skin flaps 102–103
  sutures 96–97

Xylocaine 382

Yellow fever 82, 366

Zephiran 392–93

Write for illustrated catalog of more than 100 outdoor titles:

The Mountaineers · Books
306 2nd Ave. W., Seattle WA 98119, (206) 285-2665

NOTES

NOTES

NOTES

NOTES